Research in Health Care

Concepts, Designs and Methods

Julius Sim
Primary Care Sciences Research Centre
Keele University

Chris Wright
School of Health and Social Sciences
Coventry University

Stanley Thornes (Publishers) Ltd

First published in 2000 by:
Stanley Thornes (Publishers) Ltd
Delta Place
27 Bath Road
Cheltenham
Glos.
GL53 7TH
United Kingdom

00 01 02 03 04 / 10 9 8 7 6 5 4 3 2 1

A catalogue record for this book is available from the British Library

ISBN 0-7487-3718-9

Typeset by Acorn Bookwork, Salisbury, Wiltshire
Printed and bound in Great Britain by Martins The Printers Ltd, Berwick upon Tweed

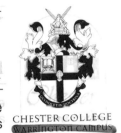

CONTENTS

ACKNOWLEDGEMENTS

We would like to thank those who have read and commented on various parts of the manuscript: Nadine Foster, Gilbert MacKenzie, Janice Sheasby, Jackie Waterfield and an anonymous reviewer. A special thank you is due to Alistair Hewison, who has provided a most helpful commentary on virtually all of the text. The shortcomings that remain in the book represent our failure to profit fully from our colleagues' advice.

We are grateful to Tony Wayte and Catherine Shaw at Nelson Thornes for their help and patience during the long gestation of this book. Additionally, J.S. would like to thank Norma Reid for encouraging and supporting his original foray into research methods teaching, and C.W. is grateful to Julie Barlow for support during the writing of this book. Lastly, a thank you to Jackie, Martin and Suzanne for their inexhaustible support, patience and understanding.

PART ONE

FUNDAMENTALS

1 INTRODUCTION

This text has been written for health care researchers and health professionals, such as nurses and therapists, who are engaged in empirical research in health care, whether as students or as qualified practitioners. Although a number of fundamental concepts and principles are explained in the text, its content has primarily been pitched at an intermediate to advanced level, and familiarity with the terminology and rudiments of research has been assumed. It is hoped, therefore, that the book will be helpful for undergraduate students in the latter part of their course of study, postgraduate students, and those working as researchers or practitioner-researchers.

1.1 CONTENT

As its title suggests, the book addresses three principal aspects of health care research: the *concepts* underlying various methodological approaches to research, the *designs* that may be used to answer specific research questions, and the *methods* through which such designs are realized. Hence, the material in the book spans both theoretical and practical issues.

The rationale for this approach is as follows. Any piece of research is conducted to answer one or more research questions. A particular research question dictates a particular structural framework for the study – the study design. However, the research question will be located within a certain theoretical perspective; hence, the choice of design for a study will depend not simply on the nature of the research question, but also on its conceptual and theoretical basis. Meanwhile, the specific methods of data collection and analysis used in a study are dictated by the design that has been chosen, and thus also have their origins in conceptual and theoretical considerations.

Hence, concepts, designs and methods are interdependent (this idea is examined in more detail in Chapters 2 and 3). In an attempt to reflect this interdependence, much of the content of the book is based on three hypothetical case studies, which are introduced in Chapter 3 and summarized in Appendix I. Based on three broad categories of research question – exploratory, descriptive and explanatory – these case studies are developed throughout the course of the book, in an attempt to unify concepts, methodology, design and methods. Most, though not all, of the examples used in the book relate to the case studies.

We hope we have given due weight to each of the main methodological approaches to health care research, and that an appropriate balance has been struck between the material relating to qualitative and quantitative data. Ethical as well as methodological considerations have been addressed. Although acknowledging the importance of professional, social, political or other contextual issues in health care research, we have not tried to cover these topics in this text; they are discussed in detail elsewhere (e.g. Daly *et al.*, 1992; Colquhoun and Kellehear, 1993; Ong, 1993). Although the material presented will be relevant to the process of critical reading and research appraisal (Hammersley, 1990; Greenhalgh, 1997; Clarke and Croft, 1998), the book does not specifically address this topic. However, an attempt has been made in Chapter 17 to explain some of the concepts and measures widely used in the literature of evidence-based health care. Moreover, the cornerstone of critical evaluation is a sound understanding of designs and methods, and we hope that this book will provide this understanding.

Similarly, we have not considered in detail the business of writing up and disseminating research. Although recognizing the importance of this topic, we have chosen to devote the space available to us to the *doing* of research, leaving a

Table 1.1   *Structure of the book*

Part	Chapters
1. Fundamentals	1. Introduction
	2. Basic concepts and principles
2. Formulating ideas for research	3. Posing research questions
3. Designing and executing a study	4. Basic elements of research design
	5. Designing an exploratory study
	6. Designing a descriptive study
	7. Designing an explanatory study
	8. Sampling
	9. Validity, reliability and allied concepts
4. Presenting and analysing data	10. Recording and organizing data from exploratory studies
	11. Analysing data from exploratory studies
	12. Presenting data from descriptive and explanatory studies
	13. Analysing data from descriptive and explanatory studies: principles
	14. Analysing data from descriptive and explanatory studies: procedures
5. More specialized issues	15. Issues in questionnaire design and attitude measurement
	16. Single instance research
	17. Systematic reviews, meta-analysis and measures of treatment effect
	18. Analysing data from descriptive and explanatory studies: further principles and procedures

discussion of writing and dissemination to other texts (e.g. Wolcott, 1990; French and Sim, 1993; Day, 1998; Jenkins *et al.*, 1998).

1.2 STRUCTURE

The book is divided into five parts, as indicated in Table 1.1. Each chapter opens with a summary of the main points to be covered. Thereafter, the content is divided into numbered sections and subsections, so as to facilitate cross-referencing. Each chapter also includes a number of boxes. These mostly contain discussions of terminology, details of specific methodological points, or further discussion of issues introduced in the main text. Although this material is not unimportant, it is not usually vital to an understanding of the central content of each chapter.

Less advanced readers may therefore wish to skip some boxes.

The chapters in Part Five cover some of the more advanced or specialized topics in health care research, and are aimed at readers with a specific interest in, or requirement for, such material. Hence, the statistical analyses addressed in Chapter 18 are aimed at readers who have a specific interest in this area, rather than those wishing to gain a general overview of both qualitative and quantitative data analysis.

Suggestions for background or further reading have not been made for the book as a whole, nor in general for each chapter as a whole, but relevant sources have been identified at numerous points within the text in relation to particular topics.

2 BASIC CONCEPTS AND PRINCIPLES

SUMMARY

This chapter explores the following topics:

- the nature of research and its relationship to evidence-based health care and audit
- the distinction between methodology, design and methods in research
- the philosophical assumptions underlying various approaches to research

In order to develop a critical understanding of research in health care and to make a reasoned and judicious choice of various designs and methods, it is necessary to consider some of the conceptual and contextual issues that underlie the processes that occur in research. This chapter will examine some of these more abstract issues, and will focus in particular on the theoretical and philosophical bases of different approaches to research. Although we recommend that this chapter be read in its entirety at the outset, particularly for more advanced readers, some may prefer to return to the theoretical issues addressed in Section 2.3 after reading some of the more applied material in Chapters 4 to 7.

2.1 THE NATURE OF RESEARCH

Lately, there has been an increasing emphasis on research in health care. Most recently, this has manifested itself in calls for 'evidence-based practice' in health care (Rosenberg and Donald, 1995; Dixon *et al.*, 1997; Gray, 1997; Bury and Mead, 1998). Basic to this movement towards greater use of existing evidence is an acknowledgement that relying on personal experience, clinical intuition, and traditional practices and procedures does not necessarily provide a sound basis for effective professional practice. It has been argued that although these 'unsystematic' approaches to professional knowledge may have some role to play, they may easily mislead the clinician and perpetuate unfounded or mistaken practices (Sim, 1995a; Gray, 1997).

The education of health professionals also reflects this concern for a research-based body of professional knowledge. Most students in the health professions are provided with a thorough grounding in the skills of critical appraisal and research appreciation, and many gain first-hand experience of carrying out a research project, even if on a small scale.

What, then, is the nature of evidence-based health care, and what relationship does it have to research? Evidence-based health care has been defined as 'the conscientious, explicit and judicious use of current best evidence in making decisions about the care of individual patients' (Sackett *et al.*, 1996, p. 71). Although evidence-based practice has recently assumed a high profile in professional discourse, there are signs that it has been an issue in health care for over a century:

> *Respecting the physiological action of Massage, it is necessary to speak with caution. Here, as is so often the case, practice has preceded theory ... We find that we cure our patients, but hardly know exactly how these results are obtained. It is easy to theorise, but we want carefully observed facts and accurately recorded experiments.*
>
> (Murrell, 1889, p. 72)

Advocates of evidence-based health care point out with some concern that many current health care interventions have not been subjected to proper evaluation in terms of their effectiveness. An allied point of concern is that even where research evidence exists for specific interventions, clinicians' daily practice may effectively disregard such evidence (Carter, 1996).

The evidence required to sustain an evidence-based mode of practice needs to be:

- up to date
- objective (i.e. not subject to the influence of individual biases and presuppositions)
- verifiable
- relevant and applicable to practice
- intelligible.

It is apparent that each of these criteria is also applicable to research. In particular, research is often put forward as an objective source of knowledge, in that it does not depend wholly upon the opinions, preferences, values or expectations of the researcher. We will later have reason to question this as a portrayal of research. However, it is reasonable to argue that whatever is to count as evidence for practical decisions in an area such as health care should be capable of being judged as either valid or invalid by the professional community at large. In this context at least, personal opinion is not a sufficient basis for professional practice. Research and evidence-based health care are therefore interdependent activities. Moreover, evidence-based health care provides a meeting point for research and clinical practice. Thus, Sackett *et al.* (1996, p. 71) argue that the 'practice of evidence based medicine means integrating individual clinical expertise with the best available external clinical evidence from systematic research'.

The close relationship that exists between evidence-based health care and research has implications for the sorts of skills required by the clinical practitioner:

> *An occupational therapy practitioner cannot engage in evidence-based practice without the problem-solving skills associated with competence in research.*
>
> (Abreu *et al.*, 1998, p. 751)

2.1.1 Research and audit

Alongside the move to evidence-based practice, there has been growing interest in the process of audit. This has in common with research that it involves the systematic collection of information – in particular the outcomes of professional intervention – and the systematic analysis of the resulting data in a way that will inform future professional practice.

Audit is often regarded as taking place in a cyclical manner, and the key components of the audit cycle are illustrated in Figure 2.1. The beginning of the audit cycle is the identification of *audit criteria*, which are specific aspects of care often expressed in terms of structure, process and outcome which are considered to be important to the quality of a service (Øvretveit, 1998). Identifying audit criteria is usually achieved by a process of consensus among professional peers, and through consultation with service users (Rigge, 1995). On the basis of these identified criteria, specific *audit standards* are drawn up. These are the desired characteristics or values of these criteria (e.g. if service response were an audit criterion, the corresponding standard might be that a patient or client should be seen within 14 days of initial referral). Service delivery is then evaluated in terms of how well it achieves these standards of care. If this reveals deficiencies in the service, appropriate changes are made and the service is re-evaluated; hence audit is a cyclical, iterative process.

Audit is, therefore, not the same as research (Wilson *et al.*, 1999). Both processes measure

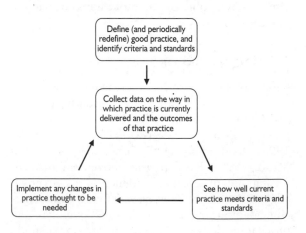

Figure 2.1 *The audit cycle.*

changes in a patient's status in the light of certain structures and processes of care, using specified outcome measures. However, research seeks to answer the question 'What should we do to the patient in terms of future practice?', whereas audit seeks to answer the question 'How successful are we in what we are already doing to the patient, compared with a predetermined standard of hoped-for results?' Audit findings focus on the relationship between intended and achieved outcomes; they do not tell us whether changes in patients' health status are the *result* of our clinical interventions. Research findings, on the other hand, often seek to test the link between aspects of care and various clinical outcomes; they tell us whether particular structures or processes of care produce outcomes superior to those of certain other structures or processes.

There are, however, important links between research and audit. In particular, audit standards should, where possible, be based on research findings (Barnard and Hartigan, 1998).

2.2 METHODOLOGY, DESIGN AND METHODS

The principal purpose of this book is not to examine in detail the role of research in professional practice or other aspects of its external relationships (though these will, of course, be touched upon where appropriate). Comprehensive accounts of such issues can be found elsewhere (e.g. Daly *et al.*, 1992; Colquhoun and Kellehear, 1993; Ong, 1993). Our aim is rather to look at the internal workings of empirical health care research; i.e. the specific methods by which it is planned and executed. Before proceeding any further in this direction, it is necessary to define a few terms.

2.2.1 Methodology

Methodology describes the overall approach taken in a piece of research. In particular, it refers to the general *principles* of investigation that guide a study, based on its underlying theoretical and philosophical assumptions. These principles will dictate that certain designs and methods are appropriate, and other designs and methods inappropriate, in order to answer a particular research question. The focus of methodology is on logical, conceptual and philosophical issues.

The term 'methodology' is sometimes also used to refer to the study of research procedures, just as 'sociology' refers to the study of society, but in this book the term will be used in the previous sense.

2.2.2 Design

The term 'design' describes the overall plan and *structure* of a piece of research, in particular the logical relationships between various steps in the research process. A design can be regarded as the framework into which particular methods are fitted. A methodological approach or perspective may embrace a number of different designs. Hence, research based on experimental methodology may adopt different designs depending on the nature of the research question and the factors that may require to be controlled or manipulated (see Chapter 4). Whereas methodology has to do with principles, designs are concerned with more concrete operational aspects of a study.

2.2.3 Methods

Research methods are the specific *techniques* employed in the execution of a piece of research, e.g. the way in which subjects or participants are sampled, the construction and use of a data collection instrument, the specific processes whereby data are analysed. Although certain methods tend to be associated with certain designs, the same methods may be found in more than one design. Accordingly, specific techniques used to measure respondents' attitudes might be used in both a psychological experiment conducted under near-laboratory conditions and in a descriptive survey carried out in a more natural setting.

2.3 PHILOSOPHICAL MODELS OF RESEARCH

All approaches to research embody a particular

philosophical perspective on reality and on the ways in which knowledge can legitimately be gained from the world. The philosophy of knowledge is known as *epistemology*, and thus a particular research approach will be based on a specific epistemological perspective. In addition, a research approach will embody a particular logical structure whereby inferences are drawn from data. The branch of philosophy which addresses such questions, and which overlaps with epistemology, is known as the *philosophy of science* (Bechtel, 1988). The debate between rival research approaches centres as much on differences of opinion about their respective underlying epistemological and logical bases as on more practical questions as to how research should be carried out.

Studying epistemology may seem to be a rather abstract enterprise, far removed from the immediate task of conducting practical research in the everyday world. However, an understanding of the epistemology of research is crucially important for the researcher who wishes to carry out research in a critical and reflective way, for the choice of a particular methodology (and, in turn, particular designs and methods) will be driven by a number of fundamental epistemological assumptions (Ackroyd and Hughes, 1992). It follows from this that a misunderstanding of these assumptions may lead to an inappropriate choice of methodology, and an attitude whereby particular research methods are employed in a mechanical and unreflective manner; a sort of 'toolbox' approach to research. Research conducted in such a manner is likely to fall foul of a number of conceptual and logical shortcomings and inconsistencies, and will consequently fail to achieve its intended purposes.

Therefore, as a basis for further and more detailed discussion of different research approaches, brief sketches will be provided here of three philosophical perspectives on research. Inevitably, these will be simplified somewhat for purposes of clarity, and some of the issues raised will be developed more fully in subsequent chapters.

2.3.1 Positivism

As a conceptualization of research, positivism rests on the assumption that the methods used to study the physical world can also be used, with some modification, to study the social world: a principle known as the 'unity of method'. Another central tenet of positivism is that there is a single objective reality, which is the same for all of us, irrespective of our individual values, attitudes or perspectives: this is the principle of value neutrality. Our task is to make contact with this external reality in an objective and scientifically rigorous manner, with as little interference as possible from our own subjective values.

Positivism further argues that the only sound basis for knowledge is experience; i.e. data that are apprehended by the senses from the outside world, with minimal participation of the researcher's subjective processes. Consequently, positivists are distrustful of concepts that cannot be observed or otherwise experienced, and thus

Box 2.1   *'Empirical' and 'empiricist'*

Research that is 'empirical' is any research that involves the collection of data from the physical and/or social world about us. These data may be either quantitative or qualitative, or indeed a mixture of the two. Empirical research can be contrasted with theoretical research, which operates by means of conceptual analysis and theoretical argument, and does not require the collection or analysis of data from the external world. The term 'empiricist' relates to *empiricism*, which is a particular philosophical view of research whose basic contention is that only knowledge that stems from first-hand observation and other forms of sensory experience is valid. Empiricism is dismissive of research that relies on notions of insight, intuition, interpretive understanding, and the like. Empiricism contrasts with *rationalism*, which holds the view that valid knowledge can be gained through reason alone.

adopt an *empiricist* view of science (Hughes, 1990; see Box 2.1). Indeed, a branch of positivism, known as *logical positivism*, went so far as to argue that any statement or proposition that could not be verified by observation is meaningless.

The hostility of positivism to any non-observable entities makes it suspicious of theory and theoretical concepts (O'Hear, 1989). For the positivist, 'metaphysical notions about which it is not possible to make any observations, have no legitimate existence except as names or words' (Blaikie, 1993, p. 14). Explanation in the positivist perspective takes the form of general laws that express empirical regularities and relationships (e.g. that a certain class of event always precedes, follows or is accompanied by another class of event). More abstract theoretical notions, such as 'cause' and 'effect', tend not to feature in these general propositions. Positivists are distrustful of explanations that go beyond the observable features of the world. Their concept of explanation rests at the level of empirically verifiable patterns and relationships in the observable world, rather than at the level of theory or other metaphysical notions.

Positivist scientific method is characteristically *inductive*. That is, it proceeds from the gathering of particular observations to the framing of general propositions or laws, rather than a deductive approach that seeks to examine existing laws in the light of observations that are made subsequently. Induction and deduction are discussed further in Section 2.4.

2.3.2 Critical rationalism

Positivism in its fairly pure form, as described above, has drawn considerable criticism. One philosopher who departed from the positivist tradition, though he is often erroneously labelled as a positivist, is Karl Popper (1972, 1979). Although he supported some of the arguments of positivist philosophers of science – such as their insistence on generalizable, objective knowledge and the notion of a single reality – Popper was very critical of their inductive approach to

knowledge and their use of verification as a means of testing propositions. Instead, he advocated a form of critical rationalism, which acknowledges the importance of theories and abstract theoretical concepts in scientific explanation and tests their adequacy by a process of attempted falsification. In this process, theories are taken as the starting point of scientific knowledge, but are then rigorously tested against observations in a process of trial and error, based on a deductive rather than an inductive logic.

Theories are thus selected as explanations of reality on the basis of 'survival of the fittest'. The best explanation is the one that has survived the most rigorous attempts to falsify it through a hypothetico-deductive method of theory testing (see Section 2.4.1). Indeed, Popper went so far as to argue that any theory that is not potentially falsifiable cannot be described as scientific; falsifiability is the hallmark of a scientific theory.

2.3.3 Phenomenology

Phenomenology is a philosophical perspective that stands in stark contrast to the preceding two. In particular, it takes a very different view of the relationship between experience and knowledge. For positivists, and for post-positivists such as Popper, experience is a means of accessing an objective reality that lies outside the individual who is experiencing it. In phenomenology, however, the world as experienced by individuals, or by a group of individuals, *is* the real world. Social reality is constructed by individuals in the process of interacting within a particular context (Anderson, 1991). There are, therefore, multiple realities, rather than a single objective reality, and reality is to a large degree relative rather than absolute (i.e. it is relative to the individual perspectives of social actors and to the particular contexts in which they interact). Accordingly, '[t]he phenomenologist is one who tries to understand social phenomena or human activity from the viewpoint of the person being studied' (Shepard *et al.*, 1993, p. 89). In addition, phenomenology recognizes the fact that social phenomena are rooted in a specific context. Phenomenology is concerned to understand such a context in both its uniqueness and its entirety, with as little interference on the part of the researcher as possible. More orthodox approaches to research often take a more reductionistic approach, and specifically abstract phenomena from their context.

In order to gain access to the world as it is perceived and experienced by individuals, a degree of cognitive and even emotional rapport is necessary between the investigator and those whom he or she is studying. Phenomenology, therefore, rejects the calls made by positivists for a high degree of objectivity and detachment on the part of the researcher. As Doyal puts it,

> *According to this view, those in pursuit of knowledge were analogous to spectators in a position to have the truth revealed about the world or society, provided that they did nothing to distort their observational links with the realities concerned. ... Anything that might distort the experience of these facts through the creation of bias or prejudice was viewed with anathema. The pursuit of truth was seen much as Mr Spock of* Star Trek *sees it, as a task much more appropriate for almost any beings other than unobjective, emotional humans.*
>
> (Doyal, 1993, p. 4)

The objective of phenomenology is not so much to _explain_ as to _interpret_ the world (Blaikie, 1993). Moreover, it is generally concerned with the uniqueness and individuality of human experience, and unlike positivism and critical rationalism, does not seek to generate inferences with a high degree of generality. Similarly, phenomenology deals primarily with the 'micro' rather than the 'macro' features of social life (Lassman, 1974). Hence, ethnography and similar interpretive approaches to research find their philosophical roots largely in a phenomenological perspective (see Chapter 5).

2.4 THE ROLE OF THEORY IN RESEARCH

Generally speaking, research can be said to have as one of its main purposes the enrichment of theoretical knowledge. This may occur by building upon our knowledge of an existing topic, or by extending our understanding into hitherto unexplored areas. In either case, our theoretical knowledge is enhanced and developed. The distinctions that may be discerned between different models of empirical research can often be analysed in terms of the different roles played by theory. As theory is such a central element in research, it is important to clarify what a theory is.

Essentially, a theory can be regarded as an explanatory conceptual framework that provides an understanding of a particular class of phenomena:

> *A theory is a set of interrelated constructs (concepts), definitions, and propositions that present a systematic view of phenomena by specifying relations among variables, with the purpose of explaining and predicting the phenomena.*
>
> (Kerlinger, 1986, p. 9)

A theory will contain within it a number of theoretical *propositions*, and these propositions generally state a relationship between certain theoretical *concepts*. For example, the theory of cognitive dissonance contains within it a number of propositions concerning two basic psychological concepts: beliefs and behaviour (Festinger, 1957). One of these propositions states a particular relationship between these concepts: viz. people are troubled by a perceived mismatch between their beliefs and their own behaviour. Another proposition states that people will more often resolve this tension by changing their beliefs than by changing their behaviour. Similarly, a theory on the psychology of pain might contain within it a proposition to the effect that the affective dimension of pain is related to the individual's knowledge of the origin and likely course of the pain-giving experience.

These concepts and propositions are at a higher level of generality and abstraction than the phenomena that they seek to explain, and are not themselves observable entities. Although it is possible to witness particular behavioural actions in the real world, we cannot 'see' behaviour as a concept. Equally, we cannot see, feel or touch an attitude, even though we may hear or observe what we take to be the expression of that attitude. Theories deal with the observable (empirical) world, but are not themselves observable. Hence, a theory goes beyond the facts to a higher level of abstraction (Trusted, 1979; Fawcett and Downs, 1992).

There are two broad ways in which research may concern itself with theory: it may set out to test an existing theory or it may seek to build a new theory. These processes will be examined in turn.

2.4.1 Theory-testing research

The starting point for the theory-testing model of research is an existing theory that the researcher wishes to test (Figure 2.2). The foremost advocate of this model of research is probably Popper, who dubbed it the 'hypothetico-deductive' approach. This model of

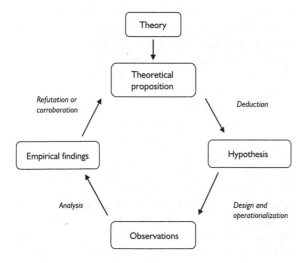

Figure 2.2 *Theory-testing research in the hypothetico-deductive model.*

research forms the logical basis for experimental research design, to be considered in Chapter 7.

More specifically, the researcher draws certain predictions from theoretical propositions contained with the theory and then collects data to see if they support these predictions. It is important to note that the propositions themselves cannot be directly tested because, as already noted, they are framed in terms of largely unobservable concepts. Rather, a prediction is *deduced* from the theoretical proposition (hence this model of research is referred to as a deductive one). For example, based on the proposition that pain affect is related to knowledge of the underlying cause of pain, a prediction such as the following could be deduced:

> *Patients suffering from pain who are told that the underlying cause of their pain is self-limiting will show lower levels of distress that those to whom such information is not provided.*

This prediction is what is known as a *research hypothesis*. A hypothesis is a type of research question, except that it takes the form of a statement rather than a question *per se* (Box 3.3).

To say that a hypothesis is deduced from a proposition is to say that the hypothesis follows as a matter of logical necessity from the proposition; if the proposition is a true one, then the hypothesis will also be true. It will be noticed that the hypothesis is stated in more concrete terms than the proposition from which it was deduced; it describes a situation that we could envisage observing in the real world of clinical experience. Thus, as we go from theories to theoretical propositions to hypotheses, we are steadily moving from the abstract and general to the more concrete and particular (Figure 2.3).

It is on the basis of the research hypothesis that the study is designed; it must be optimally suited to testing this particular hypothesis. In the process, the hypothesis is *operationalized*. That is, the elements in the hypothesis are

Box 2.2   *'Proof' and 'disproof'*

In the deductive model of theory-testing research, it is possible to disprove a theoretical proposition, but not to prove one. There are several reasons why this is the case. First, the logic of deduction dictates that where one proposition (the 'consequent') follows deductively from another (the 'antecedent'), if the consequent is shown to be false this in turn requires the antecedent also to be false (e.g. if it rains, the path will get wet; the path is not wet, therefore it cannot be raining). The opposite is not the case, however. The consequent may be true without this guaranteeing the truth of the antecedent (e.g. If it rains, the path will get wet; the path is wet – but this does not necessarily means it is raining, for the path could be wet for reasons unconnected with rain). Hence, a 'positive' outcome from an experiment does not establish the truth of a proposition. Indeed, it can even be argued that increasing numbers of 'positive' experiments do not even make it more *probable* that the alternative hypothesis is true (Chalmers, 1982). Second, there are a large number (probably an infinite number) of hypotheses that can be deduced from a given proposition. Clearly, a study that shows one of these hypotheses to be true does not ensure the truth of the original proposition, because when another hypothesis derived from this proposition is tested in a subsequent study, this hypothesis might well be shown to be false. Thirdly, there is an important philosophical principle known as the *underdetermination of theory by data* (Quine, 1964). This states that any set of data can always be explained by more than one theoretical account. Whatever theoretical explanation is proposed, there will always be at least one other that will also be consistent with the data (Dancy, 1985). Hence, the data from a study will inevitably 'underdetermine' a particular theory, and cannot therefore establish the truth of one hypothesis to the exclusion of certain other rival hypotheses. Consequently, a set of empirical findings cannot decisively establish, or prove, one theoretical explanation over another, because these other explanations will always be viable alternatives. For all these reasons, hypotheses must be subjected to a process of attempted disproof, not one of attempted proof (see also Section 13.4.8).

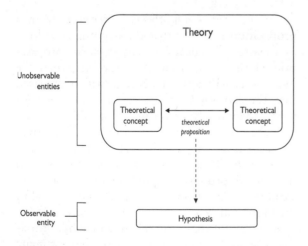

Unobservable entities

Observable entity

Figure 2.3   *Relationships between theory, theoretical concepts, theoretical propositions, and hypotheses.*

rephrased in terms of specific actions or operations. The researcher decides precisely who will qualify for the purposes of this study as a 'patient suffering from pain', determines the way in which information as to the cause of their pain will be transmitted to them, and identifies a procedure by which their pain affect will subsequently be measured.

Once the process of operationalization has been carried out and the design and methods of the study have been established, the process of data collection can take place. These data can be analysed to produce the *empirical findings* of the study. In the present case, these findings might be that the patients to whom the explanation had been given showed lower levels of distress than the group from whom the explanation had been withheld. This would corroborate the hypothesis, and the theoretical proposition from which it was drawn would therefore 'pass' the test. Alternatively, it might transpire that there was no difference in levels of distress between the two groups, or even that distress was more pronounced in the group that had received the explanation; in both cases, the hypothesis would be disproved by the empirical findings, and the corresponding theoretical proposition would be refuted (see Box 2.2).

In the deductive model of research, therefore, theory is the starting point and the research proceeds to the collection of data as a means of testing this theory. In the process, there is a move from the general (theory), to the particular (data), and then back to the general (the return to theory); in this way the process is cyclical. This model of research will be developed further during the discussion of experimentation in Chapters 4 and 7.

2.4.2 Theory-building research

A theory-building model of research operates in essentially the reverse direction to that of theory-testing research. Whereas theory-testing research follows a deductive logic, theory building research operates in terms of an inductive logic. The essence of induction is that particular observations are gathered and general statements are then derived from these observations. In contrast to deductive research, the movement is from the particular to the general (Figure 2.4). The role of this model of research is to generate a theoretical framework of understanding where none previously existed (or at least where only a poorly formulated body of theory existed), and to derive this understanding from the data. Research that is exploratory in purpose and involves the collection of qualitative data tends to follow a theory-building model of research (see Chapter 5).

It was suggested earlier that positivism espoused an inductive mode of inference of a very pure form. However, this use of induction has been largely discredited as naïve (Chalmers, 1982), and what will be described below is a more complex and judicious use of inductive

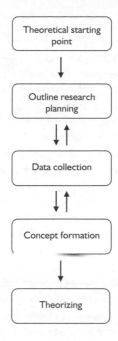

Figure 2.4 *An inductive model of theory building.*

logic as it appears in much interpretive research based on qualitative data.

Whereas in deductive research a theory or a theoretical proposition *per se* is the starting point, in inductive research there is usually only what might be called a theoretical starting point, i.e. a collection of theoretical ideas or assumptions. Without such a theoretical starting point there would be no basis on which to plan the study or decide what observations or other data would be relevant to the research question. However, this theoretical starting point falls short of constituting a fully formulated theory (Box 2.3). Further, as there is no theory at the outset, it is not possible to derive any hypotheses. Inductive research, unlike deductive research, is not a process whereby hypotheses are tested.

The next step in the process is research planning. However, it is likely that only a very preliminary and provisional research design will be laid down at this stage, because it is characteristic of inductive research that the research design unfolds and develops during the process of data collection. Thus there is often an

Box 2.3   *Theory and data*

The idea that data can ever speak for themselves has been thoroughly discredited. In order to decide what is to count as data, the researcher needs to have taken some sort of prior theoretical standpoint, even if only a very tentative one. For example, if it is intended to record the actions of a group of people in a certain situation, the observer needs a theoretical account of what an 'action' is. Such an account is likely to differ considerably between researchers operating with either a behaviourist or an interactionist perspective. Accordingly, the aspects of human behaviour that will qualify as data will differ in each case. Ackroyd and Hughes (1992, p. 34) point out that 'data materials, whatever else they may consist in, have to be "read" through, in terms of, a theoretical framework to exist as data'.

iterative movement between research design and data collection (as indicated by the fact that arrows go in both directions between these two boxes in Figure 2.4).

Data analysis in an inductive study is conducted in a way that allows concepts and themes to emerge from the data. More specifically, the researcher looks for patterns across the data, and thus establishes points of commonality or contrast within the dataset as a whole. This need not wait until all data have been collected, but may occur during the data collection process

(again, the movement between the corresponding boxes in Figure 2.4 is bi-directional). In this way, more general themes are created out of the particular observations that constitute the dataset. Relationships between these themes can then be identified, and theoretical propositions can be generated in a process of theorizing or theory building.

Although the underlying inductive logic of this model of research is in principle the same as that of positivism (Section 2.3.1), the purpose for which it is employed is radically different. Whereas induction was used by the positivist purely as a means of establishing empirical generalizations about the observable world, in the model of research that has just been described, induction is a means of moving from empirical data to the theoretical concepts and propositions, with little concern for generalizations at a purely empirical level. The inductive model of research will be considered further in Chapters 5 and 11.

2.5 CONCLUSION

This chapter has examined some of the fundamental theoretical and conceptual aspects of health care research, which will underpin much of the discussion in subsequent chapters. The following chapter will examine the issues surrounding the identification of a research question and its relationship to various aspects of study design and methods.

PART TWO

FORMULATING IDEAS FOR RESEARCH

3 POSING RESEARCH QUESTIONS

SUMMARY

This chapter explores the following topics:

- the definition and key features of a research question
- sources of research questions
- the distinctions between exploratory, descriptive and explanatory research questions
- the relationship between research questions, theory, methodology, designs and methods
- criteria by which a potential research question can be judged

The core of any study is a research question (or in some cases, a set of research questions), which identifies the gap in existing knowledge that the study seeks to fill. Not only is the answering of a research question the overall objective of a study, but it also guides the design and methods utilized during the course of the study. Research methods are only good or bad, or appropriate or inappropriate, in terms of the research question to which they are applied. This chapter will examine more closely the nature of a research question and will consider ways in which research questions may be classified and evaluated in terms of their adequacy.

3.1 THE NATURE AND ORIGIN OF A RESEARCH QUESTION

A research question may spring from a number of sources. On occasions, it may simply stem from curiosity: a desire to satisfy an intellectual query that comes out of the blue. Alternatively, a research question may be based on observations that have been made during clinical practice. For example, a nurse may have noted that the post-operative recovery period of a category of apparently similar patients undergoing the same procedure differs considerably from patient to patient, and may wish to examine the reason for such variation. More often in health care, perhaps, a research question is the result of particular barriers or problems that have confronted the practitioner in the course of his or her practice. For example, an occupational therapist may wish to find a more effective means of controlling ulnar deviation of the fingers in patients with rheumatoid disease, and may wish to test the relative effectiveness of a number of corrective orthoses. In such a case, answering a research question is not just a means of acquiring knowledge, it is also a problem-solving process through which professional practice is evaluated and improved.

Another important source of research questions is previous research, especially as published in the professional literature. By reading reports of others' research, a practitioner may identify unanswered questions or recognize ways in which a previous study can be taken further (Portney and Watkins, 1993). Further, studying the literature has a very important role to play in refining and adjusting research questions from other sources. It is also a means of checking that the proposed research question has not already been answered (see Section 3.2.3 in relation to the 'originality' of a research question).

A research question does not exist in a vacuum. It must be viewed within a particular theoretical context. The very fact that this question, rather than some other, has been deemed worthy of investigation reveals certain theoretical concerns on the part of the researcher. Similarly, the concepts in terms of which the question is framed will derive their meaning from a particular body of theory. In the case of theory-testing research (Section 2.4.1), this theory will be at a relatively high level of development and refinement. In the case of theory-building research (Section 2.4.2), on the other hand, the theoretical context of a research question may be at a very early stage of development; however, some sort of theoretical starting point will still be present. Thus, in all forms of research the researcher will approach his or her research question with theoretical presuppositions of some sort.

Figure 3.1 illustrates the complex relationship between theory, a research question, research methodology, research design and research methods (as defined in Sections 2.2.1 to 2.2.3). Notice that there are both direct and indirect lines of influence. Although theory will determine methodology through the particular research question chosen, it will also influence methodology directly. A methodology will be significantly dictated by a theoretical perspective, regardless of the particular research question (Ackroyd and Hughes, 1992). This reinforces the argument that a study must have a theoretical

context; you cannot choose designs and methods without already having taken some sort of theoretical stance. Similarly, a research question will cause a particular design to be chosen, but this design will also be determined by the chosen methodological approach. The same applies in terms of the influence of methodology and design on specific research methods.

A word or two should be said about how research questions should *not* originate. A common mistake is to develop a liking for a particular method of research and then look for a question to which it can be applied. A question arrived at in this way is unlikely to fulfil the criteria for a good research question (Section 3.2). Similarly, Robson (1993) warns against studies that are undertaken purely in response to funding opportunities or with a view to the publications that may result.

3.1.1 Types of research question

One way in which research questions can be classified is in terms of their purpose, i.e. the question they set out to answer (Box 3.1). On this basis, research questions can be divided into three broad categories: exploratory, descriptive/ normative and explanatory (Babbie, 1989; Robson, 1993). As much of the material in this book is based upon this distinction, it is important to differentiate these types of research question.

Exploratory questions

Exploratory questions are characteristically very broad questions, framed with reference to an area that is as yet poorly understood. Such a question is appropriate where the topic concerned has been only partially explored, if at all, and where there is not yet an established body of theory to explain it. According to Robson (1993, p. 42), an exploratory research question has one or more of the following purposes:

- to find out what is happening
- to seek new insights
- to ask questions
- to assess phenomena in a new light.

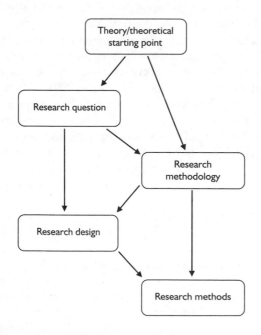

Figure 3.1 *Relationships between theory, research question, methodology, design and methods.*

Box 3.1 *Classifying research*

In this book, *studies* will be classified primarily in terms of whether the research question they address is exploratory, descriptive or explanatory – thus, an explanatory study is simply one that seeks to answer an explanatory question. Studies are also sometimes categorized as being either quantitative or qualitative, based on the nature of the data to be collected. It would seem more logical, however, to classify a study according to its research question, as this drives virtually all other aspects of the study and is thus a more fundamental characteristic of the study. It is reasonable, however, to speak of quantitative or qualitative *approaches* to research, since an approach is a much wider notion than a particular research question. The terms 'quantitative' and 'qualitative' are not really appropriate to classify research in terms of its *design*, however, since it is probably more helpful to categorize designs in terms of their underlying logic – experimental, quasi-experimental, non-experimental.

Exploratory research questions often serve to prepare the ground for descriptive research questions, which in turn may generate explanatory research questions. Because exploratory research questions are usually concerned with the uncharted territories of research, it may not be possible to determine in advance the precise methods that will be appropriate. The research design in such cases is therefore *emergent*; i.e. it develops during the course of the study as preliminary findings make it clear what specific methods of data collection are required. Consequently, there may be a degree of overlap between stages of the research process (e.g. data collection and data analysis may occur in parallel, rather than sequentially). In much the same way, exploratory research questions may not be formulated in detail at the outset of a study, but may be developed and refined from a broad initial idea during the early stages of the study (Maxwell, 1996).

The data to be collected are generally qualitative, since in most cases the concepts and phenomena being investigated are not sufficiently well understood to permit quantification.

Babbie (1989) points out that exploratory research questions may also function to test the feasibility of undertaking a larger and more systematic study, and to develop the methods to be employed in such a study.

Descriptive and normative questions

A descriptive research question, as its name suggests, provides a descriptive account of a phenomenon within an established framework of knowledge. It is likely that the fundamental concepts and variables of the topic will already have been identified, partly by means of studying the existing literature in the area (see Box 3.2). However, the researcher will want to produce a fuller account of these phenomena by describing them in greater detail and perhaps quantifying some of the key variables. Additionally, the researcher will probably wish to identify some relationships of potential theoretical interest. The primary purpose of descriptive research may therefore be to develop a theory or body of knowledge in more detail; putting flesh on the bones, as it were.

The fact that the basic framework of understanding is likely to exist means that the descriptive research question itself and the design and methods to be employed to answer it can usually be specified fairly completely in advance. Survey methods such as self-completed questionnaires are often used in descriptive studies, and the nature of such instruments requires that they be fully specified before data collection begins. Phases within the research design tend to be sequential, with little overlap.

Normative questions are similar in their purpose to descriptive questions, of which they may be regarded as a subtype. However, they include an additional objective, in that they compare the data gathered with a criterion or standard (Hedrick *et al.*, 1993). Hence, a study that sought to establish the mean range of knee motion of patients three weeks after a total knee

Box 3.2   *Reviewing the literature, or not?*

Conventional wisdom is that a thorough search of the literature should be undertaken in order to develop and refine a research question. This is important simply to establish that another worker in the field has not already answered the question. It is probably safe to say that a literature search of some form should precede any study. However, the scope of the search is a matter of debate. Some writers argue that a comprehensive literature search may actually detract from an exploratory study. Strauss and Corbin (1998) argue that if the researcher enters a study with a list of theoretical themes and categories derived from the existing literature – which may or may not apply to the area under investigation – this may impede the inductive generation of themes and categories from the data. They comment that, in inductive approaches such as grounded theory (which will be examined in Section 11.1.1), the researcher 'does not want to be so steeped in the literature that he or she is constrained and even stifled by it' (Strauss and Corbin, 1998, p. 49). Glaser (1992) shares this concern about preconceived theoretical perspectives, but takes a slightly different approach to the issue. He advocates an initial literature review, so as to develop the researcher's sensitivity to theoretical issues, but suggests that this should be in subject areas unrelated to the researcher's own. Hence, whereas a full review of literature related to the intended topic of research is usually appropriate at the outset of a descriptive or explanatory study, this is not necessarily the case with respect to an exploratory study.

replacement would answer a descriptive research question. However, if the study also sought to determine the proportion of patients who were discharged with a specified range of motion required for everyday activities (for sake of argument, 105 degrees of flexion), this would constitute a normative research question.

Explanatory questions

Explanatory questions tend to be more specific than the preceding types of question, and frequently serve to test a hypothesis. Indeed, explanatory research questions generally take the form of a hypothesis. As indicated in Section 2.4.1, a hypothesis is a prediction that the study sets out either to reject or to retain, usually by means of statistical analysis (see Box 3.3). A hypothesis can therefore be regarded as a form of declarative research question, rather than an interrogative research question (Cormack and Benton, 1996). That is, it takes the form of a proposition rather than a question. Explanatory research questions characteristically deal with quantitative data.

Box 3.3   *Research questions and hypotheses*

If a research question aims to determine whether a particular relationship between two or more variables exists, it is generally framed as a hypothesis. A hypothesis is a prediction, to the effect that the relationship in question does exist, which is then tested against the data gathered in the study. This hypothesis is known as the 'research hypothesis', or the 'substantive hypothesis'. In Section 13.4.4 it will be seen that two further hypotheses are constructed from the research hypothesis for the purpose of statistical inference – the null hypothesis and the alternative hypothesis. Studies that are based on exploratory or descriptive research questions do not generally seek to test hypotheses. It follows, therefore, that whereas all hypotheses are research questions, not all research questions take the form of a hypothesis.

An explanatory study is seeking to answer a fairly specific question, formulated at the outset of the study. However, there will be a number of other possible answers to such a question, and it is important that these alternative explanations are in some way eliminated from consideration in the course of the study. The research design will therefore have to be carefully planned and tightly structured before the study begins, in order to control for these competing explanations. Explanatory studies tend, therefore, to follow a predetermined sequence of rigorously controlled steps, without room for the flexibility and impromptu changes of tack that may be seen in exploratory studies. It is unusual for the steps in the research process to overlap in explanatory research in the way that may occur in exploratory research. Similarly, the research question is normally fixed at the outset, and is not modified during the course of the study.

The key characteristics of these three types of question are summarized in Table 3.1. An example of each type of question will be used as a case study subsequently in this book (Box 3.4).

Box 3.4   *Introduction to case studies*

Much of the subsequent material in this book will be based on three hypothetical case studies, corresponding to the three types of research question described in this chapter. These case studies will be unfolded in increasing detail in subsequent chapters, and summaries of the studies are given in Appendix I. However, the research questions on which the case studies are based are stated below.

Case Study 1 – exploratory research. What do health care students understand by 'self-inflicted' illness in terms of the notion of responsibility for health? (The 'Student Attitudes Study', carried out by Dr Teresa Ganz.)

Case Study 2 – descriptive research. What are the characteristic patterns and modes of practice of therapists in respect of clients with rheumatoid arthritis? (The 'Rheumatoid Arthritis Study', carried out by Angela Carella.)

Case Sudy 3 – explanatory research. Is there a difference in effectiveness between an individual-based and a group-based cognitive-behavioural approach to the management of low back pain? (The 'Low Back Pain Study', carried out by Dr Joseph Buckley.)

Table 3.1   *Key characteristics of exploratory, descriptive and explanatory research questions. Distinctions between different forms of research have been somewhat simplified for clarity, and there may be a degree of overlap (e.g. there may be an element of theory testing in a study whose purpose is principally descriptive)*

	Exploratory	Descriptive/ normative	Explanatory
Nature of research question	General and provisional	Fairly specific and largely definitive	High specific and definitive; usually a hypothesis
Research design	Flexible, overlapping, and emergent	Structured, sequential, and largely predetermined	Highly structured, sequential, and predetermined
Data collected	Usually qualitative	Usually quantitative, but may include qualitative	Usually quantitative
Relationship to theory	Seeks to build theory	Seeks to develop or elaborate theory	Seeks to test theory

3.2 CRITERIA FOR A RESEARCH QUESTION

Within the context of empirical research, a research question should fulfil the following criteria.

3.2.1 Feasibility

A research question should be feasible in two respects. First, it should be feasible at a conceptual-empirical level; i.e. the concepts and proposition(s) within the research question should be susceptible to empirical investigation. For example, compare the following two questions:

1. Is withholding the truth from terminally ill patients morally wrong?
2. Do nurses in critical care feel that withholding the truth from terminally ill patients is morally wrong?

In the first case, collecting data from the real world will not on its own provide an answer to the question; what people may *consider* to be wrong will not determine conclusively what *is* wrong. The answer to this question depends ultimately on philosophical analysis at a theoretical level, not on the measurement of attitudes (Pellegrino, 1995). In contrast, the second question can indeed be answered by collecting data on individuals' opinions.

Second, a research question must be practically feasible. It must be possible to provide an answer to the question within the constraints of time, financial resources, subject accessibility, available expertise, cooperation from other agencies, and so forth. There is a tendency to underestimate the various practical barriers and difficulties that may be encountered in research, and studies addressing a research question that is unduly ambitious in terms of the practical demands that it imposes are likely to fail.

3.2.2 Interest

Research requires sustained commitment and imagination on the part of the investigator. If the research question is one in which the investigator is uninterested, it is likely that this commitment will be lacking. In addition, the interpretation of research findings often draws upon the creativity and intuition of the researcher, especially when dealing with qualitative data. It is difficult to be creative and imaginative on an uninspiring topic.

3.2.3 Originality

The criterion of originality should be interpreted carefully. To say that a research question must be original does not mean that it cannot have been previously investigated. There is a valuable role to be played by research that replicates previous investigations (Ross *et al.*, 1998). In this way, methodological shortcomings of the original study may be remedied, or the topic may be examined in relation to a different population and/or at a different time. What matters is that the findings that result from the study should make a new contribution to existing knowledge. There is little point in re-establishing what is already well known, but it may be useful to clarify existing knowledge that is in some respects unclear or incomplete.

There is an exception to this, however. Research is sometimes undertaken as a learning exercise, rather than with a view to generating new knowledge. This may be the case in research projects that form part of an undergraduate degree. Here, it is accepted that the findings of a study may not make any new contribution to knowledge (though it is, of course, an added bonus if they do), because the main purpose of the study is to provide the student with practical experience and training in the process of carrying out research.

3.2.4 Relevance

A key requirement of a research question is that it should be relevant. What is meant by 'relevant' will differ between basic and applied research (Hedrick *et al.*, 1993). In basic research (i.e. research undertaken with the purpose of enlarging knowledge and understanding for their own sake), a relevant question is one that sheds new light on the theoretical processes and relationships within a particular body of knowledge. In applied research, on the other hand, a relevant question is one that addresses particular issues and provides solutions to practical problems.

Within applied health care research, questions that might be considered of little relevance are those that do not relate to the sphere of practice of a particular group of practitioners, or are likely to produce findings that will have little influence, direct or indirect, on the way in which practice is carried out. Discussions with professional colleagues are a valuable means of clarifying the relevance of a proposed study (Bird *et al.*, 1995; Seale and Barnard, 1998).

3.2.5 Theoretical basis

As was argued earlier in this chapter, a research question should be set in the context of existing theory. In exploratory research, this body of knowledge may be very sketchy and undeveloped, but a theoretical framework of some sort should nonetheless exist.

3.2.6 Ethical legitimacy

A research question should be ethical in three senses. First, it should not require designs or methods that are likely to threaten the rights or welfare of research participants (e.g. methods that involve unjustifiable deception or are likely to cause physical, psychological or social harm). Second, it can be argued that a research question should not be pursued if it is reasonably foreseeable that the findings will be used to the detriment of certain individuals, particularly if

there is no countervailing benefit to others. It is on such grounds that some people oppose research into behaviour modification, eugenics and cloning (Penslar, 1995). Third, the choice of one research question rather than another can have ethical ramifications. Certain groups of people can be disadvantaged by being consistently excluded from research (Sapsford and Abbott, 1996). Thus, some unglamorous medical conditions might be overlooked by researchers, and the health of certain minority groups might attract little scientific inquiry. Some basic concepts and issues in research ethics are outlined in Section 4.4.

3.3 CONCLUSION

The success of an empirical study hinges on the research question on which it is based – in two senses. First, the question must be coherent and relevant. These qualities should be judged in terms of the relevant body of professional knowledge and theory, and underline the importance of basing empirical research on a clear and well-articulated conceptual and theoretical perspective. Second, the question must be appropriately translated into the structural and procedural features of the study in question. The extent to which this is achieved is assessed in methodological terms; the following chapter will examine some of the relevant issues in more detail.

PART THREE

DESIGNING AND EXECUTING A STUDY

4 BASIC ELEMENTS OF RESEARCH DESIGN

SUMMARY

This chapter explores the following topics:

- the development of an appropriate research design
- the concepts of variable and measurement
- the selection of cases for inclusion in a study
- the times at which data should be collected
- a classification of basic research designs
- the ethical issues that may arise in health care research

Three broad categories of research question and their relationship to methodology, design and methods were introduced in Chapter 3. This chapter will focus more specifically on the issue of research design, and will consider a classification of basic designs that encompasses the wide range of approaches to research available within health care. These designs have their origins in a variety of disciplines: natural science, medicine, psychology, sociology and anthropology. Judicious choice of the design to be employed in a study underpins the credibility of any findings from that research and, consequently, their ability to inform health care practice. It follows that an understanding of design principles is as important for the consumer of published research as it is for the research practitioner. A sound design also determines to a large degree the quality of other methodological aspects of a study, in particular the analysis of the data gathered.

4.1 INTRODUCTION TO RESEARCH DESIGN

A design specifies the logical structure of a research project and the plan that will be followed in its execution. It determines whether a study is capable of obtaining an answer to the research question (the focus of the study) in a manner consistent with the appropriate research methodology and the theoretical and philosophical perspectives underlying the study (Figure 3.1). In general, design is concerned with the following operational aspects of a study:

- what entities or variables to examine
- under what conditions to examine these entities or variables
- what type(s) of data to collect
- from whom (or what) to collect these data
- at what time points to collect the data
- what method to employ for data collection
- what implications ensue for subsequent data analysis
- other aspects

For explanatory and most descriptive research questions, prior knowledge enables these aspects to be considered and a detailed strategy to be specified before any data are collected. In practice, some of these aspects might be considered conjointly and in an order that develops during deliberation, which may differ from that in which they are presented above. Minor alterations may be made to the initial design and there may be refinement of the research question to produce more specific questions or hypotheses. However, in general the design of an explanatory or descriptive study tends to be determined in advance. In contrast, exploratory research questions do not require that decisions be made on all aspects of design before data collection begins – indeed, it is desirable that this should not occur, so that the study retains a degree of flexibility. Rather, the design emerges in the course of the study, in response to collected data and their analysis.

Any research design is subject to various constraints, and must therefore be a reasoned compromise between the desirable and the feasible. All studies are prone to resource constraints in terms of time, money, availability of suitable equipment or instrumentation, and the number and expertise of available researchers. These all have obvious implications for the design, as do practical factors such as limited access to sources of data or prospective participants. These issues are often particularly troublesome for students undertaking a research project as part of a course of study. However, providing that the objectives of a study are realistic in terms of the likely constraints, worthwhile findings can be generated from an apparently modest piece of research.

Given such constraints, Hakim (1987) points out that on occasions it may be necessary to trade down to a simpler and cheaper design. However, care must be taken to ensure that the objectives of the original study are not made unattainable in the process.

4.1.1 What entities or variables to consider

At the simplest level, an *entity* is something having a distinct or real existence, such that it may be examined empirically. Some entities can be apprehended directly in a fairly tangible form (e.g. weight, height, temperature). In contrast, other entities represent more abstract concepts – such entities are sometimes referred to as *constructs* to reflect the fact that they are constructed at a theoretical level, and may not be directly observable. We cannot, for example, observe the concepts of 'grief' or 'depression' directly, but we can observe behaviour or hear talk that we take to express these concepts. These are the *empirical referents* of the concept, and the process whereby a concept is translated into its empirical referents is known as *operationalization* (see Section 7.2.3).

Variable is a term applied to an entity that varies or can take on more than one value, and generally denotes entities that can be quantified. For example, in the general population, sex, age, occupation and marital status are examples of demographic variables that vary from one person to another. Range of motion of the glenohumeral joint, muscular force, blood pressure and

functional capacity are examples of physiological variables that differ from client to client, and vary across time for a given individual. Anxiety and depression are psychological variables that may also differ within and between individuals, and may be influenced by other variables such as health status and coping ability. There are instances, however, when these same characteristics and properties might be constant; that is, fixed at a specified value (or within a specified range of values). In a project investigating the problems that mothers with low back pain face when coping with a young family, gender is a constant (since only women are included) and pathology is constant (since only those with low back pain are considered).

At a more general level, a variable may be defined as a characteristic or property of a person, group, object or situation that can be observed or manipulated and that exhibits different values under different conditions or on different occasions (Portney and Watkins, 1993; Polit and Hungler, 1997).

In research, the entities or variables of interest are inherent in the research question. Perceptions of self-inflicted illness, patterns of practice, mode of practice, characteristics of clients, low back pain, effectiveness of therapy, and treatment modalities are examples of entities and variables in the case studies introduced in Chapter 3 (Box 3.4). At this stage, variables might appear vague and lacking definition. What do 'low back pain' and 'effectiveness of therapy' mean? Before they can be classified or measured in a meaningful way, these concepts must be expressed in more concrete terms, through the process of operationalization referred to above.

It might be apparent, also, that many studies involve variables that are not of direct interest to the researcher and are not obvious in the research question, but could nonetheless influence findings from the study. These are called *extraneous* variables and it is important that they are considered at the design stage (whether or not the researcher is able to deal with their influence). For example, age, comorbidity, and previous medical history with respect to low back pain will impact on the effectiveness of a therapy programme.

4.1.2 Under what conditions to consider the entities or variables

Having outlined the sorts of entities that can be studied, it is important to consider the conditions under which they can be examined. Many different terms are used to denote the variables in a study. Common terms are given in Table 4.1. Variables of direct interest can be classified as manipulated or non-manipulated. Manipulated variables are deliberately controlled or changed in a planned way by the researcher in order to determine the effect upon some measure of interest (a measured variable, which is not manipulated). In general, explanatory studies involve at least one manipulated and one measured variable. When other sources of explanation can be accounted for, observed changes in the measured variable are ascribed to the effect of the manipulated variable (see Chapter 7). For example, individuals with compulsive-obsessive disorder could be specifically allocated

to receive treatment either by behaviour modification techniques or by cognitive restructuring techniques (these constituting a manipulated variable), to determine the effect of each of these on the frequency of their compulsive-obsessive behaviour (this being a measured variable).

Non-manipulated variables fall into several categories, discussed in more detail in Domholdt (1993). Some variables are inherently non-manipulable, such as gender, age, or years of experience. Participants in a study might be classified according to specified age categories across which comparisons on some measure of interest could be made. Alternatively, actual ages might be recorded and the relationship with other variables analysed.

Some variables are manipulable but the researcher chooses to study them without any planned interference. The effect of behavioural and cognitive strategies for persons with compulsive-obsessive disorder might be investigated through the existing caseloads of therapists who routinely use one of these techniques in their clinical practice, rather than through the specific

Table 4.1 *Alternative terminology for variables within a study*

Conditions	Direction of assumed *effect* between variables X and Y X → Y	
• deliberate manipulation of the X variable • X is presumed to affect Y • control of the important extraneous variables	Manipulated variable; cause; independent variable; intervention variable; treatment variable; experimental variable; factor; stimulus variable; determinant	Measured variable; effect; dependent variable; outcome variable; response; response variable; criterion variable; consequences

Conditions	Direction of assumed *prediction* between variables X and Y X → Y	
• no manipulation of the X variable • X is presumed to predict Y • designation of X and Y might be somewhat arbitrary • some control of extraneous variables	Predictor variable; treatment variable; explanatory variable	Predicted variable; response variable; estimated variable; outcome variable

Conditions	No directional relationship posited between study variables
• no manipulation of the study variables • no control of extraneous variables	Concepts; phenomena; responses; observations

assignment of participants to one or other treatment.

Extraneous variables can be classified as controlled, randomized or disregarded. Control and randomization are two strategies for excluding extraneous variables as possible sources of explanation of variation in a measured variable. Control can be exercised in several ways. An extraneous variable might be held fixed or constant during the study, for example by explicitly including only units (e.g. persons, items, objects, institutions or countries) with some pre-specified attribute. For example, a study involving only clients newly diagnosed with rheumatoid arthritis essentially considers time since diagnosis as constant. Alternatively, the control might be on the environmental conditions (e.g. all information is collected from one clinical setting) or the conditions under which manipulation takes place (e.g. a fixed period of treatment, or treatment delivered at the same time of day for all clients in the study). This approach to controlling variables is sometimes referred to as *specification*. Alternatively, the influence of extraneous variables can be dealt with by means of randomization. This involves randomly allocating subjects to two or more groups, so that the characteristics of these subjects are, as far as possible, equalized across these groups (see Section 7.2.1).

Some degree of control may feature in designs addressing descriptive research questions. The survey conducted in the Rheumatoid Arthritis Study is, for example, restricted to physiotherapists and occupational therapists with a certain kind of clinical experience. Various statistical techniques can also be used to control for certain variables in the analysis of descriptive studies, just as in explanatory studies. However, randomization and the manipulation of variables are not characteristic features of descriptive studies.

When extraneous variables are described as disregarded, no attempt is made to control them through the design of the study, randomization, or statistical analysis. The worst situation is one in which an uncontrolled variable is completely confounded with a variable of direct interest – that is, the effects or influences of these two variables are inseparable (Section 7.2). Such a study would lack internal validity (Section 7.2.8).

In exploratory studies, the entities of interest are explored in a natural setting without interference and without any attempt to control extraneous variables – if this were to be done, the setting would cease to be a natural one (see Section 5.1). In the Student Attitudes Study, Dr Ganz wishes to observe the interaction that occurs spontaneously during teaching sessions. If steps were taken to control certain variables in the teaching situation, the reactive effects of doing so would quite probably distort the normal pattern of interaction.

The variables within a study are often named in different ways, according to the sort of analytical relationship being examined (Table 4.1). Some of the terminology used is potentially confusing (such as reference to 'independent' and 'dependent' variables; see Box 4.1). Accordingly, in an attempt to achieve greater clarity, the following conventions will be followed in this book:

1. If a relationship of association or correlation is at issue, the simple term 'variable' will be used for all variables.
2. When values of one variable are used to predict those of another, we will use the terms 'predictor variable' and 'outcome (or predicted) variable', respectively.
3. Where causal relationships are being tested, such as in an experiment, the terms 'intervention variable' and 'outcome variable' will be used to denote the cause and effect, respectively. (On occasion, it is appropriate to use the term 'factor' instead of 'intervention variable'; see Sections 7.3.1 and 18.1.1.)

In order to examine these, and any other, relationships in a meaningful way, it is necessary to collect the right type of data in the appropriate form; this will be addressed in the following section.

Box 4.1 *'Independent' and 'dependent' variables*

Variables are often classified as independent or dependent. This terminology reflects the relationship between variables within a specific type of study, in particular with regard to causal relationships. The causes are often referred to as 'independent' variables and the effects as 'dependent' variables. The value of a dependent variable is considered to be consequent upon that of the independent variable (e.g. a person's reported level of pain is a consequence of the type of treatment he or she has received). Independent variables are unrelated, in that the value of one independent variable does not influence the value of another, thus allowing them to be manipulated separately (e.g. the type of treatment received by participants in a study and the frequency with which they receive such treatment can be manipulated separately). Note, however, that although independent variables do not influence one another, they may together have a combined influence on a dependent variable, such as when

an interaction is present (see Section 7.3.1). Thus, rather confusingly, the variables themselves are independent but their effects may not be. This use of 'independent' and 'dependent' is inappropriate in studies where variables cannot be classified as cause or effect; this is the case when values of two variables are *associated*, which does not imply a causal relationship. Similarly, this terminology is best avoided when values of one variable are used to *predict* those of another variable; again, there is not necessarily a direct causal relationship between the variables. Moreover, the terms are not ideal even when referring to experimental studies. Even though experiments do address causal relationships, to say that values of one variable 'depend upon' those of another presupposes precisely the relationship that is being tested for. In sum, the terms 'independent variable' and 'dependent variable' are best avoided altogether (Hulley *et al.*, 1988b; Everitt, 1998).

4.1.3 What data to collect

Data are pieces of information collected during a study to address the research question. They contain relevant information about the entities or variables that the researcher has chosen to study and form the basis of all analyses. Data can be narrative (e.g. words describing the experiences in a work situation for a person with low back pain) or numerical (e.g. range of movement, or numbers representing work disability). Data may even take the form of material objects or artefacts (e.g. everyday utensils, pieces of artwork). Whether they are descriptive or numerical, data should possess certain characteristics, such as validity and reliability (see Chapter 9).

Narrative descriptions can be obtained through discussion with participants or observation of the participants' behaviour in a specific situation. Narrative records can be extracted from existing documentation such as diaries (see

Section 6.3.3). The data normally exist as text, but may sometimes take a diagrammatic form. Narrative data are associated with exploratory and descriptive research questions.

Numerical data are numbers obtained through measurement. Measurement can be defined as the planned process of assigning numbers to variables using an instrument that minimizes the subjectivity of the assignment of these numbers. More formally, according to Nunnally and Bernstein (1994, p. 3), measurement comprises 'rules for assigning symbols to objects so as to (1) represent quantities of attributes numerically (scaling) or (2) define whether the objects fall in the same or different categories with respect to a given attribute (classification)'.

The numbers derived through measurement may represent labels for distinct categories, or may reflect how much of an attribute is present. In The Rheumatoid Arthritis Study information on respondents' profession might be labelled '1' for occupational therapy and '2' for physiotherapy.

The numbers 1 and 2 have no quantitative meaning; they serve only to differentiate therapists with respect to profession. In contrast, the numbers representing range of motion can be any value along a continuum from 0 (no motion) to 180 (or some other value that represents full range) and reflect the amount of angular movement of a joint, with higher values indicating more movement. In this case the numbers used *do* have a quantitative meaning, since they represent the magnitude of the variable being measured.

Many instruments have been developed for use in health care research. They range from physical instruments (e.g. pressure gauges) to multi-item scales (e.g. the Aberdeen Back Pain Scale). Whatever type of instrument is used, it must have validity and reliability. *Validity* refers to the extent to which an instrument measures what it is intended to measure. An invalid instrument produces meaningless values. There are several types of measurement validity depending upon the nature of the instrument and the context in which it is used. The four principal components, which are discussed in detail in Section 9.2, are face validity, content validity, criterion-related validity and construct validity.

Reliability refers to the extent of reproducibility or consistency of values measured under specified conditions. An unreliable instrument produces values that are subject to high variability or measurement error. Reliability is assessed through measures such as inter-rater and intra-rater reliability and internal consistency. Further details on these various forms of measurement reliability are given in Sections 9.3, 15.3 and 18.3.

4.1.4 From whom (or what) to collect the data

In Chapter 8, the process of sampling is examined in detail, in relation to exploratory, descriptive and explanatory studies. In each of these approaches to research, the researcher is most usually in the position of not being able to collect data from all those cases that are of potential interest and relevance to the study. This is the situation in each of the case studies:

Teresa Ganz is unable to tap the attitudes of all student nurses and occupational therapists, Angela Carella is unlikely to gain access to all therapists working with patients with rheumatoid arthritis, and Joseph Buckley can study only a subsection of patients with low back pain.

Thus, the researcher will usually select for the study a *sample* of cases from a larger *population* of such cases. The principal criterion for selecting a sample is that it should be representative. There are, however, different types of representativeness. A sample can be *empirically* representative or *theoretically* representative, or both (see Sections 5.3 and 8.2). It is important to note that some researchers conducting exploratory studies do not intend to generalize their findings to cases beyond those that they have actually studied, and for this reason theoretical, not statistical, representativeness is the key issue in the process of sample selection. In studies such as these, a sample is selected in terms of its ability to generate important insights into the focus of the study, rather than its representativeness of a wider population of cases.

A second important criterion is the size of a sample. In many descriptive and explanatory studies, where statistical representativeness is a crucial consideration, it is important to obtain a sufficient sample size so that the study has the capability to detect clinically important differences as statistically significant, or to estimate effects/attributes with stated precision (Section 18.6). Different considerations apply, however, in studies where theoretical representativeness is the chief concern (see Sections 5.3 and 8.2).

4.1.5 At what time points to collect the data

Data might be collected at one point in time (*cross-sectionally*) or at several points in time (*longitudinally*). Data collected at one point in time can be used to describe variables (e.g. behaviour, attitudes, characteristics or functional status) for a population, or to compare attributes across more than one population. Such information represents a snapshot in time. This does not necessarily imply that all the data are collected on one day or within one hour, rather that no events that are liable to impact upon the variables of interest are anticipated or planned to occur during the period of data collection.

When interest focuses on change or trends over time, data are collected at two or more points, in the direction of either the future (*prospectively*) or the past (*retrospectively*), with respect to the start of the study. The spacing of the time points depends on the data source and the period over which it would be important to discern any change or trend. In studies that investigate the impact of an intervention, data are normally collected prospectively, that is, at a baseline (before the intervention is applied) and on at least one time point after the application of the intervention. This might be a point at which any impact is likely to have occurred, or specified times post intervention selected to investigate the rate at which any impact occurs.

In exploratory studies, the total duration for data collection might be specified at the outset, but the decision about the number of occasions on which to collect data is often made after the initial data have been collected and analysed. This reflects the characteristically emergent character of research design in such studies (see Section 5.2).

4.1.6 What method to employ for data collection

Common methods of data collection include questionnaires, interviews, focus groups, the Delphi method, observations, and instrumented measurement tools. These methods will be discussed in detail in Chapters 5 and 6 with respect to specific research questions, but are mentioned here because the choice among them is a key element within the design of a study.

4.1.7 Implications for subsequent data analysis

The research methodology and research question influence what data are collected and how, with implications for the subsequent analysis and for the generalizability or otherwise of findings. Narrative information is analysed through some form of content analysis, whereas numerical data can be analysed using descriptive or (if appropriate) inferential statistics. Later chapters cover such analyses in detail. The crucial issue is to think ahead, to plan in detail the strategy for the analysis, and to check that it is capable of producing interpretable results that address the research question or hypothesis. If this cannot be achieved, the research design and/or the research question should be revised.

4.1.8 Other aspects

Other aspects that need to be considered at the design stage include difficulties or limitations that might be encountered during the study, and actions that might be taken to circumvent or prevent such issues (Box 4.2).

Box 4.2 *Limitations and delimitations*

It is helpful to distinguish between these terms. According to Cresswell (1994, p. 110) these both refer to the 'boundaries, exceptions, reservations, and qualifications inherent in every study'. However, *delimitation* refers to a restriction of scope within a piece of research. Owing to certain practical or methodological restraints, a researcher might decide to limit a study to a certain population of respondents, or to a particular period of time. The design adopted within such delimitations should still provide an appropriate answer to the research question, even though the scope of this question may have been narrowed. A delimitation represents a reasoned response to certain issues outside the researcher's control, and is not necessarily a shortcoming within a study. In contrast, a *limitation* can be considered to be a shortcoming of a study. For example, it may not be possible to access the data most appropriate for a particular research question, or the best available instrument to collect quantitative data may not reach the desired level of reliability. The presence of limitations means that a research question is likely to be answered suboptimally, or even inappropriately.

The issues involved here are more specific to the particular design that is selected for the study and will be touched upon again in later chapters. In general terms, the difficulties that might arise include failing to secure access to equipment, clients or data, addressing too broad a research question, overlooking important variables within the study, selecting inappropriate instruments (possibly invalid or unreliable), trying to collect too much information, high attrition, running out of time, and ethical problems. Possible actions could include establishing contact with gatekeepers or consultants before starting the study, trying not to target people who are obviously too busy to help, seeking peer review or expert appraisal on the proposed design at the planning stage, running a pilot study to test the feasibility of the design and the instruments, minimizing the information collected, ensuring that the participant information sheet is friendly and inviting, and planning follow-up calls or letters for non-responders.

4.2 CLASSIFICATION OF BASIC RESEARCH DESIGNS

It is usual to label and classify the different types of research design (Reid, 1993). Identifying a broad category of design in relation to a particular study helps to clarify the types of methods and procedures that are likely to be appropriate or inappropriate within that study. Unfortunately, there is no one, universally accepted taxonomy of research designs. One approach is to classify basic types of research design according to their structural features, time frame, unit of participation and context (Table 4.2). Other designs can be considered to fall on a continuum between those described through combinations of these categories

4.2.1 Time frame

As indicated earlier (Section 4.1.5), a study in which the data are collected and/or variables are manipulated at one point in time is termed *cross-sectional*, as compared with a *longitudinal* study, in which data are collected at two or more points in time (possibly with variables being manipulated over the corresponding time interval). When the focus is on an extended period of time, the data can be collected prospectively or retrospectively with respect to the start of the study.

4.2.2 Unit of participation and context

With respect to unit of participation, data might be collected on an individual unit (a person, clinic, organization or object) in what is called a *single instance* study, or on several cases (for example, different persons or clinics) in a *group* study.

The context for data collection is the research setting: that is, the physical location in which the data will be collected. This could be a field setting (i.e. a naturalistic environment) or a laboratory setting (i.e. an artificial and controlled environment). Much health care research occurs in a context that falls between these two extremes. For example, controlled clinical trials

Table 4.2 *Basic types of research design*

Structural features	Time frame	Unit of participation	Context
Experimental	Longitudinal – prospective	Two or more groups of units	Most often artificial
Quasi-experimental	Longitudinal – prospective or retrospective	One or more groups of units, or single unit ('single system')	Artificial or natural
Non-experimental	Cross-sectional (single snapshot)	One or more groups of units, or single unit ('single case')	Most often natural

often involve the delivery of treatments within the context of fairly routine care, but may involve specialized clinical measurements conducted in a highly controlled setting.

4.2.3 Structural features

An *experimental design* involves manipulation, control and randomization (Table 4.3). It is a highly structured design whose aim is to establish the existence of a cause–effect relationship; i.e. whether the introduction of an intervention causes a change in the outcome measure(s) of interest. Other plausible explanations for this change are isolated or eliminated (as far as possible) through control, randomization or specific features built into the design. Experimental design is appropriate for an explanatory question, and utilizes a hypothetico-deductive method of theory testing (see Section 2.4.1). It is longitudinal (prospective) and may be used in a clinical, community or laboratory setting.

A *quasi-experimental design* lacks the full control of an experimental design and is used when the 'true' experiment is not feasible or is in some respect impractical (Behi and Nolan, 1996b). Such designs are commonly employed in epidemiological research. More specifically, a quasi-experimental design is one in which either there is not a *separate* control group, or if a separate control group is present, subjects are not randomly assigned to it (see Table 4.3). More than one level of the predictor variable is included in the design of the study, but this may

not necessarily occur through active manipulation. Quasi-experiments address explanatory research questions, and are longitudinal (either retrospective or prospective). Quasi-experimental studies often occur in natural contexts, where it is not possible to exert the degree of control required for a true experiment. Cherulnik (1983, p. 272) comments,

> *If we limit our research to true experiments, we stand to lose many rich opportunities to study behavior as it is influenced by real and powerful events that are scheduled and shaped by forces we cannot control.*

The drawback of the quasi-experiment is that lack of full experimental control means that there is usually at least one plausible explanation for change other than the effect of the intervention (Reichardt and Mark, 1998). Single system designs, in which a participant is used as his or her own control, are quasi-experimental. Other examples include designs for which group membership is based on the predetermined values of a particular attribute or on pre-existing groups (Table 4.4). These include cohort and case–control studies (Cummings *et al.*, 1988; Newman *et al.*, 1988a; Mant and Jenkinson, 1997); these designs are illustrated in Figure 4.1.

Designs that depart from the true experiment in further respects are often referred to as *pre-experimental* designs (Campbell and Stanley, 1963). An example of such a study would be a one-group pre-test/post-test design; i.e. one in which a single group of subjects is pre-tested on

Table 4.3 *Key characteristics of research designs classified by structural features*

Feature	Experimental	Quasi-experimental	Non-experimental
Manipulation	Variables are actively manipulated	Variables may be actively manipulated	None
Control	High degree, with a separate control group	Restricted, sometimes lacking a separate control group	None or minimal
Randomization	Random assignment to levels of the manipulated variable(s)	None	None

Table 4.4   *Some examples of quasi-experimental designs*

Type of study	Description	Key features
Case–control study	A group of cases (i.e. those with an illness) are matched with a group of controls (i.e. those without the illness) and a retrospective comparison is made of variables that are possible causative factors for the illness.	Group membership is determined by a pre-existing status (i.e. with or without the illness), rather than by randomization from a single pool of subjects. Levels of the predictor variable are pre-existing and are therefore not manipulated. Suitable for investigating the cause of rare illnesses.
Cohort study	A group of individuals with a possible risk factor for an illness, and a matched group without the risk factor are followed up prospectively. Those who go on to develop the illness are compared with those who do not to see if contracting the illness is associated with the presence of the possible risk factor. A cohort study can also be retrospective, if information on risk factors and illness relates to the past.	Group membership is determined by a pre-existing status (i.e. with or without the risk factor), rather than by randomization from a single pool of subjects. Levels of the predictor variable are pre-existing and are therefore not manipulated. In contrast to a case–control study, a specific risk factor must be selected for study at the outset. Suitable for investigating the effects of rare risk factors.
Non-equivalent control group design	Two or more pre-existing groups of subjects (whom the researcher is unable to mix up) are recruited. Each group is pre-tested on appropriate outcome variables and then subjected to a different intervention (or a no-intervention phase). The groups are then post-tested on the outcome variables to determine any difference in effect of the interventions.	A separate control group is present but group membership is pre-determined and there is therefore no randomization. Levels of the intervention variable are manipulated.
Interrupted time-series design	A single group of subjects are subjected sequentially to two or more interventions (or to a single intervention and a no-intervention phase), with intervening measurement of appropriate outcome variables.	There is no separate control group (and therefore no randomization) – the subjects act as their own control. The intervention variable is manipulated.
Single system design	As for the interrupted time-series design, except that a single subject (or unit) is used instead of a single group of subjects (see Section 16.2).	As for the interrupted time-series design.

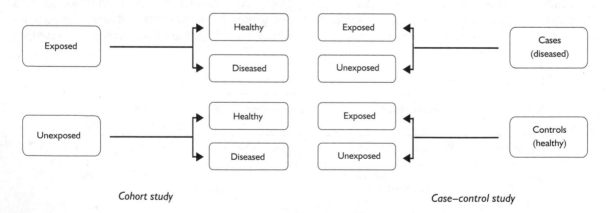

Cohort study   Case–control study

Figure 4.1   *Cohort and case-control studies. Inference of disease causation is prospective in a cohort study but retrospective in a case-control study.*

an outcome variable, subjected to an intervention, and then retested on the outcome variable. The absence of any form of control group means that such a study cannot be described as quasi-experimental and is therefore classified as pre-experimental (Cherulnik, 1983; Cresswell, 1994). The term 'pre-experimental' is not very widely used – nor are the specific designs that it describes, on account of their limited ability to eliminate alternative explanations for any effect observed.

A *non-experimental design* covers all situations not catered for by the preceding categories of design; specifically, those in which there is no attempt to manipulate predictor variables, create a control group, or randomize subjects between groups. The reason why there is no attempt to include these design features is usually not because the researcher would wish to do so but cannot, but because such features are inappropriate to the research question. It must not be thought, therefore, that there is something missing from a non-experimental design and that it is a residual category for suboptimal methodological approaches.

Descriptive and exploratory studies normally utilize non-experimental designs. Because the purpose of such studies is not to isolate cause–effect relationships, there is no need to exert a rigid influence over the design features of the study. In the case of exploratory studies in particular, the need to examine social life as it occurs naturally will preclude such influence.

A non-experimental study may be cross-sectional. In both the Student Attitudes Study and the Rheumatoid Arthritis Study, data are collected from the study participants at a particular point in time. Non-experimental studies may also be longitudinal. A researcher exploring the notion of an 'illness career' (Price, 1996) might interview a client at various points in the course of his or her illness and thus collect data prospectively. Similarly, a case study might focus on the workings of a hospital emergency room, and collect data at various points over a period of several months to gauge fluctuations in caseload and any resulting changes in practice.

Of course, a study may encompass more than one methodological approach, particularly if it addresses more than one research question (see Section 9.6), leading to a combination of designs or a hybrid research design. This situation could arise if a practitioner were interested both in comparing the efficacy of alternative treatments for low back pain and in exploring patients' perceptions of these treatments.

4.2.4 Choice of design

The research question (or hypothesis) is the focus of a study and the basis for creating a design. Designs and methods are appropriate or not in terms of the research question to which an answer is sought (Sackett and Wennberg, 1997). The operational aspects discussed in Section 4.1 and presented schematically in Figure 4.2 constitute one route for the development of an appropriate design. This figure will be presented with appropriate modifications at subsequent points in this book, to illustrate specific research designs.

4.3 ACTION RESEARCH

There has lately been growing interest in a form of research that lies somewhat outside the framework outlined hitherto in this and the previous chapter. Action research is a form of enquiry that is closely linked to the evaluation and modification of practice in contexts such as education, social services and health care (Hart and Bond, 1995). At its core is a cyclical process of evaluation, introduction of change, and re-evaluation. It is also an intrinsically cooperative and participatory form of enquiry (Box 4.3), with the researcher working in close collaboration with the users and providers of a particular service (Holter and Schwartz-Barcott, 1993; Meyer, 2000). The participants in the study are encouraged to identify an issue or problem that they consider important and, through a process of discussion and negotiation, the researcher and the participants jointly formulate and execute a plan of action to introduce change. The effects of this change are evaluated, lessons are learnt

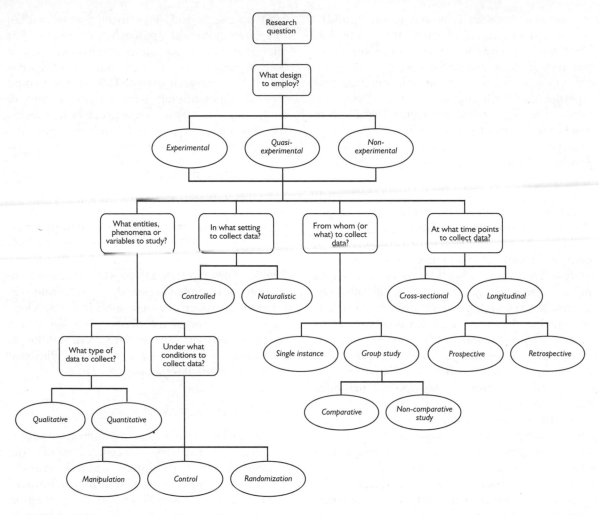

Figure 4.2 *Basic choices in research design.*

from it, and further change is introduced as appropriate (Susman and Evered, 1978). Thus, action and evaluation occur separately but simultaneously (Taylor, 1994). Action research can be regarded as a means of effecting change through the *process* of research, as well as through the *outcomes* of research.

To some extent, action research has affinities with experimental method, but differs from it in at least six ways. First, the focus of the research and the way in which it is to be conducted come from within, rather than being imposed by the researcher. Second, a wide variety of qualitative and quantitative data may be collected through informal as well as formal means. Third, the nature and structure of a study are not predetermined at the outset, but are allowed to evolve and develop as the research progresses; in this respect, the process of action research resembles that of most exploratory studies. Fourth, action research does not attempt to isolate and manipulate a single variable and control all other potential confounding variables to the same extent as experimental studies (Cohen and Manion, 1994). Although one or more specific interventions are carried out within a social

Box 4.3 *'New paradigm' research*

Action research, as commonly understood, can be located in a broader approach to enquiry which has been dubbed 'new paradigm research' (Reason and Rowan, 1981a). This model of enquiry breaks with traditional approaches to research in a number of ways. First, it rejects the claim that research is a wholly objective process, and makes room for the human, emotional and intuitive elements of everyday life; It seeks to be 'objectively subjective' (Reason and Rowan, 1981a, p. xiii). Second, it espouses a collaborative stance (Reason and Heron, 1995): new paradigm research is *with* and *for* people, rather than *on* people (Reason, 1988). Third, following the tenets of critical theory (Held, 1980), new paradigm research argues that research may move beyond being participatory and serve an emancipatory role. Hence, research may be a legitimate and effective means of counteracting patterns of oppression, discrimination or injustice within society, such as are experienced by disabled people (French and Swain, 1997). In this respect, it has affinities with feminist research, which also frequently adopts an avowedly political stance in the pursuit and application of knowledge (Webb, 1993). Further details on a number of aspects of new paradigm research are to be found in Reason and Rowan (1981a) and Reason (1988).

situation, there is normally little attempt to control other aspects of the research context. Fifth, the purpose of action research is to solve a practical problem in a particular situation, rather than to produce generalizable conclusions (Susman and Evered, 1978). Hence, Roth and Esdaile (1999) used this approach to facilitate and evaluate scholarly development in an academic department of occupational therapy, in response to a specific directive in the university. Accordingly, the concern for external validity that is present in experimental research is replaced by a focus on the particularities of a specific social or institutional context. Finally, a distinctive feature of action research is that the implementation of findings is an integral element of the research process, rather than a separate process occurring once a study has been completed (Kelly, 1985; Simmons, 1995). Similarly, it is usually the case that one of the purposes to be achieved within action research is that of empowering research participants as agents of change. Although this might be a desire of a researcher conducting an experimental study, it would normally be a subsequent process, rather than an intrinsic part of such a study.

In the light of such considerations, the research question addressed within a piece of action research would seem to be in one sense exploratory (in that the study identifies issues and problems from the participants in the course of the study, rather than in advance on the basis of the researcher's own perspective), and in another sense explanatory (in that it seeks to identify the effects of certain changes that are deliberately introduced).

Hart and Bond (1995) provide a comprehensive account of the nature and history of action research and provide a number of informative case studies. Webb (1989) and Meyer (1993) provide accounts of the methodological and ethical issues that may arise in the course of carrying out action research.

4.4 ETHICAL CONSIDERATIONS IN RESEARCH DESIGN

Nearly all research that involves human beings – whether directly or indirectly – gives rise to ethical issues. In health care, where individuals may be in a particularly vulnerable state on account of illness or disability, these issues are often all the more pressing. Some of these concern factors outside the research process; for example, the question whether a certain piece of research should be done in the first place or, once a study has been performed, what should be done with its findings. Others have to do with the specific design and conduct of a project, and may represent a tension or conflict between the methodological and moral aspects of research (Sim, 1989; Pallikkathayil *et al.*, 1998a, 1998b). The main issues to arise in this latter category are briefly defined in the following section.

4.4.1 Central issues in research ethics

Most of the specific issues and conflicts that give rise to ethical concern in health care research fall under one or more of the following headings.

Informed consent

Informed consent may be defined as 'the voluntary and revocable agreement of a competent individual to participate in a therapeutic or research procedure, based on an adequate understanding of its nature, purpose, and implications' (Sim, 1986, p. 584). It comprises four elements, each of which must be present for consent to be considered valid: disclosure, comprehension, competence and voluntariness.

Disclosure refers to the adequacy of the account provided by the researcher. This is to be distinguished from *comprehension*, which is the extent to which the research participant is able to understand what he or she has been told about a study. Whereas disclosure has to do with the details imparted by the professional, comprehension concerns the message received by the patient; disclosure relates to the *sufficiency* of information, comprehension to its *intelligibility*. The third element, *competence*, refers to the patient's ability to reach a rational, autonomous decision. Individuals with appreciable cognitive impairment are unlikely to be competent to consent. Equally, certain psychological or emotional states may impair competence. Finally, *voluntariness* refers to the absence of pressure, influence, inducement or coercion.

Privacy and confidentiality

Privacy is concerned with access to other people, or to information about them. Confidentiality is more specific. It relates to the way in which we treat information that we have gained about others (Sim, 1996). We can invade a person's privacy by gaining illegitimate access to their personal affairs, but we do not breach confidentiality unless we convey this information to others. Similarly, if information is gained from a person with their full consent, but then disseminated against their wishes, confidentiality has been breached even though privacy has not.

Anonymity

Anonymity is distinct from both privacy and confidentiality. It concerns whether or not what a person has said or done, or other personal information, is attributable to that person. Informants may happily concede a large measure of their privacy, and may be content for what they say to be quoted, so long as they are not identified as the source of the views or information expressed.

Deception

Research may involve deception in a number of ways. It may be that participants are not told the true nature and objectives of a study, such that they are led to make incorrect assumptions about its purpose (deception by omission), or it may be that a study involves communicating facts that are known to be untrue (deception by commission). In either case, deception is usually employed to satisfy a methodological requirement of the study concerned.

Risk of harm

Those participating in research may undergo harm in a number of ways (Sieber, 1992; Seale and Barnard, 1999). In studies that involve the testing of treatment, involving physical, pharmacological or behavioural procedures, there may be a risk of physical and/or psychological harm. Psychological harm may also arise in research that involves an examination of individuals' attitudes and beliefs, particularly if it uncovers sensitive issues or feelings of guilt or inadequacy. It may also result if involvement in research causes false hopes to be raised – for example, if a participant is encouraged to identify health care needs that are not capable of being fulfilled.

Social harm may also occur during research. If

sensitive information about individuals is laid open to public scrutiny, they may be subject to vilification, ostracism or discrimination. Economic harm might also come about if they are dismissed from employment as a result, or legal harm if they are revealed as having engaged in illegal activities.

Exploitation

Exploitation is a general term that may be used to cover instances in which participants are used for the purposes of research in a way that disregards their wishes, dignity or welfare. As such, it overlaps with some of the issues that arise under the headings of informed consent and risk of harm. Participants who are exploited in research, especially in the context of experimentation, are sometimes described as being treated as 'guinea pigs' (Pappworth, 1967; Farsides, 1989).

4.4.2 Basic ethical principles

One way of analysing the ethical implications of aspects of the research process is to explore their relationship to fundamental ethical values or principles (but see Box 4.4). There are five such principles (Sim, 1997), and these are shown in Table 4.5. This table also indicates the way in which the specific ethical concerns that arise in research can be linked to one or more of these basic principles.

By tracing a concrete ethical issue back to one or more of these basic principles, it is possible to explain why the issue in question is of ethical concern. This can then serve to justify a particular judgement. For example, if a research project involved deceiving participants so that they do something that they would ordinarily avoid doing, a judgement that this is morally wrong can be justified by pointing to its contravention of the principle of respect for autonomy.

Difficult decisions arise when there is some form of conflict between ethical requirements in research. Some of the specific issues that may arise will be considered in subsequent chapters in relation to particular research designs and

Box 4.4 *Approaches to ethics*

It should perhaps be pointed out that the use of these basic principles is not the only means of making decisions on ethical matters, and ethicists differ in the weight they attach to the use of principles. Whereas *deontologists* are happy to use these principles as the final arbiters in ethical decision making, *consequentialists* argue that, in the final analysis, it is the likely consequences of a course of action that matter most, rather than the fact that one or other moral principle may have been breached. Another school of thought, known as *virtue ethics*, judges human action in terms of the particular character traits that it exemplifies – its primary focus is on the sort of people we are rather than on the actions that we perform. Although these approaches may differ in the way they analyse ethical issues, they often arrive at similar conclusions. For example, the use of deception can be criticized because it breaches respect for autonomy (deontology), or because it leads to an undesirable loss of trust between patients and health professionals (consequentialism), or because it embodies the undesirable character trait of dishonesty (virtue ethics). Detailed consideration of these approaches, though important for a thorough understanding of research ethics, is beyond the scope of this book. Further discussion can be found in Gillon (1986), Johnstone (1994), Beauchamp and Childress (1994), and Sim (1997).

approaches. In most cases, certain methodological demands of the study are at variance with the requirements of ethics, with the result that the value of the research has to be weighed against the interests of those taking part.

4.4.3 Gaining ethical approval

When research involving human participants is carried out within an institution such as a hospital, formal ethical approval is normally required. An application must be made to the

Table 4.5   *Fundamental ethical principles and the specific ethical issues in research to which they can be related.*

Principle	Associated requirement	Related issues in research
Respect for autonomy	The requirement that we should protect the autonomy or self-determination of others	• the need to gain informed consent • the need not to deceive participants • the need not to exploit participants • the need to respect confidentiality and privacy
Respect for persons	The requirement that we should treat people with consideration of their individual human dignity, and not use them merely as a means to an end	• the need to gain informed consent • the need not to exploit participants • the need to ensure that research procedures do not undermine a person's dignity or self respect
Beneficence	The requirement to perform actions that will bring benefit to other people and promote their well-being	• the need to carry out research whose findings will benefit members of society • the need to disseminate such findings
Non maleficence	The requirement that we should refrain from actions that will bring harm to other people	• the need to avoid causing harm or distress • the need not to breach confidentiality or anonymity • the need not to raise unrealistic or unfulfillable expectations in research participants
Justice	The requirement that we should deal with others in a way that is fair and in accordance with their individual merit	• the need not to use vulnerable individuals in research • the need to ensure that the benefits and burdens of research are distributed fairly

relevant Research Ethics Committee (or Institutional Review Board in the USA), and the study should not proceed until approval has been granted. The specific procedures that are involved in this process will vary from country to country, and there are often variations at the level of state, region, district or institution within a given country.

It should be remembered that approval from a research ethics committee or institutional review board does not mean that the ethical aspects of a study need no further attention from the investigator. Ethical considerations should be given ongoing scrutiny as a study proceeds, and it should not be assumed that an ethics committee has necessarily addressed all issues of possible ethical relevance – to a large degree, the verdict of the ethics committee concerns what is *permitted*, not necessarily what is *permissible*.

Further discussion of the process and procedures of ethical review can be found in Sieber (1992) and Evans and Evans (1996). Levine (1988) and T Smith (1999) provide a comprehensive guide to ethical issues in clinical research. Kimmel (1988, 1996) and Homan (1991) cover issues arising in social research. Specific ethical questions will be addressed in relation to particular research approaches in Sections 5.8, 6.7, 7.5 and 16.2.2.

4.5   CONCLUSION

This chapter has emphasized that credible findings are dependent upon the research design that is employed in a study. It takes time to develop a design that has the optimum capability of achieving the required objectives, through an approach that is compatible with the desired research methodology. One approach is to consider the operational aspects appertaining to the information (or data) to be collected. This should guide a researcher towards an appropriate design. Once developed, the resultant design might then be classified – a possible taxonomy has been presented in this chapter. For any study, there is normally no one correct design. Many alternative designs could be developed; each will possess advantages and disadvantages. It is the researcher's task to choose wisely, and in the following chapters we aim to assist such choices.

5 DESIGNING AN EXPLORATORY STUDY

SUMMARY

This chapter explores the following topics:

- the relationship between exploratory research questions and qualitative data collection
- basic elements of research design in exploratory studies
- sampling in exploratory studies
- accessing the research setting and managing the researcher role
- principal methods of collecting qualitative data
- the general approach to analysing qualitative data
- ethical issues that arise in exploratory studies

An exploratory study is one that addresses one or more exploratory research questions, as defined in Section 3.1.1. Its purpose is to shed light upon a topic that has not yet been described in detail and is likely to be poorly understood at the level of theoretical explanation. This has important implications for the types of design that may appropriately be employed to address such questions. The purpose of this chapter is to examine some of these design features in more detail. Some of the epistemological presuppositions of exploratory studies will be outlined; these presuppositions will also be considered in Section 6.2, by way of contrast to those underlying descriptive studies.

The processes of design, data collection and data analysis tend to overlap in exploratory studies. Consequently, the issues presented in this chapter should be considered in conjunction with those addressed in Chapters 10 and 11. The division of material between these chapters

is for ease of exposition only, and should not be taken to imply that these elements of the research process are separate.

5.1 THE NATURE OF EXPLORATORY STUDIES

Exploratory research questions are most often answered by the collection of qualitative, rather than quantitative, data (Robson, 1993). The nature of the concepts and phenomena in terms of which such questions are framed are such that they are more appropriately captured by data that seek to *describe* and *categorize* than by data that seek to *quantify*. Why should this be the case? In order to quantify data at more than a very basic level (such as simply counting occurrences), two conditions must be met:

1. The nature of the phenomenon in question must be fairly well defined and agreed upon.
2. Common units of measurement must exist that can be applied to all instances of this phenomenon.

Hence, we can measure blood pressure and heart rate because we more or less agree what blood pressure and heart rate are, and we have developed at least one way of measuring each of these in different people. If we attempt to measure blood pressure in more than one person, we are confident that we are measuring the same thing – pressure readings in one person are commensurable with pressure readings in another person.

In contrast, the sorts of concepts or phenomena that form the subject of exploratory studies tend to be ones that are recognized and understood in only general and tentative terms. Indeed, it is quite likely that, at this stage, no names or labels will have been attached to these concepts and phenomena. In these circumstances, the purposes of data collection tend to be those of description and categorization, rather than of quantification.

To say that exploratory research tends to involve the collection of qualitative data is not to say that qualitative data can play only a preliminary or preparatory role, prior to a more structured investigation dealing with quantitative data. Indeed, qualitative data may usefully be collected after a quantitative study, so as to add depth and further insight to the data already gathered.

In Section 2.3, three of the fundamental philosophical perspectives underlying research approaches were considered. Research that concerns itself with the collection of qualitative data is likely to adopt a perspective akin to phenomenology; i.e. one that stresses the perceptions and interpretations of the world held by an individual or a social group (see Box 5.1). The accent within this perspective is on the individuality, even the uniqueness, of each person's or group's set of perceptions, which are located in a specific social context (Shepard *et al.*, 1993). These perceptions are therefore not commensurable, and this precludes the possibility of a common scale of measurement which can be applied across individuals.

It is important, however, not to define exploratory studies solely in terms of features that they do not possess. Maxwell (1996, pp. 17–21) outlines the purposes of research based on qualitative data as follows:

- to understand the meanings that people draw from the situations and activities in which they are involved;
- to understand the particular context within which people act and interact;
- to identify unanticipated or hitherto unknown phenomena;
- to gain insight into the processes underlying social life;
- to develop causal explanations of human activity and interaction.

The last of these purposes requires some clarification and qualification. To uncover an objective cause–effect relationship, one potential causative factor has to be tested while all other such factors are held constant; this is the role of the experimental or quasi-experimental design, rather than an exploratory study based on qualitative data. However, as Maxwell goes on to indicate, an exploratory study may provide insights into the *processes* by which an established cause–effect relationship operates. Similarly, Guba and Lincoln (1981) point out that such a study may also shed light on the contexts in which cause–effect relationships occur. Moreover, qualitative approaches can uncover the reasons and motivations to which people ascribe their own actions and behaviour: what one might call a subjective causal explanation. Insights gained in this way play an important part in understanding the processes of lay decision making underlying the uptake of health care interventions (Green and Britten, 1998).

Another important characteristic of exploratory research is that it tends to be *naturalistic*. That is to say, it is conducted in a natural setting and with as little control and influence as possible on the part of the researcher (though it would be a mistake to think that a natural situation can ever be *wholly* uncontaminated by the activity of the researcher). Hence, data collection in such studies is often referred to as 'fieldwork'. Exploratory studies are not the only ones that can be carried out in natural settings, of course. Experiments and, especially, quasi-experiments can be conducted in real-life settings as well as in laboratory situations (hence the term 'field experiment'), and much experimental research in health care is of this nature. However, although the setting may be natural, there remain the essential elements of experimental control and manipulation of variables.

As well as being naturalistic, exploratory research tends to be *holistic*, in that it seeks to understand a phenomenon in its entirety. This is in contrast to some approaches to research based on the collection of quantitative data, which tend to be *reductionistic*, i.e. to study phenomena at the level of their basic elements or constituents.

Box 5.1 *Terminology*

A number of potentially confusing terms are used in discussions of research based on qualitative data. *Phenomenology* is a particular perspective in philosophy initially developed by German philosophers such as Hegel (1770–1831), Husserl (1859–1938) and Heidegger (1889–1976), and carried over to sociological theory by Schütz (1899–1959). As indicated in Section 2.3.3, phenomenology sees human experience and consciousness as the basis of human reason and understanding: 'the capacity of the human mind to understand meaning is more basic than either formal logic or the mode in which knowledge is articulated or structured' (Mitchell, 1979, p. 141). Phenomenology is thus a theoretical perspective rather than a particular research methodology (Holloway, 1997). However, a number of methodological approaches to research are based firmly on the principles of phenomenology (Parry, 1991; Benner, 1994; Smith, 1996). *Hermeneutics* is a perspective that emphasizes the notion of interpretation and understanding, and argues that there is an essential interaction between the interpreter (with his or her particular cultural background), the object of interpretation, and the author or creator of this object (the 'hermeneutic circle'). Hermeneutics has considerable overlap with phenomenology (Plager, 1994; van der Zalm and Bergum, 2000), but has some specific differences of emphasis (see the discussion of *epoché* in Section 11.1). The term *ethnography*, originally used in anthropology, refers to the first-hand study of a human culture, and the social practices and interaction that occur within it (Hammersley and Atkinson, 1995). Ethnography can be regarded as a methodology (Schmoll, 1987; Baillie, 1995), and the methods of data collection most commonly employed within it are participant observation and interviewing. In so far as it seeks to understand a culture on the basis of its members'

own social meanings, ethnography frequently adopts a phenomenological perspective. The term can also be used to denote the product of a study (Hughes, 1992); e.g. 'an ethnography of critical care nursing practice'. Despite its name and the fact that some describe it as such, *ethnomethodology* is not strictly a research methodology. Rather, it is a sociological perspective on the processes of everyday life, first developed by Garfinkel (1967), and centred in some of the core tenets of phenomenology (Cuff and Payne, 1984). Ethnomethodology sees social interaction as a communicative process in which individuals rely on shared common-sense knowledge in order to construct and make sense of everyday interaction (Benson and Hughes, 1983; Holstein and Gubrium, 1997). The way in which social order is established and the rules and rituals that are utilized to this end are key concerns of ethnomethodology (Denzin, 1971; Zimmerman, 1971). Conversational analysis and participant observation are the principal methods of investigation adopted by ethnomethodologists. Finally, *symbolic interactionism* is, like ethnomethodology, a sociological perspective. Based on the work of the Chicago sociologist G. H. Mead (1863–1931), symbolic interactionism regards social life, and the social identity of the individual, as things that are created in the process of social interaction (Swingewood, 1984). In everyday life, each participant is constantly interpreting the symbolic communication – both verbal and non-verbal – of other participants. Through formulating and reacting to such interpretation, the participant creates his or her own social identity and attaches meaning to the social activity in which he or she is engaged (Denzin, 1971). The method of participant observation is closely associated with research conducted from a symbolic interactionist perspective (Ackroyd and Hughes, 1992).

Leininger (1985a, p. 5) sums up the essential purpose of exploratory research as 'to document and interpret as fully as possible the totality of whatever is being studied in particular contexts from the people's viewpoint or frame of reference'. This quotation highlights another important feature of research based on qualitative data: its detail. Studies taking this approach are generally concerned with generating descriptions and accounts that are in-depth and rich in detail; they are often described as providing 'thick' description (Box 5.2).

Box 5.2 *'Thick' description*

A 'thick' description is one that possesses more specificity of detail than a 'thin' description (Ryle, 1947; Geertz, 1973). For example, to describe an action as 'ungenerous' or 'callous' gives a more detailed account of that action than merely to describe it as 'bad', and to characterize a patient as being 'intensely frustrated by a sense of powerlessness in the face of relentlessly increasing disability' provides a richer description than simply to describe him or her as 'distressed'. Schwandt (1997, p. 161) argues, however, that it is not just a matter of the degree of detail in an account: 'to thickly describe social action is actually to begin to interpret it by recording the circumstances, meanings, intentions, strategies, motivations, and so on that characterize a particular episode. It is this interpretive characteristic of description rather than detail per se that makes it thick.' Denzin (1989a, pp. 83–84) argues that thick descriptions create a sense of verisimilitude; i.e. they 'produce for readers the feeling that they have experienced, or could experience, the events being described'.

5.2 THE PROCESS OF RESEARCH IN EXPLORATORY STUDIES

The strategy adopted in designing an exploratory study differs from that usually followed in descriptive or explanatory studies. Whereas a survey or an experiment is likely to be planned in considerable detail at the very outset, with each step in the research process clearly mapped out, a researcher may begin an exploratory study with only a general idea of how the study is to be executed. Since the topic of an exploratory study is, by definition, one that is understood only in very general terms, it is simply not possible to specify in advance the precise means by which data should be collected. The researcher must, of course, have a general idea of the methods to be used, but it is unlikely that he or she will have drawn up a precise step-by-step plan. As noted in Section 3.1.1, research design in exploratory studies is usually emergent, during the course of data collection and analysis. In this and the following two sections, some more specific aspects of exploratory research design will be examined, with reference to the Student Attitudes Study (see Appendix I for a full description of this study).

In this study, Teresa Ganz sought to examine health care students' understanding of putatively 'self-inflicted' illness in the context of the notion of responsibility for health. She hoped to gain an understanding of the nature and the source of students' perceptions and attitudes, and initially considered using a questionnaire for this purpose. However, on reflection it occurred to her that she was unable to predict what sorts of issues her informants would consider relevant on this topic, and that she could not specify in advance the dimensions on which their attitudes might lie. The issues on which the study would focus might be identified only in a tentative and provisional way at the outset. It would therefore have been very hard to predetermine the appropriate structure and content of a questionnaire, and had she attempted to do so, it would have reflected her own understanding of self-inflicted illness rather than her informants'. Instead, Dr Ganz identified three principal methods of data collection to be employed in her study:

- individual interviews with health care students;
- non-participant observation of small-group teaching sessions on relevant areas of the curriculum;
- a review of core texts used by the students.

These methods are highly typical of those used in exploratory studies. Through their use, Dr Ganz was able to explore the topic of her study from various perspectives. The individual interviews provided information on the students' beliefs and attitudes in respect of 'self-inflicted' conditions. The observation of the teaching sessions gave information on the way in which these attitudes and beliefs manifest themselves in the interaction that occurs in the teaching situation, and students' psychological, emotional and intellectual responses to the taught material presented. Finally, accessing and analysing key texts used by the students indicated whether the students' perceptions are in accordance with the images of 'self-inflicted' illness present in the academic and professional literature to which they are likely to be exposed. At this stage, however, she cannot predict precisely what sorts of data are likely to be produced in each of these sources, nor the strength with which they will emerge. For example, there are various ways that students might express their attitudes in the context of an interview, and equally there are a number of ways that students' underlying attitudes might become apparent during classroom interaction. Consequently, the techniques used for collecting data in this study will have to be responsive to the issues that emerge in the research situation, rather than being finalized in advance of entering the field.

This last point emphasizes the adaptability that is often required of the researcher in exploratory studies. Although there may be clear thoughts in the researcher's mind as to how he or she intends to conduct a study, in reality research in natural settings tends to be a messy business. Factors and circumstances that the researcher cannot, and might not wish to, control often upset the best-laid plans (anticipated sources of data turn out to be inaccessible, expected issues or responses do not arise, informants do not turn up for interviews, etc.). Consequently, procedures that might seem optimal in terms of textbook accounts (such as the present one) may need to be adapted or even abandoned in favour of others, in response to the demands of the immediate situation.

5.3 SAMPLING

The sample chosen for this study was a convenience sample (Section 8.4.2) of nursing and occupational therapy students at a university, numbering approximately 15 in total. Two professions are represented in the sample because the researcher anticipated that there might be points of comparison and contrast between these groups of students, given their rather different patterns of professional education and socialization. Thus, the students were chosen for study on the basis of their particular experiences, and for this reason also constitute a judgemental sample (Section 8.4.1).

Dr Ganz is not unduly concerned about the likely representativeness of the sample with respect to the wider population of students in these professions. This is a preliminary, exploratory study, and she is not seeking to arrive at any definitive conclusions that might be generalized beyond the context of this investigation. The principal focus is on identifying and exploring the themes and issues that emerge from the data rather than on establishing their strength, prevalence or typicality.

Researchers who have been brought up on more quantitative approaches to research may find it hard to accept the apparent lack of external validity of the findings from qualitative approaches. In studies that employ inferential statistics, the representativeness of the study sample with respect to the study population is often crucial, and even in surveys that seek only to generate descriptive data the question of external validity is an important one. Altman and Bland (1998, p. 409) argue that 'the usefulness of research lies primarily in the generalisation of the findings rather than in the information gained about those particular individuals'.

In exploratory research, however, the whole idea of generalization may not be among the purposes of the study, and the statement made above by Altman and Bland will often be strongly contested. Many such studies are *idiographic*; i.e. they seek to construct an in-depth picture of a single case or a handful of cases, with no pretension to establishing general patterns or similarities. This is in contrast to *nomothetic* research, which seeks to establish law-like generalities (the word 'nomothetic' means 'law-creating'). Hence, it is not so much that researchers dealing with qualitative data *cannot* produce generalizations from their findings (which is to some extent the case), but that they do not *intend* to do so. In this connection, Sandelowski (1996, p. 525) warns against adopting what she calls a variable-oriented approach to qualitative data:

> *In the rush to find core variables, recurring themes, and transferable concepts, analysts of qualitative data too often miss the idiosyncratic, unique and nonfungible features of cases that give them their integrity and make them valuable for study.*

A 'nonfungible' feature is one that cannot be replaced by a more general term or description. Hence, an attempt to use such generic categories to describe qualitative data will exclude some measure of their essential individuality of meaning.

The sort of understanding that is aimed for in exploratory research is one of depth rather than breadth. A detailed description of one or a few cases is constructed, rather than an aggregated profile across a large number of statistically representative cases. Dr Ganz will not, therefore, be seeking statistical representativeness in her chosen sample of 15. However, she is likely to look for theoretical representativeness in terms of the concepts, themes and issues that emerge from her findings (see Section 8.2 for the distinction between statistical and theoretical representativeness). At the conclusion of the study, it is most probable that she will wish to extend the conceptual and theoretical insights gained from the study to other contexts or settings, but it is unlikely that she will attempt to generalize her specific empirical findings. Extrapolation beyond the specific context of the study is at a theoretical, not an empirical, level (Sim, 1998).

Indeed, researchers working with qualitative data often reflect their departure from orthodox views of generalization by avoiding the use of terms such as 'generalizability' and 'external validity'. Instead, they tend to refer to findings as 'transferable' rather than as 'generalizable', and speak of 'fittingness' instead of 'external validity' (Guba and Lincoln, 1981; Lincoln and Guba, 1985). These issues are discussed further in Section 9.4.

The criterion for sample size in this type of research is different from that in most descriptive and explanatory studies. In explanatory studies, it is necessary to obtain a sample that is sufficiently large for clinically important differences to be detected as statistically significant, or for effects or attributes to be estimated with a stated minimum degree of precision (see Section 18.6). In exploratory studies, however, the sample needs to be of such a size that it will generate a volume (and perhaps also a diversity) of data that will provide meaningful insights. Such a volume of data may be gained from just a few cases – or even a single case.

Sandelowski (1995, p. 179) argues that the key issue is 'the quality of information obtained per sampling unit, as opposed to their number per se'. If too few cases are studied, there may be insufficient variety in the information gathered, and certain important concepts or perspectives may be unrepresented (compare the notion of saturation discussed in Section 11.4.1). On the other hand, if the sample is large, it is hard to grasp the detailed specificity of each informant's response and the individual meanings that underlie it (Parker, 1994). Accordingly, it is not possible to give any meaningful guidelines on sample size in studies based on qualitative data. All that can be said is that a certain sample may be either too small or too large for a given purpose (Sandelowski, 1995).

5.4 GAINING ACCESS AND MANAGING THE RESEARCHER ROLE

As was suggested in Section 5.1, exploratory studies usually take place in a natural setting. According to Jorgensen (1989), such a setting may be either *visible* or *invisible*, and either *open* or *closed*. A visible setting is one about which information is generally available to the public (such as a hospital or a university), whereas an invisible setting is one that is largely closed to public scrutiny (such as meetings of certain marginal or outsider groups). An open setting (such as a waiting room in a hospital) is one to which access is more or less freely available and requires little if any negotiation, whereas access to a closed setting (such as a hospital management committee meeting) requires a considerable degree of negotiation (Jorgensen, 1989). Invisible settings tend to be closed settings. Correspondingly, visible settings tend to be open settings, though this is not always the case. Thus, the institution in which Dr Ganz proposes to conduct her study is visible, but access to it will certainly require negotiation.

Obtaining access to closed settings may present certain practical and methodological problems:

- It is sometimes unclear who the appropriate gatekeepers are for a particular research setting, and different gatekeepers may be appropriate for different aspects of a study.
- Permission to enter a setting may be difficult to obtain.
- Seeking such permission may require the researcher to reveal details of the study which, once public, may influence or even bias the data to be collected.
- Access may only be permitted on conditions that may undermine the purposes of the research.
- The researcher may be perceived to be a representative of, or to have taken the side of, the gatekeepers and may thus encounter barriers from other groups within the institution.

The precise way in which access is gained will to a large degree be influenced by whether the research is to be carried out overtly or covertly (Hornsby-Smith, 1993). Covert research is conducted in such a way that participants are unaware that they are being researched.

Accessing a closed, invisible setting for the purposes of covert research may be very difficult, and will usually only be achieved through some degree of deception (see Section 5.8).

In some cases, the researcher may need to adjust the objectives of a study in order to gain access to a setting. Grady and Wallston (1988) suggest that in order to gain the cooperation of a physician in a study that does not have immediate practical relevance, a more clinically oriented strand may have to be built into the project. In this way both the researcher and the collaborating professional benefit from the research. Roper and Shapira (2000) provide further discussion of the practical and methodological issues associated with gaining access.

Even once access has been gained, the researcher has to give careful thought to the identity that he or she will present to respondents or participants, and consider the details of the study that will be explained to them (Burgess, 1984). How the researcher is perceived may exert a major influence on the data available. In a study of perceptions and experiences of spinal injury, Carpenter (1997) found during a pilot study that her informants inferred from her identity as a physiotherapist that her primary interest was in aspects of their rehabilitation. This was not in fact her principal topic of interest, and in the main study Carpenter presented a rather different image to her informants in order to explore other aspects of their experience. Smith (1996b), Melia (1987) and Sword (1999) recount similar experiences. In her study of the occupational socialization of student nurses, Melia was concerned to present herself as a 'non-establishment' figure, and downplayed her professional identity as a nurse:

Throughout the research I emphasized whichever side of my dual role of research associate and postgraduate student at the university was most expedient at the time. I freely told the students that I was writing up the study for a doctoral thesis. This often created a feeling of comradeship, in the 'we are all students together' sense. It was also a useful means of creating the informal atmosphere which was desirable for the interview.

(Melia, 1987, p. 194)

The researcher may have to present different personae to different research participants within a study (Arksey and Knight, 1999). Whatever persona is presented to other participants in a study, there is always a danger that the researcher may lose sight of his or her own role as a researcher. In the course of a study, the researcher may become deeply immersed in the setting being studied and highly engaged, psychologically and emotionally, with the feelings or experiences of those within it. Although this form of engagement can be a valuable part of data collection (see Section 5.5.1), there should nonetheless be some degree of separation in the researcher's mind between the role of researcher and that of participant in the situation being studied (see Box 5.3). Foster (1996, p. 78) refers to this as the problem of 'managing marginality'.

If a balance between the insider and outsider roles is not achieved, there is a danger of 'going native'. This describes the process whereby 'researchers adopt the values and perspectives of the people they study, and identify with them so much that they are unable to sustain their previous identity as researchers' (Holloway, 1997, p. 79). One way in which researchers try to counteract this potential problem is to keep a reflective diary or journal (Section 10.1.3), in which they record their own reactions, feelings, insights and perceptions during the process of data collection (Maykut and Morehouse, 1994). This allows them to reflect upon and audit their involvement with the research setting once they have left it (Lincoln and Guba, 1985).

5.5 DATA COLLECTION METHODS

In the Student Attitudes Study, three methods of data collection were proposed: interviews, observation, and documentary analysis. These are

Box 5.3 *Emic and etic perspectives*

A distinction is sometimes made between 'emic' and 'etic' perspectives. These terms originated in anthropology, and have caused much debate on the appropriate stance of researchers *vis-à-vis* those whom they are studying (Headland *et al.*, 1990). An *emic* perspective is that of the insider in a particular culture or social setting, and reflects the particular beliefs and values that are associated with such a setting. According to Fetterman (1998, p. 20), 'an emic perspective compels the recognition and acceptance of multiple realities', which are central to phenomenology (see Section 2.3.3). An *etic* perspective, by contrast, is that of the outsider; i.e. the researcher (Leininger, 1985b; Holloway, 1997). The interpretations or explanations that researchers generate will tend to correspond to these perspectives. An emic perspective will tend to produce an explanation framed very much in terms of the participants' framework of values and meanings, whereas an etic perspective will generate an account that is expressed in terms of the theoretical concepts of a particular academic discipline. Boyle (1994) argues that the ethnographer should attempt to assimilate both perspectives when seeking an understanding of situations and behaviours.

probably the most commonly used means of gathering qualitative data, and will be considered in turn. The use of focus groups will also be addressed.

5.5.1 Unstructured interviews

There are two main varieties of interview. First, there is the *structured* interview, in which a series of scripted questions, mainly requiring closed-ended answers, are put to a respondent. The structured interview characteristically seeks to gather relatively superficial information on a wide range of topics, and is essentially equivalent to a questionnaire administered face to face. The way in which the interview is conducted is standardized as far as possible, so that each respondent is presented with a nearly identical set of stimuli (Ackroyd and Hughes, 1992). Consistency on the part of the interviewer, and the avoidance of bias or ambiguity, are the principal concerns here (Fowler and Mangione, 1990). Structured interviews are discussed in Section 6.3.2. Second, there is the *unstructured* interview, in which questions are not scripted in advance, but are based on a list of provisional topics and allow for a considerable degree of flexibility and spontaneity (Britten and Fisher, 1993). Accordingly, Grbich (1999) describes this type of interview as a 'guided' interview. The term 'semi-structured interview' is sometimes used to designate an interview that falls somewhere between these two extremes (Arksey and Knight, 1999), though some writers use this term to refer to what has been described as an unstructured interview. We will not use this term. The unstructured interview is not, of course, totally unstructured, since any verbal interaction between two people will develop a certain structure, and an interview without any structure could not achieve a specific intended purpose (Britten, 2000). Rather, it is minimally structured, with the researcher relinquishing control over the form and content of the interview to the maximum extent feasible (Rose, 1994).

Interviewing allows the researcher a considerable degree of flexibility, since the informant can be asked to reflect on both present and past experiences. Observational methods, in contrast, focus on the 'here and now' (Erlandson *et al.*, 1993). Indeed, some researchers use the interview as a predominantly retrospective tool, in what is known as *life history* research (Tagg, 1985; Hagemaster, 1992; Admi, 1995; Plummer, 1995). The informant is asked to describe and reflect upon his or her past experiences – usually in a chronological sequence – and place these within their historical and cultural context. In this way, insight may be gained into the way that people's lives may be structured around and influenced by their experiences of health and illness.

The unstructured interview is useful 'where highly sensitive and subtle matters need to be covered, and where long and detailed responses are required to understand the matters the respondent is reporting on' (Ackroyd and Hughes, 1992, p. 104). A key element in the unstructured interview is therefore the establishment of rapport and even empathy between interviewer and interviewee (Massarik, 1981). Without some degree of psychological and even emotional engagement with the informant's perspective, it is unlikely that the interviewer will be sufficiently sensitive to the often complex and subtle issues that may emerge (Oakley, 1981). Hence, Cannon (1989) regarded the friendship she had formed with women diagnosed with breast cancer as vital to the quality of the data gathered when interviewing them (Box 5.4).

Box 5.4 *Identification, neutrality and feminist research*

Much feminist research is premised on the notion that the researcher should identify with those being studied. Hence, Mies (1993, p. 68) calls for 'conscious partiality' rather than 'neutrality and indifference', on the part of the researcher. The idea that this partiality should be 'conscious' indicates that it is more than just empathy, and embodies a certain critical distance from the object of study. On some interpretations, including that of Kremer (1990) and Mies's own, this view would require that only women can meaningfully research the lives of other women, as only they would have the necessary experience and insights to understand the social situation of other women. However, this is not a view held by all feminist researchers (Harding, 1986), and the emphasis is often placed more upon the idea that feminist research should be *for* women, rather than necessarily *by* women. Issues such as these are discussed more fully by Millman and Moss Kanter (1975), Webb (1984, 1993), Scott (1985), Harding (1986), Blaikie (1993) and Burman (1994b).

Unstructured interviews are usually conducted in as naturalistic a way as possible. The setting chosen for the interview is one that will be familiar and comfortable to the informant. Hence, when interviewing student nurses about their experiences, Melia (1987) chose to conduct the interviews in the nurses' homes rather than in the more formal setting of the ward. The mode of communication adopted in an unstructured interview is also as natural as possible. In contrast to the strictures of survey research, which urge the researcher not to provide information to the respondent or to reveal his or her own opinion, the interviewer may feel it is appropriate to answer questions and even to share feelings with the informant (Oakley, 1981; Wilde, 1992; Bailey, 1996).

The degree of active participation by the interviewer must be delicately balanced against a more passive persona. On the one hand, the expression of views or ideas by the interviewee may heighten rapport and act as a stimulus to disclosure by the interviewee. On the other hand, the underlying purpose of the interview is to gain the informant's perspective, and there is a danger that active participation on the part of the interviewer may prompt or influence the views expressed by the interviewee. Where the balance is struck on the active–passive continuum will largely depend upon the topic and context of the interview and the identities of the participants. However, a false sense of 'objectivity' should be guarded against. Instead of being a source of bias, personal involvement may be 'the condition under which people come to know each other and to admit others into their lives' (Oakley, 1981, p. 58). The notion of objectivity in relation to qualitative data is discussed further in Section 9.4.

Conducting the unstructured interview

Hammersley and Atkinson (1995) describe unstructured interviewing as *reflexive*, in contrast to the *standardized* interviewing characteristic of survey research. They elaborate on this as follows:

Ethnographers do not usually decide beforehand the exact questions they want to ask, and do not ask each interviewee exactly the same questions, though they will usually enter the interviews with a list of issues to be covered. Nor do they seek to establish a fixed sequence in which relevant topics are covered; they adopt a more flexible approach, allowing the discussion to flow in a way that seems natural.

(Hammersley and Atkinson, 1995, p. 152)

Thus, to a large degree the precise topics on which the interview will focus, and the way in which it is conducted, emerge in the process of the interview, and are responsive to the perceptions, concerns and priorities of the informant (Box 5.5). Control of the data collection process is surrendered partially (though not wholly) to the informant. The approach to interviewing that is to varying degrees characteristic of unstructured interviews is sometimes also referred to as being *recursive*. This approach is one in which the line of questioning is predominantly steered by the interaction occurring in the interview, and in particular by the informant's response to the previous question (Minichiello *et al.*, 1990). In contrast to the formal *interview schedule* employed in structured interviews (Section 6.3.2), the unstructured interview is conducted according to an *interview guide* (Arksey and Knight, 1999).

Topics in an unstructured interview may be raised in different ways or in a different order with different informants, and some topics may not even be touched upon at all if it appears that they are not of interest or relevance to the informant concerned. Since the intention in this form of interview is to gain insight into a topic from the perspective of the informant, it is important that the agenda for the interview is not imposed by the interviewer, but is negotiated between interviewer and interviewee (Jones, 1985a). Rubin and Rubin (1995) describe such interviews as 'guided conversations'. This is relevant in the present example. As a health psychologist, Dr Ganz may have particular views

Box 5.5   *Two approaches to the interview*

Not only the structure but also the purpose and approach of the sort of interview conducted in an exploratory study are likely to differ markedly from more traditional models of interviewing. Kvale (1996) expresses this through the analogies of the miner and the traveller. The traditional interview is seen in terms of a search for knowledge. This knowledge is regarded as 'buried metal and the interviewer is a miner who unearths the valuable metal' (Kvale, 1996, p. 3). In the more exploratory interview, however, the interviewer is likened to a traveller, who enters upon a journey in an unfamiliar territory. The traveller 'wanders along with the local inhabitants, asks questions that lead the subjects to tell their own stories of their lived world' (Kvale, 1996, p. 4). Holstein and Gubrium (1997, p. 114) take a similar approach: 'Respondents are not so much repositories of knowledge – treasuries of information awaiting excavation, so to speak – as they are constructors of knowledge in collaboration with interviewers.' In this model, the interview is not a process by which information is transmitted by or elicited from a respondent, in the manner of survey research (Section 6.3.2), but is one whereby knowledge and understanding are created through the interaction of researcher and informant.

on the notion of 'self-inflicted' illness which may well differ from those of the students she proposes to interview, and it is important that she does not impose her own perspective on the data collection process.

Some of the specific techniques advocated within this approach to interviewing include the following:

- It is important to demonstrate active listening. The way in which the interviewer responds, verbally and non-verbally, to what the informant says conveys understanding, encourages further disclosure, and provides cues for elaboration or clarification (Arksey and Knight, 1999).

- For the most part, *open-ended* questions (i.e. those that do not specify the range of possible answers; Section 15.1.6) should be used, to prompt the informant to provide detailed answers and to minimize the extent to which these answers may be influenced by the interviewer's own views or perceptions. Closed-ended questions do, however, have a role in unstructured interviewing (Hammersley and Atkinson, 1995).

- Very general questions can sometimes be successful as stimuli to disclosure. However, some informants may find such questions too vague to relate to their experience, and more focused questions may be more successful. Hence, Arksey and Knight (1999) report that asking family carers to identify three changes that they would make to the hospital discharge process was more fruitful than posing the question 'What do you think makes for an effective hospital discharge?'

- Specific examples should be requested where appropriate in order to clarify the informant's meaning: people usually find it easier to enlarge on their initial answer in concrete rather than abstract terms.

- The use of *probes* (supplementary questions, comments or non-verbal behaviour that seek clarification or further disclosure) is an important means of fulfilling three functions: to indicate the level of detail wanted from the informant; to encourage the informant to conclude a particular answer; and to demonstrate attentiveness and understanding on the part of the interviewer (Rubin and Rubin, 1995).

- The interviewer can paraphrase or summarize what the informant has said by way of seeking confirmation. However, it is important to be alert to any tendency towards automatic acquiescence on the part of the informant. Excessive paraphrasing or summarizing may also irritate some informants, or even make them feel that the interviewer is dubious about the answers being given (Minichiello *et al.*, 1990).

- Silences need to be managed carefully. An expectant silence on the part of the interviewer may stimulate further disclosure or elaboration by the informant. If the informant is silent, this may indicate lack of comprehension, or that the topic is one on which the informant is reluctant to speak. Equally, it may just be a natural process of deliberation prior to responding (Grbich, 1999). The interviewer should not be too quick to fill gaps in the dialogue.

- Assuming an air of ignorance or naïveté may encourage the informant to give fuller and more detailed responses. However, the opposite may also apply: interviewees may open up to an interviewer whom they perceive to be knowledgeable and well informed (Strong and Robinson, 1990).

- The informant is more likely to confide in the interviewer if the latter demonstrates *unconditional positive regard*, i.e. positive feelings that do not need to be earned and will not be affected by what the informant may say or may have done. This is particularly important if the interview is to cover sensitive or taboo subjects, where the informant should be made to feel that the interviewer will not be shocked or react judgementally. This may even require the interviewer to lead the informant to a small degree, to show that it is acceptable to report behaviour or express attitudes that are potentially embarrassing or stigmatizing. This is in contrast to the view of leading questions which would normally be taken in survey research (Table 15.5).

- By being somewhat disingenuous (but without being unduly dishonest), the researcher may elicit fuller and more forthcoming responses. For example, a question may deliberately be made to lead in the opposite direction to that anticipated ('I

imagine you were pleased to find that …'), and thus prompt the informant to provide a detailed correction. Similarly, Rubin and Rubin (1995) suggest that the researcher can deliberately misstate certain details when summarizing what the informant has said, again with a view to eliciting a detailed corrective statement.

- By repeating or rephrasing questions (sometimes referred to as *mirroring*), the interviewer can steer the interviewee back on track if there is some degree of deviation from the central topic. One should be cautious, however, about labelling responses as 'irrelevant'. Field and Morse (1996, p. 84) comment, 'The dross rate may be high if the participant is an elderly person who is inclined to wander off the topic, or if the researcher permits himself/herself to be tempted into listening to irrelevant stories or lacks the ability to focus the interview.' Setting aside the rather stereotypical view of elderly people, this may seem reasonable advice, and there is clearly a need to maintain some form of agenda in the interview. However, it should be remembered that exploring what is relevant to the *informant* is central to the phenomenological approach that underlies many exploratory studies. Moreover, a seemingly 'irrelevant' response may in due course prove to be an important source of insight if it is given a hearing.

- In some instances, rich data can be gained through minimizing the questions asked and letting the informant speak in the manner and the pace that he or she chooses. Oppenheim (1992, pp. 73–74) suggests that the interviewer 'may merely suggest a topic with a word, or an unfinished sentence left trailing, and the respondent will "take it away" and will produce a rounded and personalized response, punctuated by sounds of encouragement from the interviewer'.

- Distress and other displays of emotion in the course of the interview need to be handled carefully. Arksey and Knight (1999) argue that it is inappropriate to change the subject immediately, but equally one should not automatically assume that the informant wishes to pursue the topic in question further. They point out that eye contact should be maintained, and that offering tissues to a tearful informant serves to legitimate his or her distress. The ethical implications of this issue are considered in Section 5.8.

It is important to note that the appropriateness of some of these techniques may depend crucially upon the identity and personality of the informant, the topic of the interview, and the context in which it occurs. What may work in one situation may be counter-productive in another. Prescriptive rules are usually not applicable to this form of data collection. Issues surrounding the recording of interview data are considered in Section 10.1.1.

5.5.2 The focus group

There has recently been an upsurge in interest in the focus group as a means of collecting data in exploratory and descriptive studies. A focus group can be defined as a group interview, centred on a specific topic and facilitated by a moderator, which generates primarily qualitative data by capitalizing on the interaction that takes place in the group setting (Sim and Snell, 1996). The method can be used for a variety of purposes within health care:

- to study service quality and consumer perspectives (Peters, 1996; Dolan *et al.*, 1999);
- to generate questionnaire items and patient-defined outcome measures (Hyland *et al.*, 1994; Sim and Snell, 1996);
- to explore health beliefs (Morgan and Spanish, 1985);
- to explore behaviour and subjective experience in illness or disability (Nyamathi and Shuler, 1990; Strong *et al.*, 1994; Kitzinger, 1994a);

- to explore professional decision-making processes (Fulton, 1996).

A focus group normally consists of between eight and 12 participants (Stewart and Shamdasani, 1990; Krueger 1994). In their seminal text, Merton *et al.* (1956, p. 137) state that the group 'should not be so large as to be unwieldy or to preclude adequate participation by most members nor should it be so small that it fails to provide substantially greater coverage than that of an interview with one individual'. It is generally considered that the composition of a focus group should be relatively homogeneous. If a group contains a mix in terms of social status, educational background, professional role and the like, this may inhibit the participation of those who see themselves to be in a minority or subordinate status. Reed and Payton (1997) describe a group in which one participant was in a managerial capacity relative to the others; this individual contributed some 95% of the transcribed proceedings. Furthermore, if a heterogeneous group is used, the commonality of knowledge and experience that is normally required for a fruitful discussion is likely to be missing.

A number of groups are often conducted within a study. This allows a broad cross-section of participants to be studied, with each group being made up of a homogeneous subgroup.

The focus group has a number of advantages and disadvantages as a means of generating data (Table 5.1). Crucial to the success of the group is the interaction occurring among participants (Kitzinger, 1994b). This interaction distinguishes the focus group from the group interview, in which questions are usually posed to participants in turn (Kitzinger and Barbour, 1999), and from methods such as the Delphi method and the nominal group technique (Morgan, 1996; see Section 6.3.5). The chief merit of this interaction is that it allows the way in which attitudes are constructed, developed and modified to be explored dynamically (Morgan, 1988). Examining the sequence of discussion is particularly important in this respect (Reed and Payton,

Table 5.1 *Principal advantages and disadvantages of the focus group*

Advantages	Disadvantages
• Group interaction may stimulate the expression of attitudes • An economical way of tapping the views of a number of people • Provides information on the dynamics of attitudes and opinions • Can provide a supportive forum for the expression of views by participants, who may feel empowered by the group setting	• Group dynamics may distort the expression of attitudes • It may be difficult to know if a consensus is genuine • Much depends upon the skills, identity and personality of the moderator • Collecting data concurrently on both the verbal and the interactive elements of the group can be difficult • Data are of limited depth, and the complexity of the issues that can be explored is limited

1997). It is doubtful, however, that topics can be explored in the depth possible in a one-to-one interview, and the focus group is not well suited to topics of great complexity. The focus group is also prone to a consensus effect, whereby the group dynamics operating encourage and highlight the dominant view and suppress divergent opinions (Carey, 1994; Carey and Smith, 1994; Sim, 1998). An apparent consensus may reflect unanimity among the participants, or it may reflect the way that group dynamics have amplified consensus and dissuaded dissent; the researcher may have difficulty deciding which is the case. In fact, it may be more appropriate to seek to assess consensus *across* groups rather than *within* a group (Sim, 1998).

In this connection, it is important to note that the findings that emerge from a focus group are not readily separable from the group context; they should not be seen merely as the sum of the attitudes of the individual participants. Accordingly, one should be wary of seeking to assess the strength of opinion that may seem to emerge from a focus group. This too may be at least partially an artefact of group dynamics. Furthermore, it should be remembered that the frequency with which an attitude is expressed within qualitative data is not necessarily a valid indicator of its overall strength (see Section 11.6).

Kitzinger (2000) notes that some seemingly diffident or unresponsive informants may respond to the group setting and make contributions that they might not have done in a one-to-

one situation. The group may also empower participants in the disclosure of sensitive issues or personal information. However, Williams (1999) argues that the semi-public nature of the focus group and concerns about confidentiality may restrict the extent to which participants will reveal intimate or potentially incriminating information (see Box 5.8).

Morgan (1996) provides a helpful discussion of the merits of the focus group relative to those of the one-to-one interview and survey methods. Krueger (1994, 1998) and Vaughn *et al.* (1996) provide helpful accounts of the conduct of focus groups.

5.5.3 Observation

Observational method can be used in many styles of research, including the structured quantitative observations that are made in some laboratory experiments, or in naturally occurring social settings in which standardized data are required (see Section 6.3.6). In exploratory studies, however, a different form of observation is usual, involving the collection of qualitative data in a systematic but far less structured manner (Pope and Mays, 2000). This type of observational method can broadly be divided into two forms: *participant* observation and *nonparticipant* observation (see Box 5.6).

As its name suggests, participant observation involves the researcher actively in the way of life he or she is studying, engaging in the normal activities and communication processes of the social group concerned. In non-participant

Box 5.6 *Two senses of 'observational'*

In the present context, an 'observational' study is one in which observation is used as the means of data collection. The term is also used, however, to describe descriptive, non-experimental studies conducted in areas of study such as epidemiology. Abramson (1990) argues that methods other than observation – such as questionnaires and documentary sources – can be used in an observational study, and Gray (1997) contends that surveys, cohort studies and case–control studies and research based on the collection of qualitative data are all examples of observational studies. This use of the term 'observational' would seem to be rather too broad to be useful, and it is probably best reserved for studies in which the predominant means of data collection is observation in its literal sense.

observation, however, the researcher keeps a distance – often literally as well as metaphorically – from those who form the subject of the study, and does not attempt to take part in the interaction that he or she is observing. Two classic studies illustrate the difference between these two strategies. Julius Roth's book *Timetables* (Roth, 1963) describes the experiences of patients in a tuberculosis hospital. Roth was himself a patient in the hospital at the time of the study, and did not disclose to most of those around him that he was studying the hospital and themselves. Members of staff who saw him making field notes assumed that this was in pursuit of his academic studies. *Sickness and Society* (Duff and Hollingshead, 1968) is an account of a large-scale study of patients' experience in a USA hospital. The researchers in this study were concerned not to participate in the activity they were observing, and were careful to make their role as researchers evident to the patients and medical staff in the hospital. Although one of the researchers was a physician, he distanced himself from any type of service role within the hospital.

This basic distinction between participant and non-participant observation has been elaborated by Gold (1958) into a fourfold classification:

Complete participant – the researcher adopts full participation in the social situation being studied, tries to behave as naturally as possible, and carries out observation covertly; Roth's (1963) study falls into this category.

Participant as observer – the researcher participates fully, but makes his or her role as a researcher known and carries out observation overtly.

Observer as participant – the researcher similarly adopts an overt stance as regards his or her role as a researcher, but participates minimally in the social situation; Duff and Hollingshead's (1968) study falls into this category.

Complete observer – the researcher plays no part in the action or communication that is being studied, but adopts a 'fly on the wall' role; some psychological studies involving covert, structured observation take this form.

Which of these roles the investigator assumes will depend on the nature and purposes of the study. In her study, Dr Ganz wishes to observe the interaction in the teaching situation, but there is no obvious role into which she could place herself. Moreover, in contrast to many social situations, her remaining fairly unobtrusive in the teaching room does not depend upon her joining in the activity taking place. It would, however, be difficult to conceal the reason for her presence, particularly if she had previously interviewed any of the students. Her role is therefore likely to be that of observer as participant.

The choice of role may also be influenced by the method required to gain access to the research setting. If, for example, the explicit permission of the subjects of the study is required in order to carry it out, it is clearly impossible to carry out the research covertly. In contrast, if the permission of research participants cannot be obtained – perhaps because the identity of the individuals to be studied cannot be determined in advance of data collection – covert observation remains a possibility.

Whatever role is adopted, the researcher should consider the reactive effects of observation. This topic is considered in Section 5.6. Issues surrounding the recording of observational data are addressed in Section 10.1.2.

5.5.4 Documentary sources

Various forms of documentary data can be used in exploratory studies (Box 5.7). These may come from a number of sources, and can be classified in terms of whether they are created for *formal* or *informal* purposes, and whether they were intended for *public* or *private* consumption. Figure 5.1 shows examples of different sources of documentary data in terms of these distinctions. Note that although documentary sources are usually textual, the term 'documentary' is also sometimes applied to oral narratives and certain non-textual objects, such as works of art (Plummer, 1983; Macdonald and Tipton, 1993).

Box 5.7   *Secondary sources and secondary analysis*

Documentary sources of a retrospective nature are sometimes considered under the heading of 'secondary research', on the basis that the material that is treated as data was created or assembled in advance of the research currently being conducted. In many cases, however, such material may not previously have been accessed for research purposes, and was not created specifically for such a purpose. These are secondary sources of data, but a primary analysis is carried out on them. In contrast, existing studies or datasets are sometimes re-analysed, often after they have been synthesized or aggregated (see Section 17.2). Again, the sources are secondary, but so also is the analysis. Accordingly, primary data are always subjected to a primary analysis, but secondary data may be the subject of either a primary or a secondary analysis.

	Consumption	
	Public	**Private**
Formal	Archives Textbooks Academic journals Curricula Official public reports	Minutes of meetings Legal documents Official confidential reports Medical case notes
Informal	Magazines and newspapers Advertisements Television and radio broadcasts Autobiographies Cultural artefacts	Diaries, journals and memoirs Letters

with **Purpose** labelling the left rows (Formal / Informal).

Figure 5.1   *Examples of documentary data sources*

Documentary data are most often historical; i.e. they were created before the time at which the research is taking place. Documentary sources of this sort may play an important part alongside interviews in life history research (see Section 5.5.1). However, documentary sources may also be used prospectively. A researcher often uses a diary or journal after it has been written, as a means of accessing information about a person's past life. However, a researcher may ask participants to keep a diary of their future experiences or reflections (Burgess, 1984; Gibson, 1995). A longitudinal profile of patients' symptoms may be constructed in this way (Francis, 1997). In such a situation, a diary becomes rather less of a private document. The use of diaries as a structured method of data collection is considered in Section 6.3.3.

Within an exploratory study, documentary sources are not merely seen as *containing* data, they *constitute* data. Hence, an understanding of the documentary medium is an important part of the analysis of these sources. Crucial to the interpretation of documents – particularly those that portray the more personal aspects of human experience – is recognition of the social and cultural context in which they were created. Stanfield and Katerndahl (1994, p. 83) argue that '[e]very human document is culturally constructed and is a culture-bound artifact defined through status filters such as class, age, ethnicity, religion, race and gender'.

Despite the richness of the data they yield, and their relative cost-effectiveness as a means of collecting data, documentary sources have certain potential drawbacks (Platt, 1981a, 1981b; Stewart, 1984; Scott, 1990; Reed, 1992; Stanfield and Katerndahl, 1994):

- The social context in which they were created may be unclear.
- The purpose for which they were produced may be uncertain, and may not be discernible from the data themselves.
- Some items of information may be given in a somewhat abbreviated or incomplete form that was adequate for the original purpose of the document but is insufficient for later analysis.
- The passage of time since their creation may make documents difficult to interpret; meanings, definitions, terminology, values and practices may have changed in the interim.
- Documentary sources may have been subject to editing, censoring or other influences since they were originally produced, and some documents may have been selected for retention whereas others may have been discarded or destroyed.
- Deliberate distortion or misrepresentation may have taken place, possibly in an attempt to protect, or sometimes even to tarnish, the reputations of individuals or institutions.

Assessing the validity and reliability of documentary sources is often difficult. Auxiliary sources of information, which might clarify or validate the details given in documentary sources, are often not available. Even if such additional sources of information can be found, it may be difficult to decide which source should act as the standard or criterion for validity (Section 9.2.3). Aaronson and Burman (1994) point out that, when dealing with sources such as health records, an investigator should be concerned with not only the reliability of data

extraction from the records, but also the reliability of the initial process of data inputting.

In Dr Ganz's study, the documentary sources she is analysing are professional textbooks. These are formal, public documents in terms of the typology outlined above. Hence, they are likely to represent a professional orthodoxy on the topics in question (more so, perhaps, than papers in professional journals, which may be more heterodox in their stance) and will probably be framed in ostensibly objective terms. Dr Ganz may therefore have to read beneath the surface in order to tap the latent attitudes contained in these texts (see Box 5.8).

5.6 REACTIVE EFFECTS OF INTERVIEWING AND OBSERVATION

'Reactivity' is a term used to describe the way in which people react to the presence of a researcher, or to the simple fact that a form of research is taking place. It is often referred to as the *Hawthorne effect*. This expression originates from a study by Roethlisberger and Dickson (1939) of worker activity in the Hawthorne plant of the Western Electric Works in Chicago. When the working environment was made more conducive to work, such as by improving the lighting conditions, productivity was seen to increase. However, the researchers discovered that when conditions were reversed – e.g. the lighting was dimmed again – productivity improved further. The conclusion they reached was that the workers were responding to the attention that they were receiving as participants in the experiment, rather than to the specific nature of the experimental intervention. Although this phenomenon was first identified in the context of experimental research, it is applicable to any form of research in which participants are aware that an investigation is taking place (see Table 7.2).

Thus, informants may express certain attitudes because they are aware that their views are the object of inquiry, and individuals' behaviour may change because they know they are being observed. The situation is no longer a

Box 5.8   *'Public' and 'private' accounts*

Documentary sources highlight the important distinction between 'public' and 'private' accounts when considering qualitative data. A public account is, as the term suggests, one given in a situation in which an informant feels open to public scrutiny, whereas a private account is directed at a more restricted audience and creates less of a sense of public disclosure. Accordingly, a private account is likely to be more detailed and frank than a public account, in which informants are concerned about the impression that they give of themselves, and may feel constrained about revealing personal or intimate facts or feelings that may be deemed to be socially unacceptable. This distinction is of equal importance when analysing interview accounts. The setting in which the interview occurs is an important issue here; informants are likely to be more circumspect about what they say in a semi-public forum such as a focus group than in a one-to-one interview. The nature of the topic is also a factor, and a potentially sensitive subject such as epilepsy may cause informants to give a public account, even in a one-to-one situation (West, 1979). Cornwell (1984) notes that, when health and illness are the topic of research, a public account given by lay respondents is likely to conform with what they perceive to be orthodox professional perspectives. When examining a public account, there may therefore be a greater gap between its manifest and latent meanings than when dealing with a private account. It is important to remember, however, that even an apparently 'private' interview consists of data that are 'social constructs, created by the self-presentation of the informant and whatever interactional cues have been given off by the interviewer about the acceptability or otherwise of the accounts being presented' (Dingwall, 1997, p. 59). Even the most seemingly naturalistic interview is never wholly natural to the informant.

wholly natural one. Generally, the more obtrusive the research process is with respect to the normal course of activity or interaction, the greater the reactive effects. Where reactivity is marked, there is a danger that the data gathered will be at least partially artefacts of the research process.

There are a number of ways in which the researcher can minimize reactive effects. In interviewing, the researcher can reduce reactivity by putting the informant at ease and creating a natural, relaxed and non-threatening setting for the interview. The content of the questions asked can also influence reactivity. For example, questions that are prone to a social desirability bias should be phrased very carefully, or avoided (see Section 15.4.2).

In observational studies, the researcher can spend some time in the research setting before collecting any data, so that the participants become habituated to his or her presence (Bogdewic, 1992). If the researcher is continuously, rather than intermittently, present in the observational setting, this is likely to assist habituation (Smith, 1996a). If observation is to be videotaped, a similar period of habituation is advisable so that participants become accustomed to the presence of the recording apparatus, and behaviour can resume a more natural form (the same applies if interviews are to be tape-recorded). The way in which data are recorded can also be geared to reduce reactivity. Outline notes can be made during the process of observing behaviour and then expanded once the researcher has left the scene. In some instances, it may even be advisable to delay all note making until after the activity has finished. In one sense, a non-participant observer appears to influence the nature of the interaction taking place less than would a participant observer. However, Smith (1975, p. 224) notes that 'the nonparticipant observer role often makes the observer conspicuous since our society has no norms for relationships where a nonmember is present but nonparticipating'.

There are, however, some potentially reactive aspects of observation or interviewing that are less easy to influence, such as the sex, age, ethnic background and perceived social identity of the interviewer. Moreover, excessively enthusiastic attempts to control reactivity may themselves be reactive, since the context for the research may become a somewhat unnatural one.

Finally, the possibility of reactive effects may be avoided altogether by the use of *unobtrusive measures*. This term is applied to any form of data collection that does not rely on the presence of those studied, or that utilizes data without those who generated the data being aware of its use for this purpose (Webb *et al.*, 1966). In this connection, the term 'measure' does not necessarily connote quantitative data.

Retrospective documentary sources (see Section 5.5.4) are an example of such measures (prospective documents may not qualify, since the individual may be required to cooperate in their creation). Physical traces are another form of unobtrusive measure. The famous example used by Webb *et al.* (1966) was the amount of wear on the floor in front of various exhibits in a museum, as a reflection of their relative popularity with visitors. Other examples of the use physical traces might be:

- examining the wear of a library book (in relation to its age) and/or counting the number of date stamps as an indicator of its use by students in a university;
- collecting discarded shopping receipts from a local store to gauge patterns of food consumption in a community;
- examining the bottles and cans thrown out from a public place such as a bar or night-club to gauge the type and quantity of alcohol consumed by its customers;
- counting at regular intervals the number of hits on an internet health education site, so as to estimate its rate of use (many sites display a cumulative total of visits).

5.7 PLANNING THE ANALYSIS OF DATA

The methods used to analyse qualitative data generated by an exploratory study differ funda-

mentally from those used for quantitative data. They will be covered in detail in Chapter 11. To a large extent, the steps to be taken during the analysis process will be dictated by the data gathered. However, because the precise nature and form of the data cannot be predicted in an exploratory study, it is not possible to formulate a precise plan of analysis before entering the process of analysis itself. Nonetheless, it is important to have a general idea of the likely analytic procedures at the outset, since these will influence the methods of data collection selected. For example, if Dr Ganz were proposing to carry out a detailed analysis of not only the verbal communication but also the non-verbal interaction occurring in teaching sessions, this would almost certainly require her to notate this interaction by a system of symbols as well as audiotaping the sessions. Similarly, if she were intending to carry out a linguistic analysis on the interview data, this would necessitate a verbatim, audiotaped record of what her informants said to her. If, however, the analysis were to be purely thematic, it may be that hand-written notes would suffice. Methods for recording interview and observational data are discussed in detail in Sections 10.1.1 and 10.1.2.

There is, therefore, a reciprocal relationship between data collection and analysis: the nature of the data governs the way they should be analysed, but the methods of analysis partly determine the data collection methods used, and thereby influence the nature of the data. Indeed, all of the phases in an exploratory study are likely to have this sort of relationship to one another (Figure 5.2). As was suggested in Section 3.1.1, the precise nature of an exploratory research question may be refined in response to the design and data collection phases of the study, and the early stages of data analysis may determine the sorts of data subsequently gathered and the way in which this will be carried out:

The qualitative research process is thus inductive and iterative, consisting of a preliminary premise that is shaped and

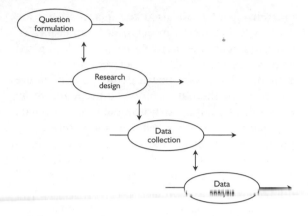

Figure 5.2 *Schematic representation of the interchange and overlap that characteristically occur between the phases of an exploratory study.*

> *refined through the research process itself. Repeated returns to collected data for reanalysis are the rule, and additional data are gathered as needed.*
>
> (Peters, 1996, p. 145)

The cyclical process of collecting and analysing qualitative data will be considered in more detail in Chapter 11.

5.8 ETHICAL ISSUES IN EXPLORATORY STUDIES

A number of ethical issues may arise when one is conducting exploratory studies. Those most likely to be at stake are informed consent, deception, privacy, anonymity, and risk of harm.

The issue of *informed consent* is not always straightforward in exploratory studies. In some observational research, consent can be sought from the participants in advance; for example, a researcher wishing to observe a series of consultations in an oncology clinic might seek the permission of the physician and the patients due to attend the clinic. In other cases, however, it is not practicable to seek consent from everybody in a particular social situation, not least because the identity of the participants may not be predictable. If the situation is essentially a public one – i.e. one in which people would assume that what they do or say would be publicly accessible to others – it may not always be necessary to seek consent. It could be argued that people in a public environment have implicitly consented to being observed or overheard. On the other hand, if observation is carried out in a non-public environment, and especially if observation is conducted covertly, this justification is not available. Indeed, in such situations the issue of consent is closely linked to that of *privacy*, for if individuals are aware that they are part of a study they can take steps to protect their privacy. Hence, one way of judging whether lack of consent is morally acceptable is to determine whether or not it is likely to constitute a serious invasion of privacy.

In addition, the process of asking for consent might well influence the way in which individuals would behave or interact. It could be argued that seeking consent would invalidate the study. It may certainly disrupt the normal course of behaviour in a way that is contrary to the naturalistic intent of ethnographic research (Dingwall, 1980). Consequently, there may be methodological reasons not to gain consent, or to give partial information about a study. Alternatively, the researcher may give a misleading account of the study – what Seaman (1987, p. 28) calls a 'cover story'. The potential value of the findings from the research might therefore be used as a justification for failing to gain fully informed consent. Whether such a justification is considered convincing is likely to depend on the specific circumstances of the study concerned and the issues it is addressing.

Munhall (1988) and Ramos (1989) argue that the emergent nature of much exploratory research makes it difficult to explain at the outset precisely what a study will involve. Similarly, in studies that extend over a long period of time, unanticipated events may occur that would have a bearing on a participant's willingness to take part (Ford and Reutter, 1990). Ramos (1989, p. 61) suggests that a process of 'ongoing consensual decision-making, where emergent difficulties are discussed openly' may be a better model of consent for such studies (indeed, it can be argued that such a model of consent should be practised in all situations).

Exploratory studies may sometimes involve some degree of *deception* on the part of the researcher. Covert observation falls into this category, by virtue of the fact that the researcher is concealing or, in the case of a closed setting, misrepresenting the true reason for his or her presence in a situation. A more subtle issue may occur in relation to the identity assumed by the researcher. As was indicated in Section 5.4, the way in which the researcher portrays his or her identity may influence the nature and extent of disclosure by informants. There are often a range of identities available to the researcher — for example, he or she might be a nurse, an educationalist, and a psychologist – and it is important to consider the dividing line between incomplete or selective disclosure and deception. It may be that presenting a particular identity causes informants to reveal thoughts or feelings that they would almost certainly not have revealed had the researcher presented another identity. Much the same applies to the way in which the researcher discloses his or her interests and purposes within a study to participants.

Whether deception and misrepresentation are ethically justifiable is a matter of controversy (Hornsby-Smith, 1993). Those who have used such procedures generally justify them in terms of the utility of the research being carried out. Humphreys (1970, p. 173), who conducted a famous piece of covert research into male homosexual behaviour, points to the value of correcting 'the superstition and cruelty' of public perceptions in this area. He also highlights the ethical implications of *not* researching an area of social concern. A justification of a study in terms of its anticipated outcomes may not always be easy, however. Archbold (1986) points out that the exploratory nature of research using a qualitative approach may mean that it is hard to specify the benefits of a study in advance. Nonetheless, the researcher can still point to the fact that greater understanding of an important topic is likely to be gained, even if specific insights cannot be predicted.

When conducting interviews, the issue of *confidentiality* may arise. Sometimes, there may a distinction between what is said 'on the record' and what is said 'off the record'. For example, it is common practice for interviewer and informant to continue to talk once the tape recorder has been switched off. Although it is probably unrealistic to expect the researcher to disregard totally anything said after this point, it should not be specifically utilized or quoted for the purposes of the study. A more dramatic situation is where the researcher discovers information in the course of a study that has serious implications for the well-being of others. In the course of an interview with a young woman, it might emerge that her children are being sexually abused. Although assurances of confidentiality may have been given at the outset, the researcher may feel obliged to pass this information on to the appropriate authorities, and thereby break the pledge of confidentiality (McCarthy, 1998). Conversely, if the facts revealed were to do with a minor criminal offence, it might be considered unjustifiable to breach confidentiality. A parallel issue may arise when information gatthered suggests that the informant himself or herself is at risk (Pallik-kathayil *et al.*, 1998b).

When using documentary sources that can be categorized as 'private' (Section 5.5.4), it is important to seek permission from their originators, where possible. If such permission cannot feasibly be gained, the issue of confidentiality becomes a prime concern, particularly since the originators of the sources may not have anticipated the use to which these may be put during research (Procter, 1993b). There may be occasions, however, when a researcher gains access, perhaps fortuitously, to documents that have been classified as confidential, but which raise important issues of injustice, discrimination or misconduct. The ethical conflict is similar to that arising in relation to deception. Respecting the demands of confidentiality in such a case may seem to do more harm than good (Homan, 1991). Similarly, it may be felt that invasion of privacy is justified if it is the only way to expose harmful or unjust practices (Kimmel, 1988). It is often necessary to consider the wider moral implications of conducting, or of failing to conduct, a particular study (French, 1993).

The issue of *anonymity* is to a large degree separate from that of confidentiality. Strictly speaking, an interview that is confidential is one that cannot be reported as research data. This would be a futile exercise, and in any case few informants would require this as part of their agreement to participate in a study. However, most informants would insist upon anonymity, i.e. that what they say is not attributable to them as an identifiable person. This requires published data to be anonymous. It is important to guard against inadvertent violations of anonymity. For example, if an informant on the staff of a rehabilitation unit is identified as being 'a male physician with over 20 years' experience in rehabilitation medicine', it may be that only one person would fit such a description. This would breach anonymity as surely as if his name were given. It is not only in relation to published material that anonymity should be protected. Interview transcripts should be identified with a code and the list of names corresponding to these codes (if it needs to be kept) should be stored securely at a separate location from the transcripts themselves. Signed consent forms are another threat to anonymity. If participants are liable to adverse consequences for having participated in a study, it may be advisable to use another means of gaining consent (Lipson, 1994).

Respecting anonymity may require more than simply not identifying specific individuals. If a person's identity is concealed, but he or she is described as a member of a particular social or ethnic group, that person is not directly identifiable, but may be indirectly affected by the reporting of findings (Hansson, 1998). For example, if an informant from a minority group reports socially unacceptable behaviour or expresses views that others may find distasteful, the group in question, including this informant, may be stigmatized as a consequence.

Exploratory studies may also raise issues of *harm*. In research that uses methods such as interviews and observation, the harm in question is most likely to be psychological, social, economic or legal. Harm might come about in one of the following ways:

- Researchers conducting observational research may have a disruptive effect on those being observed; e.g. the researcher's presence may alter the delicate relationships of trust and cooperation existing between staff and patients in a psychiatric hospital.
- Informants may become distressed if intimate and sensitive issues are explored (Kavanaugh and Ayres, 1998); e.g. an interview with a person with a psychiatric disorder may elicit memories of past traumatic events which may trigger the return of symptoms.
- Participants may be led to reflect on past events in such a way that feelings of shame or loss of self-esteem may occur; e.g. a mother with a physically disabled child who is asked to discuss her behaviour during pregnancy may come to believe that her actions were the cause of her child's disability.
- Discussions during interviews may raise unrealistic expectations; e.g. informants may be encouraged to reflect on their health problems and to identify a need for services that are not available.
- Participants with whom the researcher has developed a close bond may experience psychological distress at the conclusion of a study; e.g. socially isolated individuals may come to regard the researcher as a friend and feel a sense of desertion when they are no longer visited as part of the study.
- If confidentiality or anonymity are violated, individuals may be exposed to adverse consequences; e.g. those identified as drug users might become stigmatized, lose their job or face arrest
- Potential harm may arise through misinfor-

mation; Kitzinger and Barbour (1999, p. 17) argue that one should not 'walk away from a group after having silently listened to people convincing each other that HIV can be transmitted by casual contact or that anal intercourse is safer than vaginal intercourse'.

- In some cases, the reporting of data may have harmful effects on others (Mason, 1996); e.g. respondents may express discriminatory or morally offensive views, or documentary sources may contain degrading images, and the researcher will need to consider whether or not reporting such data serves to disseminate such opinions.

Sometimes, a risk of harm may not result from any action on the part of the researcher, but may develop as a natural consequence of a social situation that is the focus of research. In such a case, the researcher – who may be in a non-participant role – must decide whether or not to intervene. Archbold (1986) argues that a health professional researcher should respond in terms of his or her clinical responsibility, and step out of the researcher role. Careful consideration should be given, however, to the methodological implications of intervening in this way. It may, for example, be necessary to disregard the intervention for the purposes of data collection – on the basis that it was not a naturally occurring event – and collect no further data from the participant(s) concerned.

The principle of non-maleficence is generally regarded as being a particularly stringent one, and it is therefore very difficult to justify any degree of foreseeable harm to research participants. Of course, harm may sometimes occur despite conscientious attempts to avoid it, and suitable preparations should be made. For example, if it is conceivable that some interviewees may experience psychological distress as a result of disclosing painful experiences, ready access to a clinical psychologist or a counsellor should be arranged in advance.

Finally, there is the question of *exploitation*. This issue is usually raised in the context of experimental research. However, it has been argued that the apparently equal relationship that generally exists between researcher and informant in an unstructured interview may carry the potential for exploitation (Finch, 1984). Indeed, it is the very trust that may develop in such a situation that creates the possibility of exploitation, since it is likely to encourage the informant to disclose in a free and uninhibited manner. Kellehear (1996, p. 102) argues that, in the unstructured interview,

> *Respondents who are allowed to ramble on about the simplest question, fuelled by empathy and eye contact, are later left wondering whether they disclosed too much or imposed too much on the researcher's time and patience.*

He regards the interview as a potentially intrusive form of research, and suggests that although rapport may well exist in the relationship between interviewer and interviewee, there is little scope for the development of genuine trust. This suggests that the researcher should be not only attuned to the content of the perceptions and experiences described by the informant, but also sensitive to what giving such an account means to the informant psychologically and emotionally.

5.9 CONCLUSION

This chapter has outlined the basic elements of an exploratory study centred on the collection of qualitative data. In the process, points of contrast have been identified with the approaches characteristic of descriptive and explanatory studies, and some key ethical issues have been highlighted.

When exploratory studies are being planned, it is important not to force them into the mould of more orthodox approaches to research, whose epistemological assumptions may be incompatible with those of an exploratory study.

The way in which notions of inference, validity, reliability, generalizability and so forth are used in relation to exploratory studies often differs markedly from their application to descriptive or explanatory studies, and it is important not to import criteria that are simply not relevant.

The principal design features of an exploratory study, as exemplified by the Student Attitudes Study, are illustrated in Figure 5.3.

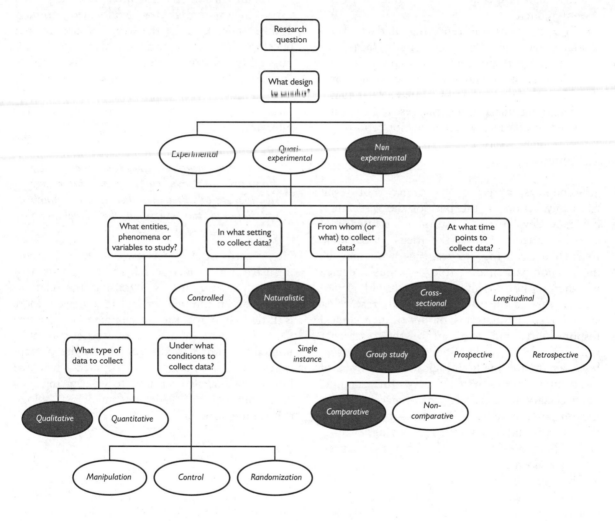

Figure 5.3 *Basic design features (shaded elements) of the Student Attitudes Study.*

6 DESIGNING A DESCRIPTIVE STUDY

SUMMARY

This chapter explores the following topics:

- the purposes of descriptive studies
- the assumptions of survey methods of data collection
- basic elements of research design in descriptive studies
- the selection of cases for inclusion
- suitable methods for collecting data
- appropriate approaches to data analysis
- ethical issues that arise in descriptive studies

A descriptive study addresses one or more descriptive research questions, as defined in Chapter 3. Its primary purpose may be to develop an existing theory or body of knowledge in more detail and, as such, it often builds upon knowledge gained from exploratory studies, or provides findings that inform explanatory studies. In general, a descriptive study is designed to collect information on areas such as the biographical or psychological characteristics of individuals, the nature of particular social structures, practices or processes, the prevalence and distribution of certain health states, or the arrangement and functioning of particular institutions and organizations.

The existence of a framework of prior knowledge enables a researcher to develop a fairly detailed design before any data are collected, in contrast to the situation that often exists in an exploratory study. A descriptive study tends therefore to be more structured and formalized than an exploratory study. This chapter discusses the basic elements in a descriptive study, in terms of design, data collection, data analysis and ethical considerations.

6.1 THE DESIGN OF DESCRIPTIVE STUDIES

Descriptive research questions are normally answered by the collection of quantitative data, or by a combination of quantitative and qualitative data; it is uncommon for a descriptive study to rely solely, or even predominantly, on qualitative data. The decision as to precisely what data to collect depends upon the purpose of the study, the philosophical perspective of the researcher (Section 2.3), and the extent of prior knowledge on the subject.

Some examples of questions that might be addressed in descriptive studies are:

- What are the characteristic patterns and modes of practice of therapists working with clients with rheumatoid arthritis? (The Rheumatoid Arthritis Study, Box 3.4.)
- Do nurses' attitudes towards performing certain routine tasks for patients with AIDS differ in regard to the extent of their knowledge about this condition and how this knowledge was acquired?
- What daily routine do children with juvenile chronic arthritis follow in relation to performing exercises and wearing splints?
- What are the general strategies used by parents with chronic low back pain when coping with a young family?
- What features are considered desirable in the design of specialist practitioner-led clinics for people with a chronic illness?
- What is the prevalence of anorexia nervosa among school-aged children?
- Within a specific outpatient clinic, what proportion of communication between a health professional and a patient is initiated by the patient?
- What is the pattern of attendance for

breast screening, after a first invitation to attend, with respect to the different districts of a particular city?

In general, specific questions such as these include descriptions of samples or situations and address more general underlying questions such as:

- For how long and/or how often do certain events occur?
- In what numbers and/or in what proportions are certain characteristics present?
- To what extent does certain behaviour take place?
- What attitudes, beliefs or practices currently exist?

A descriptive study may involve an investigation of suspected associations between variables (Box 6.1), or differences between populations with respect to variables of interest, and may therefore include research questions or hypotheses that address aspects such as:

- Is one attribute present to a greater or lesser extent than another?
- Is a characteristic more prevalent in one group of people than in another?
- Does one process occur faster or slower than another?
- Is one practice more or less prevalent than another?
- Is a phenomenon observed in a sample generalizable?

These general questions illustrate two common features of descriptive studies: the collected data are mainly quantitative, and an objective is to generalize findings to a collection of cases (called a 'target population') wider than those included in the study.

The target population is defined alongside the study objective(s) at the outset. The next stages involve specifying a design, devising a reliable and valid data collection instrument, collecting the data, analysing the data and writing the report. These basic stages are shown in Figure 6.1 and are often collectively referred to as a *survey* (Babbie, 1990; Fink, 1995a). Note that

Box 6.1   *'Correlational' studies*

A number of authors refer to a 'correlational design' (Grady and Wallston, 1988; Fawcett and Downs, 1992; Drummond, 1996; Bailey, 1997; Clifford, 1997; Hicks, 1999). Grady and Wallston (1988, p. 50) state that '[c]orrelational designs are nonexperimental designs in that there is no intervention or treatment. They involve collecting data on two or more variables and exploring the relationship between them'. Fawcett and Downs (1992, p. 9) meanwhile comment: 'Correlational studies require measurement of the dimensions or characteristics of phenomena in their natural states.' Such uses of the term 'correlational' are ill advised because a statistical relationship of correlation may not be the only one at stake. Indeed, Hicks (1999, p. 66) illustrates this fact when she describes a correlational study as one in which the researcher is 'not interested in looking for differences between groups or conditions ... but instead is concerned to find out whether two variables are associated or related'. This is misleading for two reasons. First, variables can be associated without being correlated; the association between levels of variables measured on a nominal scale (Section 14.1.1) is not strictly a correlation. Moreover, variables can be 'related' without being either associated or correlated; they may be related in terms of differences, and a non-experimental study may well wish to examine such differences. So-called 'correlational' studies are better simply described as 'descriptive'.

some authors use the term 'survey' to denote the actual design of a descriptive study (Polgar and Thomas, 1995), or the method of collecting and/ or analysing data (de Vaus, 1991; Portney and Watkins, 1993; Bowling, 1997; Fink and Kosecoff, 1998). Other authors suggest that a survey is not defined solely in terms of the methodological structure of a study, but also by the nature of the information gathered. For example, Everitt defines a survey as

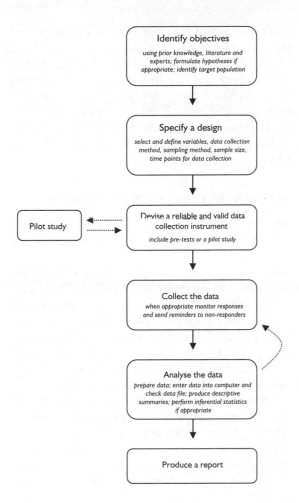

Figure 6.1 *Basic stages in a descriptive study. In some cases, there may be a process of feedback from data analysis to the method used to collect data.*

A study that collects planned information from a sample of individuals about their history, habits, knowledge, attitudes or behaviour in order to estimate particular population characteristics.

(Everitt, 1998, pp. 292–293)

Barnett (1991) extends the scope of surveys to topics such as the social environment and the economic structure of society.

Phrases such as 'survey design' or 'survey method' are also used quite frequently. The 'survey approach' defines a particular tradition of social research based on certain methodological assumptions and certain data collection methods (see Section 6.2).

The study objective is reformulated as one or more research questions (or, where appropriate, hypotheses) that can be answered using the data collected on the study variables. These variables are identified from existing knowledge, theories and the literature, and might represent attributes, behaviours, attitudes, beliefs, health status or psychological states or traits. A clear definition of each variable ensures that appropriate measurement tools are selected or devised, and that findings can be compared with those from other studies involving the same variables. It is usual to include some demographic variables (e.g. gender, age, ethnic origin) to provide a context for the study.

An important characteristic of descriptive studies is that the variables of interest are not manipulated and thus do not represent any deliberate intervention or interference with their natural state (Section 4.1.2). However, some control is exercised over extraneous variables through, for example, the use of the same measurement tool, administered by the same method, at a specified point in time, in the same environmental setting, for every participant who satisfies stated inclusion and exclusion criteria. Hence, the *setting* for a descriptive study is generally a natural one, but the *conduct* of the study may involve quite a high degree of control. Further, although the participants might constitute a random sample from the accessible population, they are not assigned to groups for the specific purpose of the study; i.e. a descriptive study may involve random *selection*, but not random *allocation*. Any comparisons that are performed in the analyses are made on naturally occurring groups (e.g. men and women; children and adults; social workers and clinical psychologists).

Descriptive studies embrace research across diverse areas of interest; consequently data may be collected through a wide range of methods, including questionnaires, interviews, diaries and observation. Focus groups, the Delphi method and the extraction of data from existing records or documentation are also used. These methods are discussed in Section 6.3. Whatever method is chosen, it is good practice to *pre-test* the instrument on a group of colleagues or other individuals experienced or knowledgeable in the area concerned. Indeed, the judicious use of experts to advise on the content of rating scales, questionnaires and other structured instruments is often of crucial importance (Grant and Davis, 1997).

As well as informal pre-testing, it is also important to test an instrument more formally in a small-scale *pilot study*. A pilot study involves a few members of the population from which the study sample is to be drawn. It is used to identify problems with the tool, such as ambiguity, poor wording, missing items, inappropriate response options, and unclear instructions. The notions of *face validity* (the extent to which the tool appears to be addressing the concepts or variables of interest) and *content validity* (the extent to which the tool covers all relevant concepts or variables) are pertinent considerations here; see Sections 9.2.1 and 9.2.2. The tool is revised in line with the results from the pilot, and in some cases may need to be re-piloted. When piloting self-completed questionnaires, it is valuable to observe participants filling them in, since there may be verbal or non-verbal signs of difficulty, and the length of time taken for completion can be directly measured. It is also important to pilot well-established, validated instruments when they are to be used on a population different from the one on which they were originally validated (Litwin, 1995).

Occasionally, a pilot study is performed in order to gain a preliminary estimate of certain variables in the population (as would be required for sample size calculations; Section 18.6). Random sampling should be used in this situation. If, however, the pilot study is for the purpose of testing instrumentation and so forth, sampling is not usually random. Rather, the researcher will normally select a few participants in each of a number of categories relevant to the main study, without regard to their proportional representation in the population (Wilson, 1996). In the Rheumatoid Arthritis Study, Angela Carella constructed a first draft of her questionnaire based on the information gained in two focus groups with local therapists. She then piloted this draft on another convenience sample of local occupational therapists and physiotherapists.

6.2 ASSUMPTIONS OF SURVEY METHODS

There is an overlap between the methods of data collection used in descriptive studies and those used either in exploratory studies or, at the other end of the scale, in explanatory studies. Some of the methods of data collection used within exploratory studies – e.g. interviews and observation – are also used to address descriptive research questions. Similarly, although questionnaires are a common tool within descriptive research, they may also be used as an outcome measure in explanatory studies. Hence, the differences between explanatory, descriptive and exploratory approaches to research lie not so much in the methods used to collect data as in the assumptions that underlie the use of these methods. This is particularly evident when descriptive and exploratory approaches are compared.

Many of the methods utilized in descriptive studies are those identified with the 'survey tradition' in social research. These are principally questionnaires and interviews, but also include more specialized methods of data collection such as the focus group (considered in Sections 5.5.2 and 6.3.4) and the Delphi method (considered in Section 6.3.5). These methods, like all others, make certain assumptions about the nature of reality (*ontological* assumptions), and certain assumptions about how best to gather information on this reality (*epistemological* assumptions). The most central of these presuppositions will be examined, and contrasts drawn with some of the presuppositions of the exploratory approach to research outlined in Chapter 5.

The first of these assumptions is that there are discernible patterns and regularities in society. Individuals are not unique, but share in broad patterns of belief, opinion, behaviour and so forth. Accordingly, although information is gathered at the level of the individual respondent (Ackroyd and Hughes, 1992), the *generality* of the data is seen as more important than their individuality. Individual responses are gathered for the purposes of subsequent aggregation. This is in contrast to the phenomenological perspective underlying much exploratory research, in which it is the *particularity* of each person's beliefs, meanings and perspectives that is commonly the focus of interest (Section 2.3.3).

Methods associated with the survey approach also assume that there is a common discourse of shared meanings among people. Meanings are fairly clearly articulated and are *intersubjective*; i.e. they are held in common across individuals and can therefore be communicated from one person to another with relative ease. It is taken for granted that there is a shared frame of reference within which these meanings can be expressed and understood. It is not assumed that these meanings are necessarily explicit, and descriptive studies may make much the same distinction between manifest and latent meanings as would be made in an exploratory study. However, the researcher does not require skills of intuition or imaginative interpretation to determine the meaning of what a person is saying in the context of a descriptive study.

A consequence of this common frame of reference is that the concepts in terms of which thoughts, attitudes and feelings are expressed are fairly well defined and commensurable. As indicated in Section 5.1, this allows these concepts to be quantified. Accordingly, survey research often seeks to reduce phenomena to quantifiable variables, in terms of which individual responses are aggregated. Furthermore, these variables can be clearly specified at the outset of a study, in contrast to the rather tentative and provisional way in which concepts are commonly identified at the beginning of an exploratory study (Section 5.2). From this perspective – often referred to as the 'variable analysis' approach to social research (Ackroyd and Hughes, 1992) – social life can be analysed in terms of relationships between a number of predetermined variables, and these relationships can be observed and quantified (Box 6.2).

Box 6.2   *Aggregating attitudes*

> A consequence of aggregating individuals' thoughts or attitudes is that they are divorced from, and thus no longer reflect, the social environment in which these individuals live and the social relationships in which they participate. Some feminist researchers find this approach unsatisfactory, since it ignores issues of social structure. Graham (1983, p. 141) argues that '[i]n obscuring the relationships that mould women's lives, the survey method masks the nature and patterns of power which derive from these social relationships. A method which blurs the political dimensions of gender and class is clearly a problematic base on which to construct an analysis of women's position.'

It is also taken for granted within the survey tradition that what people say is a direct and honest reflection of what they think or feel, and that they communicate in order to convey an accurate description of these thoughts or feelings. Exploratory research often takes a different view of the accounts people give, and draws on the idea of *reflexivity*, developed within ethnomethodology (Box 5.1). This states that, in giving an account – as in an interview, for example – a person is not merely seeking to provide a description of his or her beliefs or attitudes, but is seeking to achieve certain purposes within the social interaction occurring at the time (Benson and Hughes, 1983). The individual is 'doing' something as well as 'saying' something. Note that the term 'reflexivity' is often used in more than one sense; see Box 10.2.

The final assumption of survey methods to be considered is that information can be gathered

Table 6.1 *Types of data sought in questionnaires*

Aspect	Description
Attitudes	Affective, evaluative or conative (i.e. action-oriented) orientations
Attributes	Factual information, such as demographic or biographical details
Behaviour	Self-reported actions and activities; perceived practice
Beliefs	Acceptance of a statement or proposition, in terms of its truth or falsity
Health status	Perceived physical and functional ability, particularly in regard to activities of daily living and social interaction
Knowledge	The extent and accuracy of factual information possessed
Psychological traits or states	Information referring to emotional and mental functions (or dysfunctions)

largely non-contextually. The physical and social environment in which data are collected and the relationship between respondent and researcher are both potentially separable or eliminable from the nature of the data collected. This contrasts with the idea – drawn from ethnomethodology and conspicuous in much exploratory research – that data are situated within a specific social context and cannot be meaningfully abstracted from that context. This notion that the meaning of what people say is dependent on the context in which it is said is referred to as *indexicality* (Benson and Hughes, 1983).

The issues discussed in this section illustrate clearly the need to choose designs and methods firmly in relation to the research question and the theoretical perspective in which it is located (Figure 3.1).

6.3 DATA COLLECTION METHODS

This section will describe data collection methods that are commonly used in descriptive studies, including self-completed questionnaires and focus groups, which Angela Carella used in the Rheumatoid Arthritis Study.

6.3.1 Questionnaires

Questionnaires are one of the most frequently used methods for data collection in health and social research. They comprise a series of items that are presented in a written format in a fixed order, where each respondent is requested to answer every item (unless directed to omit

certain items). The items are constructed to elicit information on attributes, attitudes, beliefs, reported behaviour, health status, knowledge, or psychological traits or states (Table 6.1). Respondents may be asked to respond to items on a past, present or predicted timescale. Each item might provide a response that is analysed individually (e.g. gender, profession, years of post-qualification experience, the number of patients with rheumatoid arthritis seen in an outpatient clinic each week), or be one of a number of items that collectively constitute a measurement scale on some concept or variable (e.g. general health status). It should be noted that, in contrast to the measurement of physical quantities such as weight or distance, the process of measurement involved with such composite scales is indirect; this raises issues as to the correspondence between the scale and the underlying construct (see Box 15.1 for a discussion of isomorphism). There are many multi-item scales published in the literature that have been developed to measure aspects of interest to health professionals; for example, the Functional Status Index (Jette, 1987) and the Beck Depression Inventory (Beck *et al.*, 1961). McDowell and Newell discuss a range of such scales and give information concerning their validity and reliability (McDowell and Newell, 1996).

A good questionnaire takes time and skill to construct, and its content and structure should be consistent with the research questions (or hypotheses) of the study. Issues in questionnaire design and attitude measurement are discussed in detail in Chapter 15. In general, a questionnaire might comprise all *closed-ended* items (i.e. those with a list of predetermined response options), or might incorporate a proportion of *open-ended* items (i.e. those to which the individual responds in his or her own words; these items are discussed more fully in Section 15.1.6). Questionnaires produce quantitative data for the most part, though those that include open-ended items will generate some qualitative data, but of less detail and depth than that obtained by an unstructured interview. The questionnaire used in the Rheumatoid Arthritis Study consisted largely of closed-ended items, though supplementary open-ended items were used on occasions to allow respondents to provide further information or give relevant examples (Figure 6.2).

The principal alternative to a questionnaire is the interview. Figure 6.3 shows the relationship between the various types of questionnaire and interview. Questionnaires tend to be classified according to their mode of delivery, whereas interviews are generally classified in terms of their degree of structure. Although questionnaires are normally self-completed (typically administered by post), they can also be researcher-completed (conducted face to face or by telephone); this may be necessary for respon-dents who cannot read or cannot hold a pen or pencil. As indicated in Figure 6.3, a face-to-face questionnaire is essentially the same as a structured interview, and it will be considered under this heading in the following section. Advantages and disadvantages of self-completed questionnaires are given in Table 6.2.

Although typically administered by post, a self-completed questionnaire might be handed to a group of respondents whom the researcher has brought together for this purpose (e.g. in a lecture room for course evaluation), or the researcher might hand-deliver the questionnaires to the respondents' homes (Babbie, 1990).

In addition to the general strengths and weaknesses of self-completed questionnaires (Table 6.2), there are some specific advantages and disadvantages of postal administration. On the positive side, the cost of this method of delivery is about half that of telephone administration and a quarter that of face-to-face administration (Bourque and Fielder, 1995). The lack of interviewer costs (recruiting, training, and monitoring) is a particular advantage in this respect. A study using postal questionnaires takes about the same length of time to execute regardless of sample size or geographical spread – typically 8–10 weeks (Czaja and Blair, 1996). Moreover, the geographical dispersion of respondents does not

Do you have a specific treatment/management programme for rheumatoid arthritis patients (tick one)?

No ☐ 1

Yes, for rheumatological patients in general ☐ 2

Yes, specifically for rheumatoid arthritis patients ☐ 3

If you have answered 'yes', please give brief details of the content of the programme below:

Figure 6.2 *An example of a supplementary open-ended item.*

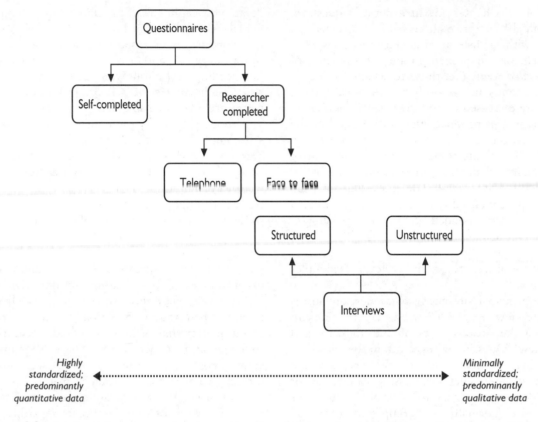

Figure 6.3   *Relationship between questionnaires and interviews. An intermediate type of interview ('semi-structured') is sometimes described.*

normally affect the cost, in contrast to methods that require telephone or, especially, face-to-face contact. A postal questionnaire can also be delivered to the whole sample at the same time. Additionally, it can be completed at the recipients' convenience, and allows them to provide information that may not be readily available (for example, a clinician may be able to look up the size of his or her average monthly caseload, but may not be able to produce this information spontaneously).

A practical drawback of postal administration is that the researcher requires a list of postal addresses, or access to respondents through a third party such as a professional body or charitable organization (in which case the researcher often has no direct control over follow-up to non-responders). A further problem is that

postal questionnaires can be subject to higher non-response rates than other means of administering questionnaires (Bowling, 1997), which may threaten the representativeness of the achieved sample (see Section 15.5.1 for a discussion of response rates). If open-ended items are included in a postal questionnaire, the answers obtained are usually shorter and less in-depth than with face-to-face or telephone interviews (Czaja and Blair, 1996).

Whatever their intended mode of delivery, all questionnaires should be piloted (Section 6.1).

6.3.2 Structured interviews

An interview may be defined as 'a conversation between interviewers and interviewees with the purpose of eliciting certain information' (Polgar and Thomas, 1995, p. 137). Structured inter-

Table 6.2 *Advantages and disadvantages of self-completed questionnaires*

Advantages	Disadvantages
• Easy to complete, if well constructed and presented in a way suited to the target population	• Developing a well-constructed questionnaire that produces valid and reliable data is difficult
• Suitable for topics for which fixed response options can be predetermined	• Of limited use for topics where the nature or form of responses cannot be predicted, or for complex issues that cannot be broken down into a series of simple questions
• Suitable for gathering much the same information from all respondents	• Less suited to situations where different categories of information are required from different types of respondent, since this would entail undue structural complexity in the questionnaire
• The form in which information is gained from each respondent is usually the same (e.g. through common response options), facilitating comparative analysis across respondents	• Participants' answers are largely constrained to fixed response options which may not be wholly appropriate or comprehensive, with limited scope to qualify their answers or introduce issues of their own
• Can gather somewhat superficial data economically from a large number of individuals	• The researcher cannot explore issues in depth by seeking clarification or elaboration
• Questions can be worded to include a retrospective time frame for the response (e.g. 'over the past 4 weeks')	• May be inappropriate when spontaneous responses are required
• Language and terminology are standardized for all respondents	• Require a minimum, common level of literacy and comprehension, and there is a potential for bias if the questionnaire has to be translated for some participants
• Anonymity of the respondent is easy to guarantee	• There is little guarantee as to where, when, by whom and in what order the questionnaire is completed
• The reactive effects of direct contact between researcher and participant are avoided (Section 5.6)	• The wording and structure of individual items may bias responses (Section 15.4.2)
• Data, particularly those deriving from closed-ended questions, are relatively easy to analyse, and a detailed analysis procedure can be determined in advance	• It can be difficult to interpret missing data, or inconsistent or ambiguous responses; there is no opportunity to query the meaning of individual responses

views are frequently used in descriptive studies. They may be carried out face to face or, as with questionnaires, by telephone (Dillman, 1978; Lavrakas, 1993; Frey and Oishi, 1995). An interviewer asks the interviewee questions in a predetermined order – in line with an *interview schedule* (Arksey and Knight, 1999) – and records the responses. In contrast to an unstructured interview, conducted according to a loosely defined *interview guide* (Section 5.5.1), a structured interview allows the respondent comparatively little chance to discuss issues that are not addressed in the prepared schedule. Structured interviews, which are really equivalent to face-to-face questionnaires (Figure 6.3),

are also referred to as 'standardized interviews' (Fowler and Mangione, 1990).

Compared with the self-completed questionnaire, the structured interview has a number of advantages (Fowler and Mangione, 1990; Bourque and Fielder, 1995; Bowling, 1997):

• A respondent does not have to possess the ability to read the questions or write the answers.
• When well-trained interviewers are used, there are fewer omitted questions and fewer errors in the use of inapplicable questions.
• An interviewer may probe for an answer, and the interviewee may seek clarification.

- When good rapport has been established, higher response rates are obtained for face-to-face interviews than for self-completed postal questionnaires or telephone interviews.
- When good rapport has been established, more in-depth responses are likely to be given to open-ended questions.

Conversely, the structured interview has a number of drawbacks compared with the self-completed questionnaire:

- Face-to-face structured interviews are more expensive in terms of travel and the time required to conduct the interview.
- If the interview takes place over the telephone, there are telephone charges (for both the initial call and any recalls necessary to obtain a specific respondent).
- As with other face-to-face methods of data collection, there may be reactive effects arising from perceived attributes of the interviewer or the nature of the interaction between interviewer and interviewee (Section 5.6); standardization of the interview and careful training of interviewers – so as to avoid verbal or non-verbal cues and create a neutral demeanour – may minimize this problem (Fowler and Mangione, 1990).
- If an interview is conducted over the telephone, there may a sampling bias in relation to those respondents who are willing or able to participate in a telephone interview; some categories of respondent may feel much more comfortable communicating over the telephone than others, and some potential respondents may, of course, not have a telephone.

The structured interview does not afford the respondent the anonymity that can be guaranteed in a postal questionnaire. This may suggest that it is less effective as a means of exploring sensitive topics. However, if some degree of rapport between interviewer and interviewee has been developed and the interview is conducted

in a non-judgemental manner, personal and sensitive issues can be explored effectively through structured interviews (Oppenheim, 1992; Bourque and Fielder, 1995). Furthermore, techniques can be utilized to permit the respondent to answer questions with minimum embarrassment. For example, in a study of sexual behaviour, a respondent could be shown a numbered list of sexual practices. The respondent only has to identify the number corresponding to each of the practices in which he or she engages, rather than state each practice in words. Lee (1993) discusses in detail the issues raised by research into sensitive topics. Dealing with displays of emotion in an interview is discussed briefly in Section 5.5.1.

Structured interviews were rejected as the principal method of data collection in the Rheumatoid Arthritis Study, since it was envisaged that they would be too costly and too time consuming. However, Angela Carella subsequently used unstructured interviews (Section 5.5.1) with a subsample of respondents to explore in more detail any unexpected or unusual results from the analysis of the self-completed postal questionnaires.

Computer-assisted methods exist for telephone and face-to-face interviews; these are described in Czaja and Blair (1996).

6.3.3 Diaries

Diaries may be used in relation to both exploratory and descriptive research questions. In an exploratory study, they are typically used to gather thoughts, reflections or reported behaviour in a fairly unstructured form. In such a situation, the term 'journal' is often used in preference to 'diary' (Ross *et al.*, 1994). In a descriptive study, a structured format for the recording of entries is usually provided by the researcher. For example, a sample of people with diabetes might be asked to record particular aspects of their symptoms, their fluid intake and their use of medications, at specified times of the day on a specially designed sheet.

Breakwell and Wood (1995) summarize the merits of diaries as follows:

Familiarity – respondents usually feel comfortable with the idea of keeping a diary.

Cost-effectiveness – if a study is carefully set up, data can be collected over a long period of time with little direct contact between researcher and respondent.

Sequencing of data – the temporal sequence of activities, thoughts, feelings and so forth is clearly represented in a diary

Intimacy – respondents may be willing to record personal and potentially sensitive thoughts or actions in a diary.

Spontaneity – when a diary was not originally kept for the purpose of research, its content is likely to be spontaneous and uninfluenced by the biases that may occur when respondents are conscious of being under the researcher's scrutiny.

Historicity – diaries may provide a detailed and contemporaneous impression of events or psychological processes that took place in the past.

There are, of course, countervailing disadvantages to the use of diaries. Their chief drawback is that the researcher can exercise little control over their use. There is only a limited amount that can be done to ensure that the entries made are those required, or even that entries are made at all. Non-completion or partial completion are serious problems, even with respondents who are initially enthusiastic and well motivated. Letters, telephone calls or visits from the researcher can offset this problem to some degree. There is also no guarantee that entries have been made at the time indicated, or in the sequence suggested by the order of entries.

6.3.4 Focus groups

Probably the most common use of focus groups in descriptive studies is to generate questionnaire items that are consistent with a study's objectives and represent the opinions, attitudes, beliefs, perspectives, activities or practices of potential participants. The procedures, advantages and disadvantages of focus groups are discussed in Section 5.5.2. In the Rheumatoid Arthritis Study, two focus groups were run to inform the response options on some of the items in the questionnaire used in the main part of the study. Members of the focus groups comprised a convenience sample of therapists from local hospitals; one group comprised eight occupational therapists and the other group eight physiotherapists.

6.3.5 Delphi method

The Delphi method is 'a method for the systematic collection and aggregation of informed judgements from a group of experts on specific questions or issues' (Reid, 1993, p. 131). As such it is a consensus method (Jones and Hunter, 2000; Box 6.3). The method was developed by the Rand Corporation in the 1950s as a method of decision making in defence policy, and has recently been used to investigate a number of subjects in health care, for example: problematic issues in the teaching of electrotherapy (Reed, 1990), identifying

Box 6.3 *The nominal group technique*

Another consensus method is the nominal group technique (Jones and Hunter, 2000). It is rather like a hybrid of the Delphi method and the focus group (Section 5.5.2). A panel of experts come together in a meeting, coordinated by a facilitator, and record in writing their initial thoughts or opinions of the topic in question. Participants then contribute their ideas to the group, as the basis of a plenary discussion. Once the list of ideas has been aggregated, clarified and tabulated, participants independently rank each idea, and these rankings are tabulated and presented back to the group as a whole for further discussion. Further rounds of ranking, tabulation and discussion are performed as required, until a consensus is reached. Although the process occurs within a group setting, the fact that all rankings are done privately and independently limits the opportunity for participants to influence one another's views.

research priorities in nursing (Lindeman, 1975; Bond and Bond, 1982; Schmidt *et al.*, 1997) and physiotherapy (Miles-Tapping *et al.*, 1990; Walker, 1994), defining the needs of critically ill children (Endacott *et al.*, 1999), identifying important educational activities in the education of radiography students (Williams and Webb, 1994).

The basic procedures followed in the Delphi method are illustrated in Figure 6.4. The topics or questions that are sent to the panel at the outset are often generated by the researcher, but may sometimes be sought from panel members themselves (Sumsion, 1998; Jones and Hunter, 2000). The cardinal features of the Delphi method are:

- Participants are chosen for their particular interest or expertise in the subject to be considered.
- Participants do not meet and are anonymous to one another, thereby preventing interpersonal factors and group dynamics from influencing the measurement of opinion.
- Attitudes are measured by seeking ratings or rankings of participants' agreement with a number of statements.
- The process is carried out iteratively, with feedback to participants, so that a consensus can be achieved in a series of stages.

The data collected in the Delphi method are normally quantitative, but qualitative data may also be gathered (Seale and Barnard, 1998). For example, participants who have provided atypical responses may be asked to describe the reasons for their views (Jones and Hunter, 2000). If, however, qualitative data are to be central to the study, Green *et al.* (1999) argue these cannot readily be subjected to usual inductive methods of analysis (see Chapter 11). Specifically, they argue that it is difficult to remain close to respondents' initial statements and also produce increasingly general formulations of these statements for the purposes of eliciting a consensus. The Delphi method would seem to be better suited to the collection of structured, mainly quantitative data.

The main advantages and disadvantages of the Delphi method are summarized in Table 6.3 (see also Goodman, 1987; Reid, 1988, 1993; McKenna, 1994; Williams and Webb, 1994; Crisp *et al.*, 1997; Sumsion, 1998; Jones and Hunter, 2000).

6.3.6 Structured observation

Observation is a useful technique when studying behaviour, especially of young children. It provides information on actual behaviour, rather than the reported behaviour obtained through questionnaires or structured interviews. Furthermore, in contrast to methods such as question-

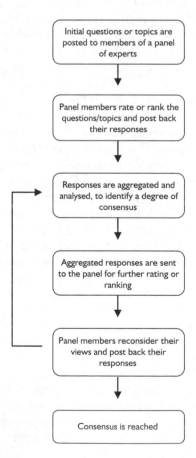

Figure 6.4   *Main stages in the Delphi method.*

Table 6.3 *Advantages and disadvantages of the Delphi method*

Advantages	Disadvantages
• Anonymity and lack of direct contact reduce interpersonal influence on opinions	• Participants' anonymity may entail a lack of accountability for the views expressed
• Participants have time to consider their responses	• The process whereby decisions are reached is not accessed
• A cost-effective method of gathering data	• Conducting a number of rounds can be time consuming
• Participants can revise, supplement and even retract their views in subsequent rounds	• There is a danger of dropout over the course of the study (though the use of experts tends to minimize this)
• It is an inexpensive method of collecting attitudinal data	• The method is prone to poor or inappropriate application
• The process of attitude measurement is responsive to the nature of emerging views	• There is a lack of clarity as to the appropriate size and composition of the panel and the appropriate number of rounds
• Qualitative data can be gathered, but are probably best used as a supplementary source of information	• The level of consensus considered acceptable may be arbitrary

naires, observational data are collected with reference to a specific social context (see the final assumption discussed in Section 6.2).

The most common form of observation used in descriptive studies is that of structured observation, as opposed to the less structured method of observation utilized in exploratory studies (Section 5.5.3). French (1993, p. 141) proposes that, in structured observation, 'researchers decide exactly what to observe beforehand and devise an observational schedule that will allow the information to be categorized in a highly specific and systematic way'. Thus, aspects of behaviour or interaction that are to be observed are predefined, and other actions that occur at the time of data collection are usually ignored. These aspects must be operationalized in such a way as to be mutually exclusive, so that there is no ambiguity about in which category to place an observation (Burns and Grove, 1997). Observers are non-participant and, in most cases, collect data overtly following informed consent from everyone concerned.

Observation takes place in a specifically chosen setting (e.g. an outpatients clinic) in accordance with the research questions. The sampling technique is therefore purposive rather than random (Bowling, 1997). Structured observation is conducted according to an observa-tional schedule that provides a checklist of what aspects to record, and might also constitute the data collection form. The detailed, systematic nature of the observational schedule helps to minimize observer bias and ensure that multiple observers all focus on the same aspects of behaviour. A large amount of data can often be collected in a short period of time – though the simultaneous observation of many different aspects of behaviour is unmanageable – and the data collected are fairly easy to code and summarize. Although the researcher may need to devise an observational schedule that is specific to the study being conducted, standardized, validated scales exist for some behaviours; for example, the Anderson Behavioral State Scale has been used in studies of infant behaviour (Gill *et al.*, 1988; Engebretson and Wardell, 1997). If the observation schedule does not have good intra-rater and/or inter-rater reliability (as appropriate) the resulting data may be meaningless.

Some limitations of structured observation are:

• Those aspects of behaviour or interaction that are not specified on the schedule might be ignored; hence, spontaneity and uniqueness of certain events may be lost (Polgar and Thomas, 1995).

- Observational methods are suitable only for aspects that are visible (e.g. movement of a limb, one person looking at another while speaking to them) or definable as an observable event (e.g. playing); the underlying motivations, perceptions or meanings of the participants are, therefore, not captured.
- It is capable of gathering data only from the location and point in time at which the observation takes place; a sampling strategy may therefore be important (Section 10.1.2).
- It might be prohibitively time consuming to obtain consent from everyone involved and to arrange convenient times to carry out the observations.
- The method is normally too time consuming to observe a large random sample of patients, professionals or organizations.

The conduct of structured observation is discussed in Moser and Kalton (1971) and Bowling (1997). Issues surrounding the collection and recording of observational data in exploratory studies are addressed in Section 10.1.2; many of these apply equally to descriptive studies. Similarly, many of the reactive effects associated with observational methods (Section 5.6) are applicable to their use in both types of study.

6.3.7 Extracting data from records or documents

A few descriptive studies use data collected from records or documents. The potential sources include patient records, case notes, and published records (e.g. cancer registrations). Some of these sources may take the form of official statistics made public by governmental organizations (Thomas, 1996). The data may exist in electronic or paper form, and may be collected retrospectively or prospectively. It is advisable to develop a clear data collection sheet, so that the necessary information is captured comprehensively and consistently. General principles relating to the use of documentary sources are outlined in Section 5.5.4. When used within a descriptive study, however, it is likely that the data extracted and the subsequent analysis will be predominantly quantitative.

6.4 SELECTING CASES

Most empirical research involves selecting a sample of cases from a larger collection of cases (the accessible population) – where these cases might be people, objects, institutions or events. Practical constraints, such as limitations on time, finances and the number of researchers who can be assigned to a study, normally prevent the inclusion of all cases that are relevant to the research question or hypothesis. The rationale for sampling, definitions of key terminology, and an account of some of the common sampling strategies are given in Chapter 8. This section considers the basic issues involved in sampling and some of the problems that might arise.

The general considerations underlying sampling are:

- defining the population
- obtaining a list of possible cases (the sampling frame)
- selecting the sampling method
- deciding on the sample size.

These considerations are closely related to each other, and to the selected method for data collection. They are discussed in the context of descriptive studies in Moser and Kalton (1971), Crombie and Davies (1996), and Czaja and Blair (1996). The underlying assumption in most descriptive studies is that we wish to generalize a study's findings to some definable population. If this is not an objective of the research, then purposive sampling (Section 8.4) may be used and issues concerning sample size are less critical.

It is appropriate at this stage to clarify which cases are deemed to constitute the target population. In the Rheumatoid Arthritis Study, the target population was all occupational therapists and physiotherapists in the UK who had patients/clients with rheumatoid arthritis. On this basis, Angela Carella decided to include in her study occupational therapists and physiotherapists from any hospital-based specialty, but to exclude those who had not seen any patients/clients with a confirmed diagnosis of rheumatoid arthritis within the previous 12 months (see Section 8.5 for a discussion of the bias introduced by this particular sampling strategy). This entailed that some therapists were excluded from the study at the outset (i.e. those not working in hospital-based specialties), whereas others were excluded on the basis of the returned questionnaires (i.e. those who stated that they had not seen these patients within the last 12 months). This process is analogous to the application of inclusion and exclusion criteria in an experimental study (Section 7.2.4).

An important question to consider here is the availability of a list of potential cases. A number of issues arise in relation to generalizing the study's findings to a population. If a list of potential cases is found, it may: (1) match the population of interest (this is the ideal situation, but is unlikely in most research), (2) include cases that are *not* members of the population of interest (so that selected cases would need to be screened for eligibility), or (3) omit cases that *are* members of the population of interest (in which case the adequacy of the list would have to be assessed against the research questions). This third problem is the hardest both to detect and to deal with – a list obviously provides information on cases that are included, but rarely gives an indication of those that are excluded. In many instances, no adequate list exists or can be constructed. This has consequences for the selection of a sampling method; for example, random sampling requires a comprehensive list of the population (Section 8.3.1).

The sampling method employed needs to fulfil two desiderata: it should be practical within the resource and time constraints of a study, and it should produce a statistically representative sample, as a prerequisite for statistical analysis of the collected data. For example, in the Rheumatoid Arthritis Study, multistage cluster sampling (Section 8.3.3) was used. This had the practical advantage that lists of occupational therapists and physiotherapists were required from 30 hospitals only, but at the same time the use of random selection helped to ensure the statistical representativeness of the sample. However, a convenience sample of 16 therapists was considered to be an acceptable sampling method for two focus groups run to discuss the content of the study's questionnaire.

Deciding upon sample size is a major consideration in any study involving inferential statistical analysis, since an insufficiently large sample may lead to inconclusive findings (Freiman *et al.*, 1978; Ottenbacher and Maas, 1999). The required sample size depends upon the sampling method and the variability of the main study variables. Its determination is based on assumptions about the role of chance in the selection of cases from the accessible population. This topic is considered in more detail in Sections 13.4.8 and 18.6. Different data collection methods are traditionally associated with samples of differing sizes, but this is a consequence of practical considerations, including ease of administration to large samples, costs and time.

6.5 PRACTICAL CONSIDERATIONS

Many practical issues in descriptive studies fall under the headings of 'documentation' or 'training'. Regularly updated, well-organized records are essential to the smooth execution of a study and allow its progress to be monitored with regard to:

- preliminary activities, such as:
  - obtaining approval from appropriate gatekeepers to run the study
  - obtaining access to potential participants
  - obtaining ethical approval for the study
  - agreeing a schedule and identifying milestones

- devising a procedure that ensures anonymity of participants

- constructing a reliable and valid measurement tool, including tasks such as:

  - literature searches on existing tools
  - developing, piloting and revising a measurement tool
  - recording reasons for decisions made

- routine tasks, such as:

  - recruiting participants
  - recording numbers of responders and non-responders (and, hence, updating the response rate)
  - taking action to follow up non-responders (recording dates of postal reminders, calling back for face-to-face interviews, or recalls on the telephone)
  - taking action to recover data on incomplete returned questionnaires
  - data coding and entry into a computer package
  - recording action points from progress meetings.

Trained interviewers, observers and participants (e.g. to make appropriate entries in diaries) minimize the potential for bias and imprecision in the collected data, but their training requires time and a budget. Resources are also required to produce high-quality photocopies of questionnaires, to pay for postage and envelopes, to provide refreshments at focus groups, and so forth.

6.6 DATA ANALYSIS

The research objectives, sampling method, data collection methods, and nature of the data determine what analyses are performed in descriptive studies. Since there is no manipulation of study variables in this type of research, the results cannot be used to demonstrate cause and effect (see the discussion of correlation in Section 14.1.2). However, the study objectives may entail an investigation of associations between different characteristics or phenomena (e.g. use of specific tools to measure pain and therapist's profession, or time since onset of a disease and confidence to cope with activities of daily living) or the testing of differences between individuals, groups of individuals (e.g. males and females), or organizations (e.g. different clinics) within a study. In many instances, analysis is limited to a description of the data; for example, the pattern of use of different tools to measure pain, the pattern of referrals from different sources to a low back pain clinic, or prevalence of a condition for people in different age groups.

The most frequently used methods of data collection – described in Section 6.3 – involve gathering data according to a highly structured format; these lead to quantitative data. A descriptive analysis of such data entails four steps: (1) preparing the data for entry into a computer package (as described for a questionnaire in Section 15.5.3); (2) entering the data into the package and checking entries in the resulting data file (Section 12.6); (3) producing summary statistics and graphs; and (4) presenting the descriptive summaries (Chapter 12). Data need to be summed across items that form a multi-item scale before any analyses are performed.

Inferential statistical methods may be used when they are in accordance with the study objectives and the data are collected using a sampling method that will secure statistical representativeness (Section 8.3). Appropriate statistical methods include significance tests for association between variables, significance tests for differences between characteristics, estimating differences between characteristics, and regression analysis (Chapters 14 and 18).

The results may be generalized when the achieved sample is representative of the accessible population (Section 8.2). This will be affected by the sampling method (Section 8.3), sampling error (Section 8.5), non-coverage, and non-sampling error. *Non-coverage* arises when some members of the population are excluded from potential selection (Crombie and Davies, 1996). This may occur because they are not accessible through the chosen method of contact (e.g. they are not on the telephone, or are not listed on an electoral register, or are homeless). More generally, non-coverage arises whenever the accessible population from which the sample is selected excludes part of the target population. This might occur if the target population consists of patients at all stages of a disease but the accessible population is located in chronic care facilities, or if the target population is the national populace but the accessible population is drawn from parts of the country in which a particular ethnic group is virtually unrepresented. Sources of *non-sampling error* include non-response, bias in the characteristics of non-responders, deliberate or non-deliberate misreporting or non-reporting of responses to certain items, and poor reliability or validity in the data collection tool (Chapter 9). Non-sampling errors may be present in data collected by any of the usual sampling methods; they are discussed in Moser and Kalton (1971), Czaja and Blair (1996) and Krosnick (1999).

A variety of factors may lead to *non-response*. The intended sample may find the subject of the questionnaire uninteresting or apparently irrelevant to their own lives, or the instrument may not have been designed so as to encourage and facilitate its completion and return (see Section 15.5.1). Those in the intended sample who do not return the questionnaire, having received it, are classed as 'non-responders'. An alternative possibility is that some of the intended sample may never have received the questionnaire, owing to factors such as their having moved or the use of an incorrect or incomplete address. The term 'ghosts' has been applied to those who fall into this category (Pope and Croft, 1996). Whereas non-coverage concerns individuals who were not included in the sampling frame in the first place, non-response refers to those who were included in the intended sample, but either chose not to respond (non-responders), or were unable to respond through not having received the questionnaire (ghosts).

There is no published minimum response rate (that is statistically based) above which an achieved sample may be considered representative. If some demographic data can be obtained on the non-responders, these characteristics may be compared across the responders and non-responders to determine whether any statistically significant differences exist. This might affect the analyses to be performed. The issue of response rates is discussed in Section 15.5.1.

If a sample has been drawn from a number of subgroups ('strata') in a population, descriptive summaries from the sample will be representative of the population if the proportion of the sample from each stratum is the same as the proportion of the population in each stratum (Section 8.3.4). Descriptive summaries computed from non-proportional sampling can be adjusted to be representative of the population. Convenience samples are unlikely to be statistically representative (see Sections 8.4.2 and 13.6).

Qualitative data might arise from responses to open-ended questions, from focus groups, and from unstructured interviews employed to explore interesting or unusual findings (as was done in the Rheumatoid Arthritis Study). The processes whereby qualitative data are handled and analysed are discussed in detail in Chapters 10 and 11 with regard to exploratory studies. In such studies, the themes and categories are generally drawn from the data, rather than being identified in advance of the process of analysis. The situation may be slightly different in a descriptive study. The analysis of qualitative data from such sources as open-ended items in questionnaires or focus group transcripts is likely to be performed in terms of previously identified themes and categories apparent in the questions that elicited the data. Hence, their analysis is much simpler than in exploratory studies.

The data in structured diaries might be summarized through proportions of occasions (e.g. days) on which respondents report some specific action (e.g. wearing splints at night), carry out an activity (e.g. performing joint strengthening exercises), or experience a problem (e.g. having a migraine). The data might also comprise values of variables such as weight (e.g. of different foods in a diet), counts (e.g. number of exercise sessions per day), or time (e.g. how long each exercise session lasted), all of which may be summarized through descriptive statistics (Section 12.4). The data are likely to be unrepresentative when the completion of diary entries is low.

A note of caution is in order. Descriptive studies may consider many variables and generate large amounts of data. The purpose of the data analysis is not to consider associations or differences between all variables in the study, but to produce results that address the specific objectives of the study.

6.7 ETHICAL ISSUES IN DESCRIPTIVE STUDIES

The ethical issues encountered in the course of conducting a descriptive study are likely to be similar to those involved in exploratory studies (Section 5.8), but usually with a rather different emphasis.

In some cases, the issues concerned are less problematic than in exploratory studies. For example, when returning a postal questionnaire, a respondent can often remain anonymous to the researcher as well as to those reading a report of the research (see Section 15.5.1 for methods of maintaining anonymity). In many exploratory studies, however, anonymity with respect to the researcher is impossible to achieve (Polit and Hungler, 1995). Similarly, the data gathered from questionnaires, structured interviews or structured observation are in most cases less detailed and intimate than those likely to be gathered in semi-structured interviews or in less structured forms of observation. Accordingly, the need for confidentiality may be slightly less urgent.

In some studies (e.g. those describing normal therapeutic practices or procedures, or addressing issues such as client satisfaction) there is no direct benefit to the participants, but the findings might inform improvement of services, practices, facilities or treatments for future users

or providers. This is consistent with the principle of beneficence (Section 4.4.2), and because participants in such studies are not likely to be disadvantaged or harmed through being involved, the objection that they are being exploited is not normally a very powerful one. On the other hand, the fact that there is not usually a specific intervention involved in descriptive studies, as there is in experiments, does not remove the need for informed consent. However, it may be easier to explain the nature and implications of a questionnaire study than those of an extended period of ethnographic research or, at the other end of the scale, a randomized controlled trial. Consent to a postal questionnaire is usually implied by its return. The information about the study accompanying the questionnaire must be exemplary in terms of detail and clarity, since there is normally little scope for the respondent to seek clarification. It should include some degree of incentive to encourage respondent participation, but not contain wording that constitutes coercion. Indirect coercion or harassment of people to participate might occur when multiple reminders are sent to non-responders.

Clumsy or insensitive items in a questionnaire can raise false hopes, cause distress, or in extreme cases prompt respondents to undertake imprudent or hazardous courses of action. A particular problem lies in the fact that the researcher is not usually in a position to detect that such effects have occurred and thus to take remedial action.

Potential problems with studies that employ structured observation as a method for data collection were outlined in Section 5.8. These included the difficulty of obtaining individual consent from all persons who may be observed, and the danger that when consent is obtained, an explanation of the purpose of the study might cause the participants to change their behaviour. However, covert observation involves some degree of deception and is potentially at odds with the principles of respect for autonomy and respect for persons (Section 4.4.2 and Section 5.8).

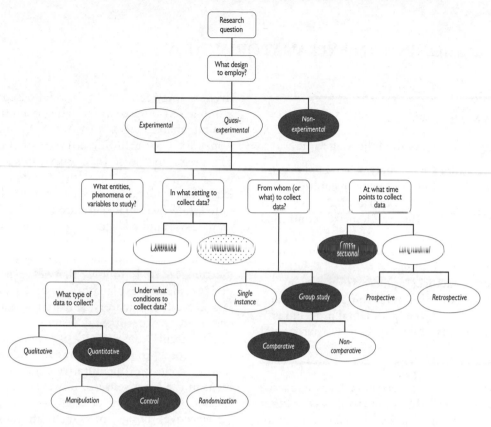

Figure 6.5   *The Rheumatoid Arthritis Study (shaded elements). It is debatable whether or not the setting for a study such as this should be classed as 'naturalistic'. Although the situation in which a questionnaire is completed may be a natural one, the process of responding to items on a questionnaire is a somewhat unnatural one (Section 6.1).*

6.8 CONCLUSION

This chapter has examined the principal design features of descriptive studies. The main features for the Rheumatoid Arthritis Study are summarized in Figure 6.5. Most descriptive studies are based on prior knowledge in an area of interest and involve a systematic approach to design, data collection and data analysis. A wide variety of data collection methods are available, each of which has advantages and disadvantages. A researcher needs to choose a method that reflects the theoretical and methodological assumptions of the area of knowledge in which the study is based, and that enables the research question to be answered within a realistic time frame and budget.

7 DESIGNING AN EXPLANATORY STUDY

SUMMARY

This chapter explores the following topics:

- the relationship between explanatory research questions and experimentation
- basic principles of experimental design, as exemplified by the randomized controlled trial
- the rationale for randomization, operationalization and blinding
- the use of factorial and crossover designs
- problems of dropout, contamination and non-adherence to experimental procedures
- ethical issues that arise in experimental research

The previous two chapters have considered the design of studies that aim to answer either exploratory or descriptive research questions. This chapter will focus on studies that address explanatory research questions, and will examine the principles of experimental design.

7.1 EXPLANATORY RESEARCH QUESTIONS

It was pointed out in Section 3.1.1 that an explanatory research question can usually be framed in declarative terms, as a hypothesis. A hypothesis is a predictive statement deduced from a theoretical proposition. Data are collected during the course of the study, and a decision is made on whether to retain or reject the hypothesis (see Section 2.4.1). The principles of statistical analysis underlying this decision-making procedure will be examined in Chapter 13.

The Low Back Pain Study provides an example of an explanatory research question (Box 7.1). Here, the researcher sought to determine whether there is a difference in effec-

tiveness between an individual-based and a group-based approach to the cognitive-behavioural management of low back pain (see Appendix I for a full description of this study). The design of choice for a question such as this is an experiment, and this design will be examined in detail in this chapter. It should be noted, however, that there are other designs that may be applied to explanatory research questions – for example, the quasi-experiment (Section 4.2.3) and the single system design (Section 16.2). It follows that all experimental designs address explanatory research questions, but not all explanatory research questions are answered by experimental designs.

The term 'experiment' is sometimes used rather loosely to refer to a range of designs that involve collecting quantitative data. An experiment in the strict sense is, however, rather more specific, and can be defined as a longitudinal (prospective) design in which an intervention variable is manipulated in order to determine quantitatively its effect on one or more outcome variables, other extraneous variables having been controlled for.

Some important aspects of experimentation can be drawn from this initial definition:

- The question that is being answered is one of cause and effect – did changes in the intervention variable cause changes in the outcome variable?
- To answer such a question, it is not enough to show that changes in the outcome variable *accompany* or are *associated with* any manipulation of the intervention variable – this does not provide evidence of cause and effect. There must be evidence that manipulation of the intervention *preceded* change occurring in the outcome variable: hence the use of a prospective design.

Box 7.1 *Explanatory and pragmatic approaches to clinical research*

When applied to clinical research, the term 'explanatory' is often used in a rather more specific sense than that in which we have used it hitherto (Schwartz and Lellouch, 1967). An *explanatory* trial in this more specific sense is one that seeks to determine whether a particular intervention works in an absolute sense. It is concerned with the *efficacy* of that intervention; here, 'efficacy' is the extent to which a treatment does more good than harm in the context of 'optimal diagnostic accuracy and compliance of both health providers and patients' (van der Linden et al., 1991, p. 2). Explanatory trials often compare a single intervention with a placebo in experimental conditions that are carefully controlled. In contrast, a *pragmatic* trial is concerned with whether or not an intervention works in a relative sense, in comparison with alternative interventions, as is the case in the Low Back Pain Study. The aim is to establish the *effectiveness* of the intervention. Effectiveness is distinguished from efficacy in that it represents the benefit of an intervention (or a package of interventions) in relation to other such interventions (or packages) in the context of everyday clinical practice, where diagnosis, compliance and overall experimental control may be less than optimal. Indeed, a considerable degree of latitude and flexibility as to how to deliver a package of treatment may be specifically allowed to participating clinicians in a pragmatic trial, so as to reflect the reality of clinical practice (Roland and Torgerson, 1998a). Pragmatic trials are usually analysed on an intention-to-treat basis (Section 18.2), and may take the form of a 'mega-trial', in which small but clinically important effects are sought in a large number of patients (Charlton, 1995; Collins et al., 1996). As a final point of comparison, whereas an explanatory trial may use just one or two measures of effect, pragmatic trials often use a wider range of outcome measures (Roland and Torgerson, 1998b). Pragmatic trials are also sometimes referred to as 'management' trials (Elwood, 1998), to reflect their focus on normal clinical practice.

- If changes in the outcome variable are to be explained by the effect of the intervention variable, it is important that other possible explanations of these changes are in some way ruled out. Hence, the influence of extraneous variables is controlled (Box 7.2).
- The change that is sought in the outcome variable is characteristically one of magnitude. Hence quantitative data are gathered.

7.2 ELEMENTS OF DESIGN IN EXPERIMENTATION

The elements of experimental design will be examined in the context of the Low Back Pain Study. The form taken by this study is that of a randomized controlled trial, which is probably the commonest type of experimental design utilized in health care research.

In the basic definition of experimental design, it was pointed out that there might be rival explanations of any changes in an outcome variable. Just as the intervention variable being tested may influence the outcome variable, so may certain extraneous variables. These are referred to as *confounding variables* or *confounders* (Box 7.3), and they are threats to the *internal validity* of an experiment (see Section 7.2.8). Many of the specific design features of an experiment – such as randomization, operationalization and blinding – serve to eliminate, or at least minimize, the possibility of confounding. These will be considered in detail in the sections that follow.

7.2.1 Randomization

An experiment is concerned with intervention variables and outcome variables, and the causal relationship (if any) that exists between these. In

Box 7.2   *Cause and effect*

Strictly speaking, in an experiment as many alternative explanations of the changes as possible are eliminated. It is not possible to eliminate *all* such explanations, and it is therefore not possible to attribute changes in an experiment definitively to a single cause. There are a number of reasons why all rival causes of change cannot be ruled out. First, as will be indicated in Section 13.4.8, even though a statistical test may be significant, this does not exclude chance factors as an explanation; it merely indicates that such factors are sufficiently improbable as to allow them to be disregarded. The play of chance can never be totally excluded, because in the long run even the most improbable outcome will eventually occur by chance. Similarly, the process of randomization (Section 7.2.1) does not wholly eliminate the influence of pre-existing intervention variables. It merely ensures that such factors can only affect the outcome by a chance, rather than by a systematic, process. The statistical test automatically takes such chance factors into account, but this brings us back to the previous point: the statistical test cannot exclude chance factors. Second, to say that all alternative explanations have been ruled out is tantamount to claiming that a particular hypothesis (i.e. the one remaining explanation) has been proven. However, as was noted in Box 2.2, it is logically impossible to prove a hypothesis. Hence, the evidence of cause and effect provided by an experiment can never be conclusive, and this should be borne in mind when considering aspects of experimental method described in this chapter.

Box 7.3   *Confounding and bias*

The effect of a confounding variable should be distinguished from that of bias (Brennan and Croft, 1994). A confounding variable is one that has an effect on the outcome variable, but exerts this effect more on one group than on the other(s). This effect is therefore 'confounded' with that of the intervention variable of interest in the study. Observed changes cannot confidently be attributed to the intervention variable, rather than to the confounding variable. Note that if an extraneous variable influences each group equally, problems may not arise – no actual confounding has occurred in respect of relative differences between groups (though the *absolute* magnitude of change within each group can no longer be attributed to the intervention variable). The degree of confounding that occurs is related to both the association between the extraneous variable and the intervention variable (i.e. the degree to which the confounder differs between treatment groups) and the association between the extraneous variable and the outcome variable (Elwood, 1998). In contrast to a confounding variable, a biasing factor is one that causes systematic error in measurement of the outcome variable; e.g. if an investigator consistently underestimated the change occurring in an outcome variable. With bias, measurement of the outcome variable does not accurately represent the true value of the outcome variable – any change is *misrepresented*. With confounding, measurement of the outcome variable may be perfectly accurate, but the source of any between-group differences is unclear – any change may be *misattributed*. Biasing is an issue for measurement, whereas confounding is an issue for study design (Brennan and Croft, 1994). Statistical analysis cannot correct for either bias or confounding, except when these have already been identified and then built into the analysis.

keeping with the basic design considerations introduced in Chapter 4, it is important to consider the conditions under which these will be examined.

The Low Back Pain Study is concerned with individual-based and group-based treatment programmes: these two forms of intervention are the *levels* of the intervention variable. In order to manipulate the levels of the intervention variable, Dr Buckley ensures that some of the patients in the study receive the individual therapy whereas the others receive the group-based therapy (Figure 7.1). Accordingly, patients are allocated to two groups (or 'arms') in the study (Box 7.4). In this way, information will be

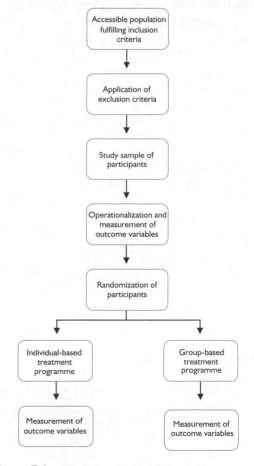

Figure 7.1 *Principal stages in experimentation, as exemplified by the Low Back Pain Study.*

Box 7.4 *'Experimental' and 'control' groups*

The groups or arms to which participants are allocated in an experiment are sometimes referred to as the 'experimental' and 'control' groups. These terms may be appropriate in a laboratory experiment, where the experimental and control groups are defined in terms of the presence and absence, respectively, of a particular intervention (e.g. an experiment on recall either with or without visual cues). However, in much clinical research, the use of these terms can be somewhat arbitrary. In the Low Back Pain Study, for example, the purpose is to test two alternative interventions. In this situation, it does not make much sense to designate either group as 'experimental' rather than 'control'. Moreover, these terms are not very helpful in cases where there are more than two groups of participants. It is probably preferable, therefore, to refer to the groups in an experiment simply in terms of the intervention they are to receive (e.g. 'group therapy arm', 'individual therapy arm'), or simply as 'Group 1', 'Group 2' and so forth. This said, when assessing the relative effectiveness of two interventions, such as by means of a risk ratio or an odds ratio, it is customary to use 'experimental' and 'control' to denote the 'novel' and 'standard' treatments, respectively (see Section 17.3.2). Sometimes, particularly in psychological research, the interventions received by the groups are referred to as 'conditions' (e.g. 'stimulus condition', 'no-stimulus condition').

provided on the relative effect of the two levels of the intervention variable.

The way in which these two groups of patients are constituted is crucial to the success of the experiment. The usual method is that of randomization; i.e. patients are allocated by a chance mechanism that will give each patient a known and equal chance of being in either group. The various characteristics in respect of which individual patients differ – age, sex, chronicity, motivation, cognitive capacity and so forth – will be distributed more or less equally between the two groups immediately after randomization, and thus any influence they may exert on the outcome variables will be more or less equalized. An important feature of randomization is that it will tend to equalize not only known confounding variables, but also unknown ones (Sackett, 1983). Moreover, it will cater for variables that, for various reasons, cannot be measured just as effectively as for those that can be measured.

Jelinek (1992, p. 85) states that, when randomizing, 'one hopes to create groups which are identical in all respects except in the treatment provided'. The word 'identical' is misleading. It is important to realize that randomization does not guarantee that the groups will be precisely the same. Although randomization will tend to distribute all patient characteristics equally across groups, there may still be chance differences between groups. Randomization does not ensure that there will be no differences in the composition of the two groups; it does ensure that any differences that arise are random (i.e. non-systematic) ones. Randomization ensures *comparability*, but not necessarily *equivalence*, of the groups.

Three further points should be made about the size of such random between-group differences. First, the randomization process ensures that large between-group differences are less likely than moderate differences, which are in turn less likely than small differences. In terms of long-run probability, therefore, groups formed through randomization can be expected (though, again, not guaranteed) to be very similar in composition. If they are not similar in composition, this is not a defect in the randomization process; randomization is designed to produce only random differences between groups, and it has achieved this. Second, the larger the number of patients randomized, the smaller the likelihood of large between-group differences (Burnand *et al.*, 1991). Third, even though long-run probability will occasionally give rise to large between-group differences through randomization, such differences are still

random, not systematic, in terms of their origin. However, it is important to note that the effect of a large random difference, in terms of confounding, will be equivalent to that of a systematic difference of the same magnitude. Therefore, the possibility of confounding should wherever possible be catered for in the design of the study, such as by using a special form of randomization (see Section 7.2.2).

It is crucial that the system of randomization employed is strictly random. Some apparently random methods of allocation may be haphazard rather than truly random, and may be open to conscious or subconscious bias on the part of the researcher (Bryant and Machin, 1997). For example, if patients are allocated according to whether their hospital number is odd or even, each patient's treatment allocation is predetermined, and is therefore not truly random (Altman, 1991b). Moreover, the researcher knows from the hospital number which treatment is destined for a particular patient, and may exclude this patient from the study if the treatment in store is not the one the researcher would have chosen. Similarly, if patients are allocated to treatments alternately, the researcher knows which treatment is to be assigned to the next patient, and has the option of excluding this patient (Pocock, 1983). Methods that preclude prior knowledge of treatment allocation, such as sequentially numbered, tamperproof, opaque envelopes, are preferable (Altman, 1991b). It is most desirable to use third-party randomization, whereby treatment allocation is taken out of the hands of the researcher and entrusted to an individual who is independent of the study (and preferably also off-site). Such a system affords better protection than any system in which the mechanics of allocation rest with the researcher (Torgerson and Roberts, 1999). The third-party approach also allows the randomization process to be monitored and evaluated (Lagakos and Pocock, 1984). In the Low Back Pain Study, patients were randomized by means of a computer-generated random number, and this was performed by a colleague who was not directly involved in the study. Thus, the process of randomization should not only be unbiased, but it should also be concealed (Altman and Bland, 1999a). The effect of unconcealed randomization may be an exaggerated estimate of treatment effect, by an average of 41%, according to Schulz *et al.* (1995).

As a final point, It is important to realize that randomization does nothing to diminish the heterogeneity of the study sample as a whole; it merely serves to reduce the heterogeneity of the groups with respect to one another (Davis, 1995).

7.2.2 Other strategies to deal with confounding variables

When it is thought that a variable may have a potentially powerful confounding influence, it is possible to carry out *stratified randomization* (Kernan *et al.*, 1999). This involves dividing the sample into strata representing the levels of the potential confounder and then randomizing from within each stratum, in a manner analogous to stratified random sampling (Section 8.3.4). For example, if it were felt that dominance (i.e. whether a person is right or left handed) and severity of impairment might influence a person's response to a cognitive retraining intervention, participants could be stratified by handedness ('right' and 'left') and severity ('mild', 'moderate' and 'severe') before randomization to two such interventions. Stratified randomization is particularly useful in multicentre trials, where the profile of patients, and other factors, may differ from centre to centre (Tate *et al.*, 1999). It is also more likely to be an important feature in a small than in a large study – in the latter, simple randomization will normally distribute potential confounders evenly between groups (Friedman *et al.*, 1982).

An important feature of stratified randomization is the use of *random permuted blocks*. This technique ensures that equal numbers of patients within each stratum are randomized to each intervention, and this is a surer way than simple randomization of distributing the levels of a particular variable equally between groups, parti-

cularly in a small study. A method of randomization that ensures equal numbers in each arm of a study (which is important for certain forms of statistical analysis) is described as *restricted* (Altman and Bland, 1999b); simple randomization may not produce equal numbers, and is therefore an *unrestricted* form of allocation. It should be noted that stratified randomization should always be restricted; if it were unrestricted, it would be equivalent to simple randomization. The implications of unrestricted randomization for statistical power are considered in Section 18.6.

It is also possible to *match* sets of participants on one or more confounding variables and then randomize (Bland and Altman, 1994c). If age were thought to be a potential confounder, each participant could be matched with another of the same age and then randomized to the study interventions. The number of matched participants will correspond to the number of arms in the trial (e.g. for a four-arm study, each participant must be matched with three others). As with stratified randomization, matching gives more surety of equalization between groups than does relying on randomization alone, but can only be done for known confounders. Matching is most easily carried out when the study sample is available in its entirety at the beginning of the study. It is harder when patients are admitted to a trial sequentially. Moreover, it is not normally feasible to match on more than approximately three variables. Matching is another form of restricted randomization. The statistical analysis associated with randomized-block and matched-subjects designs is addressed in Section 18.1.7.

A process known as *specification* may also be used (Newman *et al.*, 1988b). This involves limiting participants to a certain value, or range of values, of a specific variable. If Dr Buckley had admitted only women to the study, or recruited only patients within a very narrow age range, this would have controlled the confounding effects of sex and age. The external validity of the findings would, however, have been reduced correspondingly. Another strategy is *minimization*. As in stratified randomization, this involves identifying a number of potential confounders; it differs, however, in that group allocation is not random. Rather, each participant is specifically allocated so as to minimize the between-group differences. This involves determining the imbalances that exist between groups at a point prior to allocating the next participant, and then assigning that participant to the group in which his or her inclusion would minimize these imbalances (Pocock and Simon, 1975; Treasure and MacRae, 1998) Finally, the researcher might be able to adjust for confounding variables statistically, such as by entering them into the analysis as a covariate (see Section 18.5). In contrast to the use of random permuted blocks or matching, statistical adjustment serves both to control and to assess the effect of a particular confounding variable. Further, whereas blocking requires a variable measured on a nominal or ordinal scale, or on an interval/ratio scale divided into fairly wide class intervals, statistical adjustment can be carried out using the actual values on an interval/ratio scale; hence, it makes fuller use of the information available on the confounding variable in assessing its effect (Newman *et al.*, 1988b).

7.2.3 Operationalization

As in all forms of research, a decision must be made as to what type of data to collect (Section 4.1.3). An experiment focuses on quantitative data and an important element in the measurement of such data is the notion of operationalization.

The general idea of operationalization was introduced briefly in Section 4.1.1. It was defined as the process whereby a concept is translated into its empirical referents. Before this, it is necessary to establish a clear *conceptual* definition of the concept and, where appropriate, to identify dimensions within it (e.g. in the Low Back Pain Study, the concept of pain is separated into two dimensions – intensity and affect). This having been done, two basic procedures then need to take place:

- indicating the precise way in which the outcome variables are to be measured
- specifying the way in which the intervention variable will be manipulated (i.e. the way in which different interventions will be applied to the two groups).

The operational definitions employed by Dr Buckley in the Low Back Pain Study are shown in Table 7.1. It is important to realize that the way in which the researcher operationalizes the concepts contained in a hypothesis may have a strong influence on the way in which the outcome of a study is interpreted. Levine and Parkinson (1994) give the example of comparing individuals in terms of their cooking skill, and point out that a different ranking might arise if the dishes cooked were rated in terms of their originality rather than in terms of the speed with which they were produced.

If a concept is multidimensional, its operational definition must reflect this fact. Hence, there are operational definitions of both pain intensity and pain affect in Table 7.1. Graziano and Raulin (1993) provide another example relating to a study of disruptive behaviour in autistic children, which illustrates the potential complexity of operationalization. In this study, disruptive behaviour was defined as:

any observed, sudden change in a child's behavior from calm, quiet, cooperative, and appropriate behavior to explosive, loud, screaming and tantrums, including sudden attacks on people, smashing and throwing objects, throwing oneself into walls, or on the floor, self-abuse such as head-banging, biting, scratching, picking sores and so on, all carried out in rapid, near 'frenzied' manner.

(Graziano and Raulin, 1993, p. 82)

Behaviour that fitted the above definition was then to be rated according to its frequency (the score being the total number of occurrences), duration (timed on a stopwatch), and intensity (rated on a three-point scale: low, moderate, high).

Table 7.1   *Operational definitions in the Low Back Pain Study*

Variable	Operational definition
Intervention variable:	
Cognitive-behavioural therapy: individual and group based	An outpatient (ambulatory) cognitive-behavioural low back pain management programme run by an occupational therapist, a physiotherapist and a psychologist, delivered for a total of 3 hours a week over 5 weeks, in one of the following ways: (1) delivered to individual patients; (2) delivered to groups of 7–10 patients together
Outcome variables:	
Pain intensity (i.e. a sensory characteristic of pain)	Scores on a 10 cm horizontal visual analogue scale for 'average' pain intensity, with the ends of the scale anchored by 'no pain' and 'worst pain imaginable', and recorded by a blinded investigator (see Section 7.2.6) 1 week before and 1 week and 12 weeks after the therapy programme
Pain affect (i.e. an emotional characteristic of pain)	Scores on a 10 cm horizontal visual analogue scale for 'average' pain affect, anchored by 'pain doesn't bother me' and 'pain couldn't bother me more', and recorded as above
Disability	Scores on the Aberdeen Back Pain Scale, recorded as above
Self-rated change	Scores on a five-point scale (1 = 'symptoms considerably worse', 2 = 'symptoms slightly worse', 3 = 'symptoms unchanged', 4 = 'symptoms slightly better', 5 = 'symptoms considerably better'), recorded at 12 weeks

7.2.4 Selection of participants

In Chapter 4, one of the key questions identified in relation to research design was: from whom should data be collected? In this study, Joseph Buckley wished to compare two types of cognitive-behavioural therapy on patients with chronic low back pain. In order to be recruited, patients had to fulfil certain *inclusion criteria*, such that all eligible patients:

- were aged between 18 and 65 years
- had experienced low back pain of mechanical origin constantly for at least the last 6 months
- had stable symptoms for the last 6 weeks
- were able to attend the hospital for treatment over a 5 week period
- consented to participation in the study.

However, in addition to applying these inclusion criteria, Dr Buckley also operated *exclusion criteria* when determining patient eligibility. Exclusion criteria do not simply specify those patients who fail to meet the inclusion criteria. Rather, they specify those patients who,

though meeting the inclusion criteria, are to be excluded from the trial for other reasons. In this case, patients were excluded from the study if they:

- had serious pathology or injury
- had received surgical intervention for their back pain, or were awaiting surgery
- had received physiotherapy or other treatment other than medication or self-help measures during the last 6 weeks
- had a diagnosis of clinical depression or other specified psychiatric pathology.

The chief purpose of these exclusion criteria is to make the population of patients from which the sample would be drawn less heterogeneous. In particular, certain extraneous variables that could potentially affect the outcome of the trial, other than the type of cognitive-behavioural programme received, are excluded at the outset. These are potential confounding variables. Hence, to offset the threat of confounding, the possibility is ruled out that some alternative treatment administered in the last 6 weeks might explain any post-treatment differences in the outcome variables, or that past surgery might influence the prognosis of the condition. By the same token, the findings of the study will not be applicable to those low back pain patients who have been excluded in this way, and it follows that the greater the number of exclusion criteria, the more the external validity of the study findings will be reduced. Hence, a trade-off often needs to be made between the internal and the external validity of a study. Hedrick *et al.* (1993) argue that internal validity is a primary concern in basic research, but external validity is paramount in applied research. It should be remembered, however, that findings that lack internal validity may not be worth generalizing.

As well as deciding what sort of patient to recruit to his study, Dr Buckley must determine how many patients to recruit. He must calculate the number required in each group in order to be confident of detecting a between-group difference of a specified magnitude, at a certain level of statistical significance. How confident Dr Buckley can be of achieving this is the *statistical power* of the study. If he can be 90% sure of detecting a between-group difference of this magnitude (where such a difference exists), the study would be said to have 90% power. This topic is covered in more detail in Sections 13.4.8 and 18.6.

7.2.5 Baseline measures

In order to determine whether manipulation of the intervention variable has had any effect, the researcher seeks to detect a change in the outcome variable. This will normally require the outcome variable to be measured prior to, and on at least one occasion subsequent to, the manipulation of the intervention variable. Hence, before either group of participants entered the therapy programme, the outcome variables specified in Table 7.1 were measured for each participant. Measurements made at this stage are often referred to as *baseline measures*; they constitute the baseline against which change is assessed. In theory, these measurements can be made either before or after randomization. If they are made afterwards they serve as a check

on the effectiveness of randomization in equalizing the groups. If, on the other hand, the measurements are taken before randomization they can be made in ignorance of the individual's treatment allocation (see Section 7.2.6). This is probably the preferable approach, since the baseline measurements can always be reviewed after randomization to check on equivalence of groups.

In addition, certain other variables are measured at this point. In particular, it is important to have information on patient characteristics that might be related to the outcome variables, so that their role as potential confounders can be assessed. Such information also assists when generalizing the findings of the study. Hence, in addition to the specified outcome variables and the measures required to implement the inclusion and exclusion criteria, the following baseline measurements were made in Dr Buckley's study:

- age
- sex
- marital status
- employment status
- comorbidity
- time since diagnosis and since first recalled episode of low back pain
- previous treatment for low back pain (and perceived success)
- health locus of control

The time from baseline at which outcomes are remeasured requires careful thought. A large number of interventions produce the greatest clinical change in the short term. Hence, statistically significant change is likely to be most detectable after relatively brief follow-up. However, an effect that is shortlived may not be of great clinical importance. Moreover, long-term effects may be very different from short-term ones (Tate *et al.*, 1999). An immediate superiority of one intervention over another may subsequently disappear, or even be reversed, such that the other intervention shows superior long-term effectiveness. In the light of these considerations, it might be considered that the

12 week follow-up in the Low Back Pain Study is not quite long enough.

7.2.6 Blinding

Randomization caters for pre-existing characteristics of the participants which might act as confounding variables, and ensures that groups are comparable, for the purposes of statistical inference, immediately after randomization. However, there are other factors that may come into play after random allocation has been completed. Particular problems centre on the issue of awareness: are the participants and the investigator aware of treatment allocation (Andrews, 1991)? If participants are aware of which intervention they are to receive, they may respond differently to each treatment according to their own preferences or expectations; a form of *expectancy effect* (Table 7.2). They may, for example, have more faith in a treatment that appears to be very 'active' than in one that appears 'passive'. Similarly, if the investigator has a preference for one treatment over another and knows which patients have received which treatment, he or she may consciously or subconsciously overrate the improvement in the group receiving the 'preferred' treatment when measuring the outcome variables. Jadad (1998) refers to this phenomenon as *ascertainment bias*.

To circumvent such problems, controlled trials are usually *blinded* where possible. There are three possible stages of blinding (Friedman *et al.*, 1982; Hulley *et al.*, 1988a):

Single blinding – either the participant or the researcher (but not both) is unaware of treatment allocation

Double blinding – both the participant and the researcher are unaware of treatment allocation

Triple blinding – the participant, the researcher and another researcher recording the data are all unaware of participant allocation (a further refinement to triple blinding is also possible – the researcher who analyses the data can also be kept unaware of treatment allocation).

Ideally, blinding should ensure that the researcher is ignorant not just of which particular intervention is received by which participant, but also of whether any two participants are receiving the same or different interventions (Mead, 1988).

The extent to which blinding is possible depends upon the nature of the study. In a drug trial, in which the alternative medication can be made into pills that are identical in appearance, all parties can be successfully blinded. Moreover, a pharmacologically inert placebo can readily be incorporated into such a study. In the Low Back Pain Study, however, it is not possible to prevent patients from knowing which form of cognitive-behavioural therapy they are receiving. A placebo is also hard to incorporate, since it is difficult to engineer a comparable intervention that would not have some intrinsic psychological impact.

Whereas concealed treatment allocation (Section 7.2.1) protects the integrity of the randomization process up to the point at which interventions are delivered, blinding protects its integrity after this point (Jadad, 1998). Friedman *et al.* (1982) point out that many studies that are designed as double-blind studies may become 'unblinded' in the course of the study. They argue that the researcher should assess the degree to which blinding has been successfully maintained throughout a study. Siemonsma and Walker (1997) suggest a number of strategies for monitoring and maintaining blinding. Trials in which double blinding is not performed may lead to exaggerated estimates of treatment effects (see, for example, Noseworthy *et al.*, 1994). Schulz *et al.* (1995) have calculated that treatment effects are overestimated by an average of 17% in this way.

7.2.7 Attrition, non-adherence and contamination

Once participants have been randomized to different arms of a study, there are three problems that may arise (Figure 7.2). Each of these forms of 'protocol deviation' (Pocock, 1983, p. 179) may give rise to confounding.

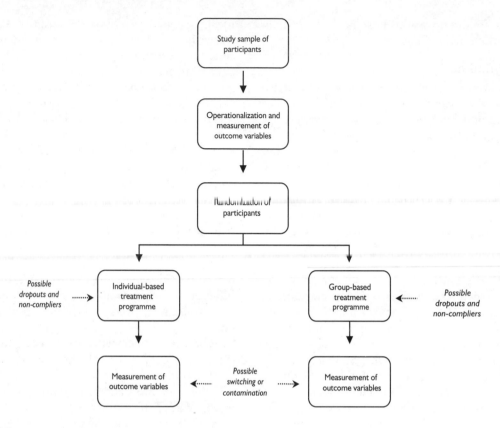

Figure 7.2   *Forms of protocol deviation.*

First, some patients may drop out of the study. In this situation, patients are effectively selecting themselves out of one or other arm of the study (*attrition*). Second, some patients may fail to follow their assigned treatment. They may simply not adhere to the treatment regime, or in some circumstances may even switch themselves to the alternative treatment (*non-adherence*). This latter eventuality is as contrary to the purpose of randomization as allowing them to select themselves into the arms of the study at the outset. When *contamination* occurs, the intervention assigned to one group comes to be received by one or more other groups in the study. This is also sometimes referred to as 'diffusion'.

Hence, some participants may fail to receive the treatment to which they were allocated, and others may experience the treatment to which

they were not allocated, either instead of or in addition to their designated treatment.

In each case, the homogeneity across arms that randomization was designed to ensure is now under threat. This threat will be realized if the effect of dropout, non-adherence or contamination is differential with respect to the groups in the study. This is likely to be the case. Participants will probably drop out from each group for different reasons, and contamination is likely to be more in one direction than another. Non-adherence too is likely to be more marked in one group than in another, because of the nature of the intervention received (it may be more onerous for the participant, have certain side effects, or be unacceptable in some other sense). Crucially, it is not merely that the *number* of participants in each group may change asymmetrically – this in itself would not be a problem in terms of confounding – but that the *nature* of the groups may change with respect to one another. What were homogeneous groups have become to some degree heterogeneous. Moreover, the researcher is unlikely to be able to determine whether participants who have dropped out or have not adhered to a regimen are in fact systematically different from others in that arm of the study, because the points of dissimilarity in question may be unknown or unrecorded. Hence, where the possibility of such confounding is apparent, it must be assumed to have occurred and an attempt should be made to correct for it at the analysis stage.

The degree of attrition, non-adherence and contamination – and the reason(s) why they have occurred, if known – should be documented. Such information might be treated as an outcome variable, or used to shed light on some of the findings that emerge from the analysis. Where possible, however, measures should be taken to prevent attrition, non-adherence and contamination in the first instance. During the process of gaining informed consent, a clear explanation of the purpose and value of the research may encourage patients to remain in the study to its conclusion (Pocock, 1983). Gilliss (1994) points out that participants in a no-treatment control group are particularly prone to attrition, and suggests that efforts should be made to maintain contact with them. Such contact should be minimal and dissimilar to the experimental intervention, so as to reduce its potential effect as a confounding variable. Similarly, steps can be taken both to monitor and to encourage adherence (Wilson and Rose, 1998). It is important, for two reasons, that such measures are not carried too far. First, there is an ethical requirement not to exert undue persuasion or influence on research participants. Second, it is important that conditions in the study should approximate those of the clinical situation to which findings will be generalized; in this respect, it is pointless to create artificially high levels of compliance with an intervention.

When contamination occurs, it is often because participants in different arms of the study come into contact with one another, and thus discover the nature of one another's assigned treatment. On some occasions, this can be at least partially prevented by randomizing participants in small groups, or *clusters*, rather than individually (Bland and Kerry, 1997; Roberts and Sibbald, 1998). In this way, participants who are likely to interact with one another are randomized to the same arm of the study. The statistical implications of cluster randomization should, however, be taken into account when designing a study, especially in relation to analysis – which is usually by a specialist method known as *multilevel modelling* (Rice and Leyland, 1996) – and sample size (Campbell and Grimshaw, 1998; sample size is covered in Section 18.6).

In a situation where there is varying adherence with the intervention being tested, it may be useful to distinguish between different levels of compliance in the analysis. If the amount of the treatment concerned can be measured for each patient, this information can be used to model the effect of the intervention in a regression analysis (Sidani, 1998). The principles of regression analysis are dealt with in Section 18.4.

If, despite the researcher's best efforts, attrition, non-adherence or contamination are found to have occurred – and particularly if they have involved more than approximately 10% of the study sample – it is important that their data should be retained in the analysis of the results of the study. That is, the data from each participant are analysed in terms of the arm to which he or she was randomized, regardless of whether or not that participant actually received the treatment associated with that arm. This is what is known as an *intention-to-treat* analysis; it is discussed in detail in Section 18.2.

7.2.8 Threats to internal validity

As was noted earlier in this chapter, confounding and bias are threats to the internal validity of an experimental study. When an experiment is internally valid, changes in the outcome variable(s) can confidently be attributed to manipulation of the intervention variable – rival explanations of the changes have been controlled or otherwise eliminated. In contrast, when internal validity has been undermined, the researcher cannot exclude other possible explanations of changes observed in the outcome variables(s); shortcomings in the design of the study have failed to cater for one or more threats to internal validity. There are a number of such threats, and they are described in detail in texts such as those by Campbell and Stanley (1963), Smith (1975), and Cook and Campbell (1979). Table 7.2 provides a brief description of the principal threats.

Behi and Nolan (1996a, p. 374) state that an experiment has internal validity 'when all possible extraneous variables have been controlled'. This should not be taken to mean that all possible extraneous variables will undermine internal validity unless they are controlled. First, some extraneous variables may have no effect on the outcome variable(s) within the experiment, or if they do have such an effect, it may be equal with respect to all groups – in both cases the internal validity of the study will not necessarily be affected. Second, it may be highly improbable on theoretical grounds that certain extraneous variables would influence the outcome variable(s). However, it may not be possible to identify some extraneous variables, and it may also not be possible to know whether or not certain identifiable extraneous variables are potentially capable of influencing the outcome variable(s). Therefore, the internal validity of a study might survive a failure to control for all extraneous variables, but the researcher may not know whether this is the case. The point to be made, perhaps, is that all extraneous variables capable of influencing the value of the outcome variable(s) should be controlled for if the researcher is to be confident of achieving internal validity within an experiment.

Internal validity must be distinguished from external validity (the generalizability of the findings from a study; see Section 8.2), and from measurement validity (the extent to which there is systematic error, or bias, in measurement; see Section 9.1.1). Whereas measurement validity has to do with the *data* gathered within a study, internal validity is concerned with the *findings* of a study; i.e. the inferences drawn from the data (Sim and Arnell, 1993). Hence, Bird *et al.* (1995) are not strictly correct to apply the term 'internal validity' to data collection techniques. However, it should be noted from Table 7.2 that measurement bias may constitute one of the threats to internal validity.

7.3 ALTERNATIVE DESIGNS

A number of adaptations or refinements to the basic experimental design are possible. Two such alternative designs are the factorial design and the crossover design.

7.3.1 Factorial designs

The Low Back Pain Study sought to establish the relative effectiveness of two levels of a single intervention variable, i.e. two methods of delivering cognitive-behavioural therapy. The study had two arms, but further arms could have been included if it had been intended to include further levels of the intervention variable. For example, in addition to the two existing groups of participants, another group could have received cognitive-behavioural therapy given in a combination of an individual and a group format, and a fourth group could have constituted a waiting list control group.

Sometimes, however, a researcher may wish to investigate the effect of more than one intervention variable, rather than multiple levels of a single intervention variable. Thus, Dr Buckley might have wished to investigate not only the mode of delivery of a cognitive-behavioural therapy programme, but also the duration of this programme, e.g. whether it lasted 1, 2 or 3 weeks. This means that two questions are being posed: (1) Is group or individual cognitive-behavioural therapy more effective? (2) Should the programme be run over 1, 2 or 3 weeks?

The most efficient way of answering these questions is to combine them in a single study,

Table 7.2 *Principal threats to internal validity*

Factor	Description	Example(s)
History effect	An event or other influence occurring at the same time as the manipulation of the intervention variable produces a change in the outcome variable.	• During a study of the effect of education on attitudes to disability, an item in the national news or a television programme portraying disability in a positive light might be an alternative explanation of any changes in attitude. • In an evaluation of nurses' job satisfaction in response to a new shift pattern in a hospital, there might be a concurrent change of personnel in senior management; this too might explain any change in job satisfaction.
Maturation	Time-related changes occurring within participants may cause a change in the outcome variable.	• In a treatment effectiveness study, there may be spontaneous recovery or remission in the condition concerned, irrespective of the effect of a therapeutic intervention. • In a study conducted on a short timescale, participants' responses may change through tiredness, hunger or boredom.
Testing effect	The initial administration of an outcome measure may in itself affect the scores recorded on the next occasion of its administration.	• Filling in an attitude inventory may cause participants to reflect on issues to which they had previously given little thought; their attitude may change as a result of such reflection, irrespective of any experimental interventions. • Repeated movement of a joint to the end of its range, for the purpose of serial measurement before an intervention, may itself change the range of movement available at that joint (Dworkin and Whitney, 1992).
Expectancy effect	Participants may respond to the perceived expectations of the investigator – the Rosenthal effect (Rosenthal, 1966) – or to the simple fact of being observed – the Hawthorne effect (Roethlisberger and Dickson, 1939: see Section 5.6).	• In a poorly controlled experiment, participants may infer that the research team have greater faith in one intervention than in another, and may respond differentially to interventions on this account (those receiving the ostensibly less favoured intervention may become demoralized and fail to improve or, alternatively, may exhibit compensatory rivalry and strive hard to improve). • In an experiment in which participants are aware that their performance or behaviour is being monitored, they may exhibit changes in their behaviour, and thereby on the outcome variable, as a result of this fact, independently of the effect of the intervention.
Practice effect	Participants' performance on a test may change simply by virtue of their having already completed it once.	• In a study using a functional assessment as an outcome measure, participants may perform better on subsequent testing by virtue of practice-based improvement on the assessment.
Statistical regression	Scores that are particularly high or low tend to 'regress' towards the mean by the time they are next measured (Bland and Altman, 1994b).	• Participants with very high scores on depression or pain entered into a study are likely to show improvements when measured again, independently of the effect of any anti-depressive or pain-relieving intervention.
Mortality	Participants may be lost differentially from the arms of an experiment, thereby undermining their comparability.	• One intervention may be more onerous than another in the demands that it places on participants, with the result that there is greater dropout from this arm of the trial (see Section 7.2.7).
Measurement bias	Biased measurement of the outcome variable may suggest that change has occurred where it has not, or that change has not occurred where it has.	• If the performance of the assessor changes over time (e.g. through practice), changes may be recorded as having occurred, and thus attributed to the intervention variable, when no such changes have in fact taken place. • A test that purports to measure state (i.e. short-term, transient) anxiety but actually measures trait (i.e. long-term, enduring) anxiety may fail to pick up a change in state anxiety when one may in fact have occurred.

Table 7.3 *A factorial design based on the Low Back Pain Study*

| | | Delivery of programme | |
		Individual based	Group based
Duration of programme	1 week	Group A	Group B
	2 weeks	Group C	Group D
	3 weeks	Group E	Group F

which is what a factorial design does (the intervention variables are referred to as 'factors' in this design; see Table 4.1). Table 7.3 shows that all levels of each of the two factors are represented in the design. The rows in the table represent the levels of the duration factor, and the columns represent the levels of the mode of delivery factor. Hence, a comparison between the data collected in relation to the rows addresses the question of the duration of the programme, whereas a comparison of the data collected in relation to the columns addresses the question of the mode of delivery of the programme. For each of these two comparisons, the other comparison is equalized, and thus controlled.

With such a design, Dr Buckley would be able to answer two research questions on a single sample. This is far more economical than setting up separate studies to answer the individual questions. Furthermore, because it incorporates all possible combinations of the levels of the two factors, the factorial design allows treatment *interactions* to be tested; i.e. whether effectiveness is affected by particular combinations of mode of delivery and duration. The required sample size for a study will depend upon whether the determination of interaction effects is an objective of the study. These issues will be covered in more detail in Section 18.1.9.

7.3.2 Crossover designs

The experimental designs considered thus far have taken the same basic form. Each arm of the study has been subjected to a different level of

the intervention variable, and the randomization process has been relied upon to create comparable groups in all other respects. The analysis of scores on the outcome variables has been *between* participants. An alternative approach is to expose all participants in the study to all levels of the intervention variable, and then analyse changes in the outcome variables *within* participants (Box 7.5).

The principal advantage of such a design is that any differences between individual participants are controlled. Because each participant is exposed to all levels of the intervention variable, the effect of that participant's individual characteristics are equalized (provided these characteristics are fairly stable and do not differ markedly within the individual as a function of time). In contrast, if participants are allocated to different arms of a study, as in the case of the Low Back Pain Study, their individual characteristics may exert a differential influence on the data derived from each arm of the study.

Another merit of a within-subjects design is that the corresponding statistical analysis is usually more powerful than the equivalent analysis for a between-groups design. An effect of a given magnitude is more likely to be statistically significant in a within-subjects design. Furthermore, as each participant undergoes each intervention, each participant counts twice (assuming there are two interventions). This is useful in terms of generating data for an analysis, but it should be remembered that it does not double the sample size for the purposes of generalization (Altman and Bland, 1997).

The main drawback of a within-subjects design is that participants are exposed to the different levels of the intervention variable in a particular sequence. An *order effect* may therefore occur, in which the effect of one intervention is carried over to, or otherwise influences, the following intervention (Levine and Parkinson, 1994). This is another example of an interaction – in this case, between the levels of the intervention variable and the sequence in which they occur. To counteract this problem, a *crossover design* can be used (Figure 7.3). This is

Box 7.5 *Terminology of experimental designs*

Various terms are used to denote experimental designs that are based on either a between-subjects or a within-subjects analysis. Seale and Barnard (1998) and Hicks (1999) refer to these as 'different-subject' and 'same-subject' designs, respectively. Coolican (1990) uses the term 'independent samples' to refer to a between-subjects design, and 'repeated measures' for a within-subjects design. Others refer to 'independent' and 'related' designs (e.g. Payton, 1994), but the term 'independent' invites confusion with the notion of an independent variable and the term 'related' is probably more appropriately used for a form of statistical analysis than for the underlying research design. Sometimes a design is based upon the randomization of participants who have previously been matched on one or more potential confounding variables. Thankfully, most writers agree in referring to this as a 'matched-subjects' design. Graziano and Raulin (1993) incorporate within-subjects and matched-subjects designs under the label 'correlated-groups' designs. However, this is a potentially misleading term, since it implies that the subsequent analysis will be of correlation, and further suggests that there is more than one group of participants, which may not be the case in a within-subjects design. A study may involve a mixture of between-subjects and within-subjects analysis. For example, two groups of participants may each pass through three different interventions. Portney and Watkins (1993) refer to this as a 'mixed' design. However, this is probably another term to avoid, since it is liable to be confused with the idea of a mixed model analysis, i.e. one based on both fixed and random effects (Howell, 1997; see Box 18.1). A preferable, if somewhat lengthier, description would be 'an experimental design with one between-subjects and one within-subjects factor' (where 'factor' is an equivalent term to 'intervention variable'). Finally, it should be noted that talking of between-subjects and within-subjects designs assumes that the sample consists of people, which of course may not always be the case.

where the sequence of interventions is randomly determined for each participant. The effect of this is that each possible sequence is equally likely to occur, thereby controlling for any order effect. A similar strategy is to ensure that each possible sequence of interventions is applied to the same number of participants; this is referred to as *counterbalancing* (Graziano and Raulin, 1993). The number of participants must be a multiple of the number of possible sequences. If just one participant is allocated to each possible sequence, a counterbalanced design is referred to as a *Latin square* (Plutchik, 1974), reflecting the fact that if each participant is represented by a row in a table and each sequence by a column, a square is produced. The number of participants in a Latin square is always the same as the number of possible sequences of interventions. However, a study may contain a number of Latin squares, such that the total number of participants allocated to a particular sequence will be more than one.

Although the basic crossover design controls for an order effect, it does not specifically diminish or eliminate the effect. In some cases, this can be achieved by incorporating a no-treatment ('washout') period between the interventions being tested (Blackwood and Lavery, 1998). This allows the carry-over effect of the first intervention to die away before the next intervention is introduced. In other cases, this may not be a realistic option, and the feasibility of a within-subjects design must be queried. It is, for example, doubtful if Dr Buckley could use a within-subjects design in his study, since the effect of prior exposure to one management programme may simply have too marked an effect on the response to the subsequent programme. For example, a patient who had undergone the group-based programme may

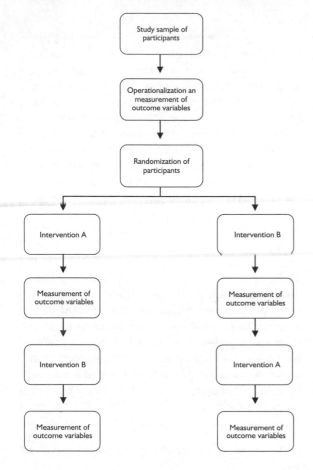

Figure 7.3 *A crossover design.*

first intervention has finished (Bland, 1995). Even when examining short-term effects, the fact that a crossover design is normally at least twice as long as a corresponding between-subjects design means that there may be a larger dropout rate (Blackwood and Lavery, 1998). Dropouts may be a particular problem in crossover studies if some patients drop out during the first intervention or before entering the second intervention (Senn, 1993). The absence of any information on their response to the second intervention restricts a comparative analysis of the two interventions. A final drawback of crossover and other within-subjects designs is that, if more than two interventions are evaluated, the appropriate statistical analysis tends to be far more complex than that used for a between-subjects design.

7.4 LIMITATIONS OF EXPERIMENTS

Although the experiment is a powerful – possibly the most powerful – means of examining causal relationships, it does have some limitations as a method of research in health care. Indeed, to some extent those features of experimentation that give it its methodological robustness are, in other respects, its shortcomings. A few of these limitations of experimentation, and in particular those relating to the randomized controlled trial, will be briefly discussed.

First, in general any shortcomings that arise through the collection solely of quantitative data, in terms of the possible lack of detail, richness and insight provided by such data, will apply to experimental designs (Wilson-Barnett, 1991). A particular concern is the nature of the information that an experiment such as a randomized controlled trial provides on the effect of an intervention. Although an experimental design may suggest that one intervention is more effective than another, it does not usually indicate *why* this is the case (Gilliss, 1994; Koes and Hoving, 1998). What is it within a particular treatment or package of treatments that was found to be beneficial by patients in the

have undergone a more or less permanent change in beliefs regarding his or her pain, and is unlikely to exhibit further response when exposed to the individual-based programme. Furthermore, mere knowledge of the nature and content of the previous intervention may influence the response to the current intervention. There are other strategies to deal with carry-over effects at the analysis stage. Nonetheless, Sibbald and Roberts (1998) express doubt as to their effectiveness and feasibility and advise against the use of crossover trials when order effects are thought to be likely.

It is difficult to assess long-term effects in a crossover design, since the second intervention cannot be implemented until follow-up for the

study? If there was poor compliance with a certain intervention, why was this (DiCenso and Cullum, 1998)? Gathering aggregate data on a limited number of outcome variables at a few points in time is unlikely to answer such questions. In order to unwrap the package of treatment (Newell, 1992b) and elucidate the mechanisms of a successful treatment, a study is required that collects fuller information. In particular, it may be important to study the pattern of change that occurs during treatment, rather than just establish that a certain mean level of change has taken place (Wilson, 1997). A single system study is likely to be a more appropriate strategy here (Section 16.2). Alternatively, if the psychosocial mechanisms of treatment are the focus of interest, qualitative data (e.g. from interviews) will probably be required.

White (1997) criticizes designs such as the randomized controlled trial for their inability to recognize the role of clinical experience and intuition in clinical decision making. However, this is an argument for the greater use of other approaches that acknowledge such issues; its force is not so much against the use of the randomized controlled trial to research clinical practice, but more against its *exclusive* use for this purpose.

Second, some diseases or clinical presentations are unsuitable for evaluation by means of an experiment. This may be due to their rarity. It may simply not be possible to find a sufficiently large sample of relatively homogeneous patients with the condition concerned to make a group study feasible. In such instances, a single system study may be more appropriate (see Section 16.2). The use of a series of small studies, analysed in terms of Bayesian statistics (see Box 13.4), has recently been suggested as another solution to this problem (Lilford *et al.*, 1995). In other cases, the heterogeneity of a clinical presentation may pose problems. In the first instance, this will reduce the effectiveness of randomization; the more homogeneous the sample is at the outset, the greater the equalizing effect of random allocation. As a further problem, if the symptomatology of a particular

condition is very variable between individual patients, it may be that only a small proportion will respond to a certain intervention. The positive response produced in this subcategory of patients will be diluted by the lack of response in the remaining patients (Koes and Hoving, 1998). Moreover, it may be hard to identify a selection of outcome measures that are appropriate for every participant. Identifying a homogeneous subgroup of patients within a diagnostic or clinical category may offset these problems, but may introduce problems of inadequate sample size in their place.

Third, certain methodological demands of the true experiment may be hard to fulfil in respect of certain conditions or situations. For example, practical considerations may effectively rule out randomization. Random allocation may not be an option when comparing two programmes of treatment, each of which is specific to a clinical unit or institution. In such a case, it would often not be possible to randomize patients to different systems of treatment within a unit, and equally it may not be feasible, for administrative or geographical reasons, to randomize patients between units. A quasi-experimental design, using pre-existing groups of patients, would be required in such a situation (see Section 4.2.3).

Features such as double blinding and the use of a placebo intervention may pose similar problems. Although these are normally feasible in drug trials, they are often not readily achievable when evaluating psychological or physical interventions (Andrews, 1991). Placebos are more characteristic of explanatory than of pragmatic trials (Box 7.1), where the intention is to compare the relative effectiveness of two or more alternative interventions. If one such intervention emerges as superior to the other within a pragmatic study, this usually provides useful guidance to clinical practice, and the lack of a placebo arm is of little consequence. If, on the other hand, no difference in effectiveness is found between the two treatments, the absence of a placebo group makes it hard to establish whether both treatments are of positive value, or whether neither treatment is better than doing nothing. In other words, it may be unclear whether the treatments are equally effective or equally ineffective. It should be remembered, however, that in the circumstances where a pragmatic trial is appropriate, established patterns of practice, or provisional evidence in support of one or both treatments viewed individually, often mean that doing nothing is not an option.

Fourth, some interventions, and also the environment in which they are delivered, may be highly complex and hard to standardize (Hicks, 1998; Øvretveit, 1998). Wilson-Barnett (1991, p. 84) claims that '[t]he more complex or varied the pattern of interaction the less likely it is that an experiment can be designed'. Many therapeutic interventions may therefore be difficult to operationalize as intervention variables, or if they are successfully operationalized, this may be at the cost of breaking them down into more basic elements that no longer represent the full nature and content of the interventions in a meaningful way. There is, therefore, a danger that the methodological demands of control and manipulation that lie at the heart of experimental method may cause complex interactive and social processes to be approached in a rather reductionistic fashion.

Finally, the results of experimental studies may be open to criticism in terms of their generalizability. This may occur through some form of selection bias, whereby some eligible patients are excluded from participation for inappropriate reasons (Jelinek, 1992). The distorting effect of selection bias on estimates of treatment effectiveness can be considerable (Herman, 1998). Even if it is possible to select a representative sample for an experiment, another difficulty may arise. A randomized controlled trial produces a measure of *aggregate* effectiveness of an intervention; it indicates that one group of patients fared better than another on average. However, some of the individual patients in this group are likely to have achieved a worse outcome than some of those in the less successful group. It may therefore be difficult to apply the findings of such a study to the management of individual

patients, unless sufficient information has been gathered to identify the responsiveness of particular subgroups of patients (Sim, 1995b; Herman, 1998).

Alternatively, the way in which an intervention is operationalized may restrict the clinical applicability of the results. For example, in an attempt to demonstrate the merits of an intervention, a researcher may test it at an intensity or frequency of application greater than that likely to be feasible in normal clinical practice. Alternatively, in order to give the potential participant a free and informed choice between two or more alternative treatments, the researcher may explain the merits of a particular intervention in a very balanced, cautious manner. In normal clinical practice, however, it might be common to give a far more positive and less circumspect account of the likely benefits of this intervention. In each of these situations, an intervention is being tested in a way that differs from that in which it would normally be delivered in the real world of clinical practice.

7.5 ETHICAL ISSUES IN EXPLANATORY STUDIES

Much of the literature on research ethics has focused on the problems that occur in human subjects experimentation, especially that conducted in health care. In comparison with the types of research considered in the previous two chapters, the issues that arise in explanatory studies differ somewhat in their emphasis. Confidentiality and anonymity are certainly a concern, though probably less so than in most exploratory and many descriptive studies, since the detail and potential sensitivity of the information collected from participants in experimental studies such as the randomized controlled trial are usually less than in interviews, focus groups, or questionnaires. Similarly, although privacy may be an issue – especially in certain psychological studies conducted in natural settings on individuals who are unaware of being experimental subjects – in most cases participants know that they are being studied. The ethical issues that are particularly pressing in experimentation are probably those of informed consent and risk of harm.

7.5.1 Consent

The necessary elements in consent – disclosure, comprehension, competence and voluntariness – were outlined in Section 4.4.1. The problem with disclosure in the context of a study like a randomized controlled trial is the familiar one: full disclosure may be perceived to conflict with the methodological demands of the study. Blinding and the use of placebo treatments usually require some degree of ignorance on the part of participants, and expectancy effects (see Table 7.2) are likely to be augmented if participants are made aware of the current state of opinions regarding the status of alternative interventions.

Comprehension raises rather different issues. Despite the best efforts of researchers to explain what taking part in a randomized controlled trial involves, potential participants often have significant misconceptions. Their recall of the technical information given during informed consent procedures may be poor (Wade, 1990; Sulmasy *et al.*, 1994). More significantly, participants may misconstrue the experimental nature of the study. Although they may have been informed that interventions are to be assigned at random, they may still believe that they will be treated on the basis of the practitioner's clinical judgment (Appelbaum *et al.*, 1987; Harth and Thong, 1995). It is clearly important to present information in as clear and accessible a form as possible, and to check that an adequate level of comprehension has taken place ('adequate' to be judged in terms of the participants' rather than the researcher's needs).

Competence to give consent may be an important consideration, especially in trials involving children or those who have temporary or permanent cognitive impairment, such as patients in confusional or delusional states or those who have had head injury or stroke. In many other cases, competence may not be an

issue. Voluntariness, however, may be a problem in all randomized controlled trials, and especially those in which potential participants are, or have previously been, in a therapeutic relationship with the investigator. A sense of vulnerability, or a feeling of indebtedness to health care providers, may simply make it hard for patients to refuse participation in a clinical trial (Hewlett, 1996). Further, some patients may feel that the quality of their ongoing care may be determined by whether or not they consent (Gray, 1975).

In view of the ethical problems that are potentially associated with informed consent, it is important that certain safeguards are taken. For example:

- Information should be tailored to the participants' level of understanding and should reflect their likely needs.
- Details of the possible benefits or dangers of participation should be presented explicitly and in a balanced manner.
- The context in which consent is sought should be as free as possible from factors that may induce or pressurize participants into giving consent, and the person gaining consent should not be in a position of power or influence.
- Assurances should be given that consent can be withdrawn at any time, for any reason, and without prejudice to ongoing care or future episodes of care.
- Even once consent has been given, continuing willingness to participate should be monitored.

Above all, informed consent should not be seen purely in terms of the administrative requirements of a consent form:

That there is a completed consent form implies only that the physician has made some effort to communicate with the patient, but its existence does not guarantee fulfillment of ethical and legal responsibilities.

(Sulmasy *et al.*, 1994, p. 193)

7.5.2 Risk of harm

In a randomized controlled trial, physical harm may arise in a number of ways (Sim, 1989):

- loss of therapeutic benefit from the novel therapy, for those receiving the standard therapy
- loss of therapeutic benefit from the standard therapy, for those receiving the novel therapy
- harmful side effects from the novel therapy, for those receiving it (such effects from the standard therapy are also possible, but less likely, since it is usually in established use)
- loss of therapeutic benefit, for both groups, from interventions other than those being tested.

Psychological harm may also be caused by certain interventions in a similar manner. In addition, any deception involved in experimental procedures may give rise to loss of self-esteem (Kelman, 1967). However, Kimmel (1996) cites evidence that many participants involved in psychological experiments in which they were deceived into behaving in a potentially discrediting manner expressed gratitude rather than resentment about having been involved.

Steps should be taken to ensure that the possibility of foreseeable harm is minimized. The choice of interventions (e.g. what treatment is compared with what other treatment), the way in which these are operationalized (e.g. the duration and intensity of treatment), and the design of the study (e.g. whether or not it is a crossover trial) are among the issues that should considered here. The researcher should ensure that the size of the sample is appropriate, so that no more participants than necessary are exposed to risk of harm (Sim, 1989; Hillier and Gibbs, 1996). Similarly, the risk of harm should be no greater in one group than in another. This is to satisfy the principle of *equipoise*:

[When] testing a new treatment B on a defined population P for which the current accepted treatment is A, it is necessary that the clinical investigator be in a state of genuine uncertainty regarding the comparative merits of treatments A and B for population P. If a physician knows that these treatments are not equivalent, ethics requires that the superior treatment be recommended.

(Freedman, 1987, p. 141)

If equipoise is not present, the researcher may knowingly disadvantage some patients by randomizing them between treatments (Lilford and Jackson, 1995).

It is also important that the possibility of harm is assessed at intervals during a study and, if it becomes clear that one arm of the trial is faring consistently worse than the other(s), consideration should be given to stopping the study early. Early termination of a study should be planned for in advance, in terms of a *stopping rule*. This is a predetermined procedure that allows a study to be discontinued if there is a sufficiently large difference in outcome between groups, as assessed by an interim analysis of the accruing data (Silverman, 1985; Ruse, 1988).

To minimize harm is not the only obligation imposed on the researcher: such risk of harm that remains must be justifiable. How this can be achieved is a thorny ethical issue that cannot be resolved here. However, three general points can be made. First, informed consent is a necessary condition for risk of harm to be justifiable, even if it is not always a sufficient condition. If consent to possible harm is not sought, both the principle of non-maleficence and that of respect for autonomy are likely to be violated (Table 4.5). Second, the likely benefits of a study, in terms of its contribution to knowledge, must be greater than the likely harm that participants may incur. Again, this is a necessary rather than a sufficient condition for justification. The fact that those who run the risk are not necessarily those who reap the benefits may mean that a study is ethically questionable, despite an apparently favourable harm/benefit ratio (Oakley, 1989;

Sim, 1989). It should also be noted that this justification requires the sample size of a study to be adequate, in order that valid findings of therapeutic benefit can be achieved in the first place. Third, there is likely to be a magnitude of harm to which participants should not be exposed, regardless of their willingness to consent or the likely benefits of the study. In other words, possible harm can only be justified up to a certain level, beyond which it is ruled out categorically.

7.6 CONCLUSION

This chapter has examined the principal design features of explanatory studies, with reference to the randomized controlled trial; these features are summarized in Figure 7.4. Variations of the basic randomized controlled trial – such as factorial designs and crossover designs – have also been considered, as have some of the ethical issues associated with this approach to research.

Explanatory research questions impose stringent methodological requirements on a

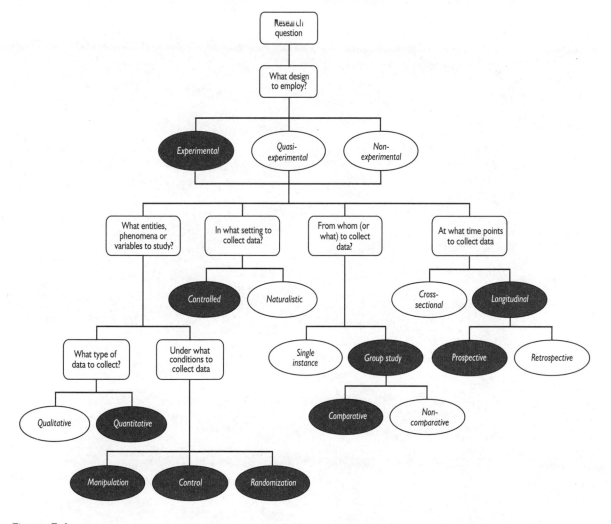

Figure 7.4   *Principal design features (shaded elements) of the Low Back Pain Study.*

study, in order to achieve internal validity in the findings. It is important to realize, however, that many of these requirements are inappropriate for studies that address exploratory or descriptive research questions. In particular, a researcher should not seek to exert the same degree of control over the research process within an exploratory study (Section 5.1).

The following chapter will examine the issue of sampling as it applies to exploratory, descriptive and explanatory studies.

8 SAMPLING

SUMMARY

This chapter explores the following topics:

- the principal terms used in relation to sampling
- the distinction between statistical representativeness and theoretical representativeness
- the nature and implications of sampling error and sampling bias
- strategies that can be used to obtain statistical representativeness in a sample
- strategies that can be used to obtain theoretical representativeness in a sample

Nearly all empirical research involves some form of sampling. The need for sampling arises because, owing to limitations of time and resources and various other constraints, not all of the cases, behaviours, contexts or situations potentially relevant to a research question can be studied. This chapter will examine the rationale for sampling, especially in relation to the notion of representativeness, and will give an account of some of the common sampling strategies available to the researcher. Fundamentally different approaches to sampling will emerge, depending upon the purpose of a study (Thompson, 1999).

8.1 INTRODUCTION TO SAMPLING

At its simplest, sampling is the selection of a group of cases from a larger collection of such cases, according to a specific procedure. These 'cases' may be persons, institutions, objects or events. Before sampling can be discussed in detail, a number of concepts and terms need to be defined (see Figure 8.1).

8.1.1 Target population

The target population is the collection of cases in which the researcher is ultimately interested, and to which he or she wishes to make generalizations. In the Low Back Pain Study, for example, the target population is patients between the ages of 18 and 65 with low back pain of at least 6 months' duration. In the Rheumatoid Arthritis Study, the target population was all occupational therapists and physiotherapists in the UK who had patients or clients with rheumatoid arthritis.

8.1.2 Accessible population

The accessible population is the portion of the target population that is accessible to the researcher for the purposes of a specific study. A sample can be drawn directly from an accessible study population but not from a target population, since you can draw a sample only from cases to which you have access. Hence the accessible population represents the *sampling frame* from which a sample is selected. On occasions, the accessible population may be the same as the target population, but is usually a subsection of the target population.

In the Low Back Pain Study, the accessible population consists of patients who meet the criteria of the target population and are current or previous attendees of three large hospitals. Note that whereas the target population includes patients who will develop low back pain in the future, these individuals clearly cannot form part of the accessible population. In the Rheumatoid Arthritis Study, the accessible population is hospital-based occupational therapists and physiotherapists working in musculoskeletal practice in the UK.

8.1.3 Sample

The sample is the selection of the accessible

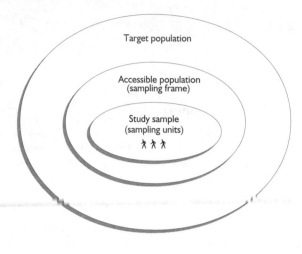

Figure 8.1   *The relationship of key concepts in sampling.*

population on which a study is conducted. The study sample may include all of the accessible population, but rarely does. More usually, constraints of time and resources dictate that only a portion of the accessible population is included. The higher the proportion of the accessible population that is included in the sample, the greater the *sampling fraction* or *sampling intensity*. If a sample does include the entire accessible population, this is known as a *census*.

There is a distinction between the *intended sample* and the *achieved sample*. For various reasons – such as subject refusal, dropout or incomplete follow-up – the sample arrived at may fall short of the sample that the researcher originally aimed to secure. In the Rheumatoid Arthritis Study, for example, 240 questionnaires were sent to physiotherapists and occupational therapists working in rheumatology, but only 150 were ultimately returned.

8.1.4 Sampling unit

The sampling units are the individual members of the sample, or cases. Frequently, these are people. However, in organizational research the sampling units might be individual hospitals or clinical units, and in research on the social impact of disability the sampling units might be families rather than individual people.

Unless indicated otherwise, in the remainder of this chapter, 'population' and 'sample' should be taken to refer to the accessible population and achieved sample, respectively.

8.2 REPRESENTATIVENESS

A central question that must be asked whenever a sample is drawn is: how representative is it? What is meant by 'representative' may, however, differ considerably between forms of research. In descriptive and explanatory research questions, the sample is usually required to be *empirically* or *statistically* representative. That is, the characteristics of the accessible population should be reflected – at the same level and in the same proportions – in the study sample. If the mean age of the population is 45 years and age is an important variable within the study, then the mean age of the sample should be at or close to this figure, and similarly for all other relevant characteristics. Generalization from the sample to the population is in terms of statistical similarities (see Box 8.1), and many statistical analyses rest on this assumption. A sample from which this type of

Box 8.1   *Statistics, parameters and estimates*

A property of a sample is known as a *statistic*, and the corresponding property of a population is known as a *parameter*. Thus the mean height of a sample of children is a statistic and the mean height of the population of children from which the sample was drawn is a parameter. Note that a parameter is not a 'boundary' or 'limit', and this erroneous use of the word (which probably arises through confusion with 'perimeter') should be avoided. A sample statistic is a single value and is thus a *point estimate* of the corresponding population parameter. Additionally, an *interval estimate* can be calculated around the point estimate, this being a range of population values with which the data in the sample are compatible. These terms will be discussed more fully in Chapter 13.

generalization can be made is said to possess *external validity*.

In exploratory research, however, a different form of representativeness may be at stake. This may be referred to as *theoretical representativeness*. Here, a researcher may derive theoretical insights from a study which are sufficiently general or universal to be projected to other contexts or situations that are comparable to that of the original study, even though these may differ in empirical terms. The generalization made by the researcher from the original situation to those to which it is related is conceptual and theoretical, and is not based on empirical or statistical similarity (Sim, 1998). Indeed, cases or situations that are quite *dissimilar* may be usefully compared in this way. Moreover, the generalization that occurs is not from the sample as such, but from the concepts, issues and themes that are elicited through study of the sample. Generalization in this sense is a logical, not a statistical, process (Mitchell, 1983).

It should not be inferred from the above comments that samples generated in order to secure statistical representativeness are not theoretically representative. It is clearly important that the population from which a sample is drawn should be defined in such a way that the resulting findings will inform the theoretical framework of a study. It is probably true to say that any sampling strategy that aims at statistical representativeness will also thereby seek theoretical representativeness, whereas a strategy whose primary aim is theoretical representativeness may not be concerned with statistical representativeness. Methods of sampling which reflect these two forms of representativeness will be examined in Sections 8.3 and 8.4.

8.3 STRATEGIES FOR STATISTICAL REPRESENTATIVENESS

Most sampling strategies that aim to achieve statistical representativeness are forms of *probability* sampling. In probability sampling, the selection of individual sampling units is left to chance (a random process), rather than to the choice or judgement of the researcher (a non-random process). Hence, the probability of selection of a particular sampling unit is known and lies between, but does not include, 0 and 1. In a *non-probability* sample, the selection of units is under the researcher's control, and is therefore influenced by the researcher's subjective judgement (Henry, 1990). The probability of selection of a particular sampling unit may or may not be known, and if known is either 0 or 1.

8.3.1 Simple random sampling

In simple random sampling, units are sampled in such a way that each unit has a known, equal and non-zero chance of being selected. Draws must be independent; in other words, the selection of one unit must not influence the likelihood of another unit being selected (Smith, 1975).

Common methods of selecting a random sample include drawing numbered balls out of a box, consulting tables of random numbers, and using computer algorithms to generate numbers at random. In order for a random sample to be selected by any of these methods, the sampling frame must be exhaustive (i.e. it must include all members of the population), and all units in the sampling frame must be individually identified. It is only through identifying all sampling units and assigning a unique identifier to each of them that you can ensure that each unit has an equal chance of selection. Moreover, it is important that units are listed only once, since duplicate or multiple listing of some units will affect their probability of selection. This might occur if the current case records of an occupational therapy department were used as a sampling frame – some patients referred for unrelated problems by separate physicians might have more than one set of records. If this situation cannot be controlled, steps should be taken to remove any repeated units from the sample before analysis begins (Maisel and Persell, 1996).

Bork (1993, p. 210) states that in a random sample 'no particular attribute has any more chance of being represented than any other attribute'. This is not strictly accurate, because attributes that are more common in the study population are clearly more likely to be represented in the sample than rarer attributes. The point to be made is that in a random sample any particular attribute has the same chance as any other attribute of being represented at its correct value or proportion (i.e. that of the population). This does not *guarantee*, however, that the attributes of any particular random sample will correspond to those of the population from which it is drawn. Sample statistics will fluctuate from sample to sample owing to sampling error.

8.3.2 Systematic sampling with random start

Systematic sampling with random start (sometimes just referred to as 'systematic sampling') offers certain practical advantages over simple random sampling, especially with large study populations. In both cases an exhaustive sampling frame must be obtained, but in the case of systematic sampling, only the first sampling unit is chosen at random; subsequent units are selected at intervals (i.e. every nth unit after the first unit selected). The sampling interval can be determined simply by dividing the population by the size of the sample required. This process does not require each sampling unit to be given a unique identifier, which may save a considerable amount of time. Moreover, the sampling frame does not need to be in the form of a list, as long as the units that it contains become available sequentially.

Imagine, for example, drawing a simple random sample of 50 from a series of 2600 hospital case notes. Each of these would have to be listed and each set of notes given a number from 1 to 2600; a random sample would then be drawn using these numbers. If systematic sampling were to be used, a list would still be required, but there would be no need to assign individual numbers to each unit and the case notes could be accessed straight from the filing cabinets. First, the sampling interval would be calculated to the nearest whole number (2600/50 = 52). A random number between 1 and 52 would be chosen – let us say 27. Starting with the 27th set of notes, every 52nd subsequent set would be drawn from the filing cabinets until a total of 50 sets had been gathered.

Systematic sampling is an efficient means of drawing a random sample. However, it is important to ensure that the sampling units are not listed or arranged in such a way that they have a regular cycle or sequence. For example, suppose a psychiatric hospital operates 14 outpatient clinics per week, making an annual total of 728 (ignoring public holidays etc.). If a researcher attempted to draw a systematic sample with a sampling interval of 7, he or she would repeatedly sample a clinic at the same point in the week. Thus, if the first clinic chosen were the one run on Monday mornings, this would also be the one sampled on every second occasion subsequently. This clinic might be in some way atypical, and the resulting sample would therefore be biased. An additional possible shortcoming is that a systematic sample will tend not to draw two consecutive units; hence, such a sample drawn from an age–sex register of patients would not include both of any pairs of twins, since these would normally be listed consecutively.

8.3.3 Cluster sampling

Cluster sampling involves the sampling of successively smaller units. This is useful when either or both of the following apply: (1) the sampling frame cannot be identified; (2) direct contact needs to be made with sample units, but these are scattered around a wide geographical area (Haber, 1994). A number of clusters of sampling units are selected, and cases are sampled from each of these clusters. Alternatively, in multistage cluster sampling, further clusters may be drawn from each of the initial clusters, and units sampled from these. Initial clusters should be as heterogeneous as possible in their content, so as not to build in biased selection. Membership of clusters must be mutually exclusive (i.e. each unit must appear in only one cluster); otherwise the same sampling unit may be selected more than once.

This form of sampling is used in the Rheumatoid Arthritis Study. In order to select a sample of occupational therapists and physiotherapists with experience of musculoskeletal practice, Angela Carella first divided the regions in the UK into three groups: predominantly urban, predominantly rural, mixed urban and rural. Two regions were randomly selected from each of these categories and, within each of the selected regions, five hospitals were selected and a list was obtained of all the occupational therapists and physiotherapists working in musculoskeletal practice who were employed within each of these hospitals. These lists formed the sampling frame from which a random sample of 240 individual therapists was drawn (Figure 8.2).

The use of this strategy obviates the need to obtain an exhaustive list of all occupational therapists and physiotherapists in the UK, which would be a near-impossible task. Furthermore, because the required sampling frame in cluster sampling is much smaller than that required for a simple random sample, the researchers can probably afford the time to ensure that it is an accurate and inclusive sampling frame. It also means that if Angela Carella wishes to interview members of the study sample, she has to travel to a maximum of 30 hospitals in six regions of the country, whereas a simple random sample might well send her off to many more hospitals in all corners of the country. A disadvantage, however, is that because this is a multistage form of sampling, random or systematic sampling error is liable to be introduced at each stage, and this error is compounded in subsequent stages (see Section 8.5 for a discussion of the bias introduced by the use of this strategy in the Rheumatoid Arthritis Study). It is wise to maximize the number of initial clusters, so as not to build too much bias in at the beginning (which would be carried on into subsequent clusters). You should not sample too many initial clusters, however,

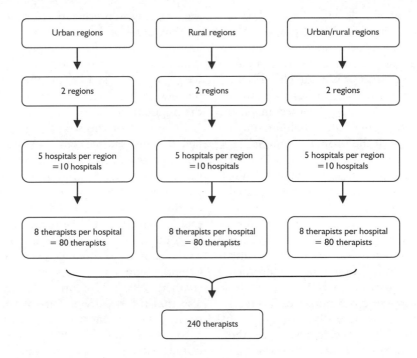

Figure 8.2 *Cluster sampling strategy employed in the Rheumatoid Arthritis Study.*

since this would mean a lot of travelling and would thus offset one of the principal advantages of cluster sampling .

In the Rheumatoid Arthritis Study, the consecutive selection of regions, hospitals and therapists is random in each case, and the resulting sample is therefore random. In some cases, however, the initial clusters may be selected non-randomly, on the basis of the researcher's judgement. In such a situation, the resulting sample would therefore be only semi-random. A further drawback of cluster sampling may arise if clusters are sampled too intensively. If a large number of individuals are selected from a given location, their proximity may mean that they share certain attitudes, beliefs and practices. Data from these individuals would therefore not be wholly independent, which would have implications for statistical analysis (Section 13.1.3). Accordingly, the number of clusters should be large enough to ensure that individual clusters are not sampled too intensively.

8.3.4 Stratified random sampling

Another variation on simple random sampling is stratified random sampling. This is where the population is divided into homogeneous subsets (*strata*) and units are then randomly sampled from each of these strata. Why might this be useful? Suppose a researcher wishes to draw a random sample of 100 nurses licensed in New Jersey, in order to gauge their opinion on a certain issue to do with the proposed rationalization of acute health care reimbursement. It would probably be important for such a study that the views of nurses at the highest managerial grade were represented, but because these are relatively few in number, a simple random sample might miss them altogether. However, if the investigator divided the population into strata based on seniority, individuals could then be randomly sampled from each of these, eliminating the risk of missing out nurses of a certain grade. In order that a numerically small grade of nurse would not be overrepresented, the researcher could sample from each subset in proportion to the composition of the population

(i.e. more junior grade nurses would be sampled than senior nurses). This form of proportionate sampling would preserve the relative representation of the various grades of nurse in the study population, and help to ensure that the attitude profile to emerge from the sample was representative of the study population.

In some cases, however, it may be preferable to conduct disproportionate stratified random sampling. This might arise if the purpose of the study were to conduct a comparison between two groups of individuals who are present in very different proportions (e.g. if the population consisted of 80% females and 20% males). If a proportionate stratified random sample were drawn, the attitude scores of those in the smaller group, the males, would be subject to a greater degree of sampling imprecision (see Section 8.5.1). Moreover, the power of any statistical test comparing males with females would quite likely be reduced by the disparity in group sizes (Campbell *et al.*, 1995; see Section 18.6). Accordingly, it would make more sense to sample males and females equally, even though their relative representation in the study population would not be preserved. Moreover, if an attitude profile of the sample as a whole were also required, this could still be achieved by weighting the scores of the males and the females in proportion to their representation in the population.

In respect of the stratifying variable, a stratified random sample will usually be more representative than a simple random sample, since it recognizes between-stratum variation and incorporates it in the sampling procedure. In contrast to the clusters generated in cluster sampling, each of which should be relatively heterogeneous in content, in stratified random sampling the strata should be homogeneous in content, but heterogeneous with respect to one another (Barnett, 1991; Trinkoff and Storr, 1997). Note also that the stratifying variable must be theoretically relevant. Most often, this means selecting a stratifying variable that is likely to be associated with the outcome variable of interest. Hence, in the example of nurses in New Jersey, it would probably not be appropriate to stratify by county of birth or even place of primary nurse education, since these variables are less likely to be related to attitudes to health care reimbursement than variables such as seniority or specialty.

8.3.5 Quota sampling

Quota sampling is an example of a non-probability sampling strategy that seeks to attain statistical representativeness. Sampling units are chosen not by a random process, but in terms of their fulfilment of specific quotas. As the following example will illustrate, this method has a number of practical advantages over probability sampling strategies.

Suppose an occupational therapy department were interested in conducting regular surveys of its clients' views on the quality of the service offered, in a quick and inexpensive manner. In order to achieve this goal, the departmental staff

decide to draw a quota sample of 50 clients. First of all, they consider in what respects it is important to achieve representativeness of their total client population, and decide that clients' age, sex and whether they receive therapy on an outpatient (ambulatory) or in-patient (hospital) basis are relevant factors (these variables become the *quota controls*). From their knowledge of their total caseload, they know that 55% of their clients are women; that 60% of their clients are aged 60 or over; and that 65% are treated on an in-patient basis. On the basis of this information, they are able to calculate the composition of the sample required to achieve representativeness in terms of the selected quota controls.

Each of the boxes in the final row in Figure 8.3 is a *quota* and each quota is given a *quota specification* in terms of the quota controls. The task that faces the department in order to obtain a representative sample is to fill each of these

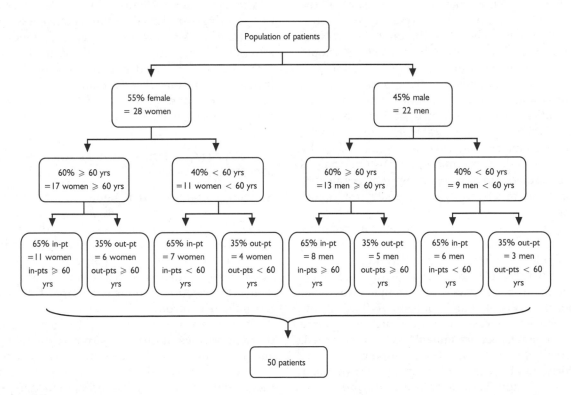

Figure 8.3 *A quota sampling strategy.*

quotas. This is done simply by approaching any clients attending the department and determining whether they satisfy any one of the quota specifications; if so, they are asked to participate. Once a quota is full – e.g. once seven female in-patients under the age of 60 have provided their views – no further clients satisfying this quota specification are approached.

The primary advantage of quota sampling is that although it is necessary to know the values of the quota controls in the study population, no sampling frame is required, since clients are approached on an opportunistic basis. Additionally, the researchers do not have to make contact with named individuals selected in advance, who might be quite difficult and time consuming to track down, but can enlist any available individual who satisfies the specification of an unfilled quota.

Against these practical advantages of quota sampling, there are a number of methodological drawbacks. The chief of these is that the resulting sample is only representative in terms of the variables chosen as the quota controls (of which it is usually only practicable to choose three or four), and may therefore be atypical of the study population in other respects (Abramson, 1990). In addition, the fact that individuals are not selected at random means that usual statistical estimates of sampling error cannot be calculated (de Vaus, 1991). By the same token, methods of statistical analysis that assume random selection (i.e. parametric statistical tests) are inappropriate for quota samples.

A further disadvantage of quota sampling relates to the way in which the researcher enlists respondents. There is a tendency to approach individuals who look as though they are likely to agree to participate – for example, those who appear to be polite and cooperative (Fife-Schaw, 1995a) – whereas those who present a more forbidding aspect are unlikely to be approached. Hence, the problem of non-response may be addressed at the cost of sampling bias (Barnett, 1991; Section 8.5). Moreover, the process of quota sampling makes it difficult for the principal researcher to monitor and control such problems during data collection (Moser and Kalton, 1971). It should also be borne in mind that some potential members of a quota are less likely than others to be available for an approach by the researcher. In the present example, outpatients who attend the department by means of their own transport are, perhaps, likely to spend less time in the department than those who are waiting for transportation, who may spend some time waiting both before and after their appointment. The opportunities for approaching the latter category of client are likely to be more numerous. There is also a tendency for cases close to quota boundaries to be undersampled; Arber (1993) points out that interviewers may not approach individuals at the extremes of an age category because they erroneously perceive them to belong to an adjacent category, or because they are wary of causing offence.

The legitimacy of quota sampling as a means of securing statistical representativeness is contentious. Although the lack of random selection is open to criticism, there are studies that have demonstrated that quota samples can in some circumstances achieve levels of representativeness comparable to that of more 'rigorous' approaches (Sudman, 1966).

8.4 STRATEGIES FOR THEORETICAL REPRESENTATIVENESS

Sampling strategies that aim for theoretical representativeness are sometimes referred to as *purposive*. This term reflects the fact that units are deliberately chosen for the sample in order to fulfil the researcher's particular purpose, rather than on the basis of a chance process in which the selection of units is removed from the researcher's control.

There is a very wide variety of terms used to describe various forms of purposive sampling, and these may be classified in different ways (Coyne, 1997). For the sake of clarity, most of these forms of sampling will be subsumed under the first of the two following categories.

8.4.1 Judgemental sampling

'Judgemental sampling' is a broad term, describing any method of sampling that is based on the researcher's judgement as to those units that will be relevant to the aims and objectives of a study. Assuming that the units in question are people, they might be included in a judgemental sample because they exhibit one or more of the following characteristics:

- They possess the necessary knowledge (e.g. a study of the development of theories and models of nursing might select academic nurses and nurse educationalists, on the basis that such individuals might be expected to be particularly well informed on this topic).
- They have had relevant experience (e.g. a study of clinical decision making in acute psychiatric occupational therapy would probably target those therapists with extensive clinical experience in this area).
- They are part of a social structure or process on which the research is intended to focus (e.g. in order to examine the interplay and conflict between clinical and managerial values in nursing, a study might sample nurses whose professional and/or institutional role places them at the intersection of these values, and therefore exposes them directly to these phenomena).

It might be asked, why doesn't the researcher simply draw a statistically representative sample of individuals who fulfil the above characteristics? There are a number of reasons why not:

- It might not be possible to construct a sampling frame from which some form of random or semi-random sample could be drawn (e.g. it might be difficult to identify cases in advance of entering the field to collect data).
- The individuals concerned might be very rare or hard to trace, restricting or eliminating the possibility of a sample large enough to be statistically representative.

- Similarly, the in-depth nature of the investigation might make it impossible to focus on more than a few cases in the time and resources available for the study.
- Statistical generalization might simply not be among the purposes of the study, thus making statistical representativeness redundant (see Section 5.3 for further discussion of this issue).

Judgemental sampling exhibits a number of features that serve to contrast it with the approach generally employed when gathering statistically representative samples. First, the sample may be recruited in parallel with the process of data collection, rather than before. An example of this is the process known as *snowball sampling* (also referred to as *chain referral sampling*). This method is often employed when sampling groups who are by their nature difficult to identify and locate. A researcher who wished to study the health beliefs of a stigmatized or 'deviant' group, such as substance abusers, would find it hard to identify such individuals in advance. Rather, he or she would probably attempt to make contact with one such individual and, during the process of collecting data, seek the names of other potential contacts known to this individual. The researcher would then make contact with these nominated people, and seek further referrals from them. In this way, a sample would be gathered in parallel with the process of data collection by a form of networking.

Second, not only may the process of sampling occur alongside data collection, but the rationale for sampling may also be determined in a similar way. In some inductive approaches to research involving qualitative data, such as grounded theory (see Section 11.1.1), there is constant interplay between data, theory and method. Data are analysed as they are collected, and modifications are made to the theory being developed in the light of this analysis. This, in turn, dictates the way in which subsequent data should be gathered, including the choice of future informants.

Third, the cases sampled may not necessarily be 'typical'. Certain phenomena may be particularly well illustrated by extreme or unusual cases (Sharp, 1998). Thus, a study into the subjective meaning and experience of limitation of mobility might deliberately focus on individuals with severe limitation – even though most disabled people are probably only moderately limited – on the basis that these extreme cases are likely to exemplify the relevant issues most vividly. Similarly, a researcher seeking to understand a professional culture in an area of health care might target practitioners who in some way fail to fit in with this culture, in the hope that such individuals might provide a particularly meaningful insight into the norms and values of this culture. In such cases, the requirement of strict representativeness is subordinated to that of obtaining meaningful and insightful data. In relation to studies such as these, Morse comments:

> *When we begin sampling, we are not interested in the 'average' response because we do not know the characteristics of the phenomenon and must first identify these. These characteristics are easier to identify in participants where these characteristics are most evident.*

> (Morse, 1998b, p. 734)

Individuals who are selected for study in judgemental sampling – particularly when unstructured interviews are used – are often referred to as *key informants* (Gilchrist, 1992) to underline the fact that they possess a high degree of insight, knowledge or experience relevant to the topic of the study.

8.4.2 Convenience sampling

Convenience sampling is just what its name suggests: the drawing of a sample in terms of the ready availability of sampling units. Frequently, constraints of time and resources may dictate that a convenience sample is used. This is often the case in student research projects, but also occurs in larger-scale studies. In many clinical trials, the study sample is drawn from those patients who happen to be attending the clinic or hospital at which the trial is based, not from a complete list of such patients.

Careful thought must be given to whether or not a convenience sample is theoretically representative. The manner in which this sort of sample is selected does not guarantee that it will be theoretically representative, but nor does it guarantee that it will not. Provided that individuals are not sampled *only* on the basis of their ready availability, a convenience sample may attain the sort of theoretical representativeness of a judgemental sample (as in the Student Attitudes Study; see Section 5.3).

A similar question arises with regard to the statistical representativeness of convenience samples. Again, the process of convenience sampling does nothing to guarantee this. Often, however, a fairly good judgement can be made as to the likely generalizability of a convenience sample. A study carried out on attitudes to mental illness among people in one state of the USA might not be readily generalized to the US population as a whole, since one would expect considerable variation in social and cultural attitudes and beliefs between, say, Maine and South Carolina. In contrast, a study of nerve conduction velocity might be expected to be generalizable across states and even countries; quite reasonably, we don't expect the physiological processes of individuals to differ as greatly as their attitudes. Payton (1994) points out that when convenience samples are used it is important to describe the characteristics of the sample clearly and in detail, so that others can make a judgement as to its external validity.

Many convenience samples are composed of volunteers, rather than individuals whom the researcher has specifically approached for inclusion in the study. This can introduce quite a serious self-selection bias (Portney and Watkins, 1993).

8.5 SAMPLING ERROR

When statistical representativeness is at issue, it is important to consider sampling precision (see

Box 8.2). No matter how a sample is drawn from a population, its characteristics will hardly ever match those of the population exactly. *Sampling error* is the degree to which the sample differs from the population (i.e. the extent to which it is unrepresentative), and it can be *random* or *systematic*.

Box 8.2 *Error and precision*

The extent to which a sample is statistically representative of a population can be expressed in terms of either *random sampling error* or *sample precision*. These are inversely related, so that the greater the precision of a sample, the less the random sampling error associated with it, and vice versa. It is probably easier to talk in terms of what one is trying to achieve (sample precision) than in terms of what one is trying to avoid (sampling error). If a sample is described as being precise, this is really shorthand for saying that it yields precise estimates of specific population parameters. It does not strictly mean that the sample *per se* is precise, since the various statistics obtainable from it may have varying degrees of precision as parameter estimates. Note that there is no set level of desirable sampling precision; how precise the sample needs to be depends upon the requirements of the particular study in question.

In systematic sampling error there is a particular pattern or trend to the dissimilarity between sample and population, owing to the fact that the chosen method of sampling favours particular sampling units over others. Hence, if a researcher consciously or subconsciously selected subjects for a study who were from a social class or ethnic background similar to his or her own (assuming that the target population is of a more varied class or ethnic composition), there would be systematic error; the sample is *biased*. Different samples selected in such a manner will be similarly biased. An element of bias has inadvertently been built into the sample for the Rheuma-

toid Arthritis Study. As was indicated in Section 6.4, the target population was physiotherapists and occupational therapists in the UK. However, since only hospitals are included in the third stage of clusters (Figure 8.2), this serves to exclude all therapists who work outside the hospital setting (e.g. in independent practice). If the mode of practice of these therapists is likely to differ from that of hospital-based therapists, the sample will be biased.

In random sampling error, dissimilarity between sample and population occurs by chance. Random sampling error is thus the fluctuation of sample statistics around the population parameters which results from the random selection process (Henry, 1990). Despite its name, it does not usually result from any sort of 'error' (i.e. mistake) on the part of the researcher (Cohen and Manion, 1994). A large random sampling error gives rise to an *imprecise* sample, but not necessarily to a biased sample (Table 8.1).

Thus, how representative a sample is depends upon the extent to which it is both precise (free from random sampling error) and unbiased (free from systematic sampling error).

8.5.1 Increasing sampling precision

There are three main factors that will serve to increase sampling precision (i.e. reduce random sampling error).

The nature of the population sampled

The more homogeneous a population, the smaller the sample required in order to secure a

Table 8.1 *The effect of random and systematic error on sample estimates (a sample that is both precise and unbiased is sometimes described as being 'accurate')*

| | | Random error | |
		High	Low
Systematic error	Present	Imprecise and biased	Precise and biased
	Absent	Imprecise and unbiased	Precise and unbiased ('accurate')

given level of precision. This becomes clear if you consider extreme cases. If every unit in the population were absolutely identical (which hardly ever happens, of course), you would need only a sample of one to get a representative sample. In contrast, if sampling units differed greatly from one another, it would need a much larger sample to capture this variability. It should be noted that the *proportion* of the population that is sampled (the sampling fraction) is not normally an important consideration in determining sampling precision. When dealing with a fairly large population, the absolute sample size, not the sampling fraction, is what matters most. The sampling fraction plays an important role in determining sampling precision only when the population size is fairly small – in other words when the sample represents a high proportion (more than about 5%) of the population (see Section 18.6.1; Moser and Kalton, 1971).

The size of the sample drawn
The larger the sample, the greater its precision. However, for many statistics, e.g. the mean, precision is related to the square root of sample size; i.e. in order to double sampling precision, you need to quadruple sample size. This means that there comes a point at which the gains in precision from increases in sample size begin to tail off. In contrast, although there are some economies of scale to be made, the cost of an increasingly larger sample tends to rise in a fairly linear fashion (Hoinville *et al.*, 1978). Specific calculations can be carried out to determine the size of sample required to estimate a parameter with a given degree of precision, or to reject a null hypothesis with a given level of probability. This topic will be examined in Section 18.6.

The method of sampling employed
Some methods of sampling are more effective in obtaining a precise sample than others. These were considered in detail in Section 8.3.

8.6 CONCLUSION

Sampling is an important stage in the conduct of almost any study in health care research. This chapter has outlined a number of different sampling procedures that permit statistical and/or theoretical generalization. Which of these two forms of representativeness is paramount will depend upon the nature of the research question and the theoretical perspective that informs it.

The issue of sample size has been touched upon in this chapter in relation to sampling precision. Further discussion of the question of sample size in studies dealing with qualitative and quantitative data can be found in Sections 5.3 and 18.6, respectively.

9 VALIDITY, RELIABILITY AND ALLIED CONCEPTS

SUMMARY

This chapter explores the following topics:

- the definitions of validity and reliability as applied to data
- the principal forms of validity – face validity, content validity, criterion-related validity and construct validity
- the sensitivity and specificity of diagnostic tests
- the principal forms of reliability – equivalence, stability and internal consistency
- the meaning of validity and reliability in relation to qualitative data
- responsiveness of quantitative measures
- the role of triangulation in relation to validity and reliability

This chapter will address issues relating to the desirable characteristics of data gathered in the course of empirical research. This is an important issue in each of the approaches to research discussed in Chapters 5–7. Particular attention will be given to the concepts of validity and reliability, and the way in which these should be distinguished. Statistical aspects of these issues will be covered in Sections 14.1.2 and 18.3.

9.1 FUNDAMENTAL DEFINITIONS

Broadly, data are said to be valid when they represent what they purport to represent, and meaningful inferences can therefore be drawn from them (Sim and Arnell, 1993). In contrast, if data are reliable this means that they are reproducible or consistent; i.e. data gathered on a particular entity will be the same when gathered by different investigators, or by the same investigator on separate occasions.

It should be noted that the concepts of validity and reliability have a different emphasis, and to some extent a difference in meaning, when applied to quantitative and qualitative data. This will be explored in more detail in due course.

9.1.1 Distinguishing validity and reliability

The definitions of *validity* and *reliability* given above are very broad ones. It is useful to distinguish between these two concepts in more detail, since they are prone to some degree of confusion. The easiest way to draw the relevant distinctions is probably in terms of an analogy. The analogy to be used is that of target shooting; the target represents the entity of interest and the shots represent the individual datapoints (i.e. measurements or observations).

If target A is examined in Figure 9.1, it is apparent that the shots are highly consistent, and thus reliable. In target B, by contrast, the shots are far less consistent, and thus less reliable. The shots on target C are as consistent as those on A, and thus similarly reliable. The difference between targets A and C, however, is that the shots on C are centred around the bull's eye, whereas those on A are towards the edge of the target: the shots on target C are therefore the more valid of the two sets.

If targets A and B are compared, it can be seen that the mean distance from the bull's eye of the shots on target B is less than that of the shots on target A (only one shot lies outside the fourth concentric ring in target B, whereas six do so in target A). Hence, although the shots on target B are less reliable than those on target A, they are more valid. Thus, target A displays scores that are reliable but not very valid, whereas target B displays shots that are moderately valid but not reliable. In each case, a different form of error is responsible for the shortfall. The poor validity shown by target A is

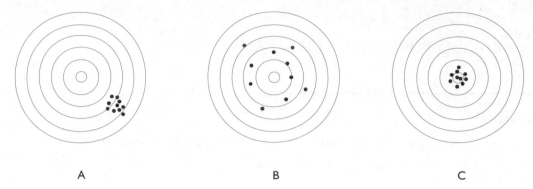

| A | B | C |

Figure 9.1   *Target-shooting analogy for validity and reliability.*

attributable to *systematic error*, or *bias*, whereas the poor reliability illustrated by target B is attributable to *random error*. Systematic error is consistent and occurs in one direction, causing the true value of an entity to be either overestimated or underestimated. Random error is inconsistent and occurs in all directions, causing the true value of the entity to be variously overestimated and underestimated (Portney and Watkins, 1993). When systematic error is known to be present, the location of a particular score on the range of its possible values may be fairly predictable, whereas the location of a score tends to be unpredictable in the presence of random error.

If targets B and C are now compared, it is evident that although the scores on target B are moderately valid, those on C are highly valid. The factor that makes the scores on C more valid than those on B is their increased reliability. This underlines a crucially important point: a high degree of validity presupposes a high degree of reliability (Wood-Dauphinee and Williams, 1989). The converse, however, does not hold: reliability does *not* presuppose validity. This can be demonstrated if one imagines that the scores on target A were all moved some distance off the target, while retaining their spatial relationship to one another (Figure 9.2). The reliability of these scores has not changed, but their validity has decreased drastically. Indeed, establishing the reliability of these shots does not require any

knowledge of where the target is: reliability is determined solely by the consistency of the shots, not by their relationship to the target. In contrast, we can assess validity only if we know where the bull's eye is (i.e. if we know the true nature or magnitude of the entity on which we are seeking to gather data).

Given that a high degree of validity presupposes a high degree of reliability, it follows that anything that undermines the reliability of data will also detract from their validity. As random error undermines reliability, it will have a further effect on validity. Consequently, the earlier statement that systematic error creates problems for validity must be elaborated slightly: although systematic error is the

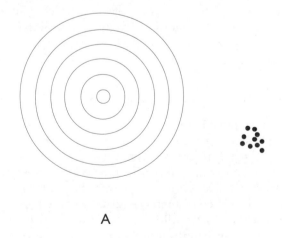

| A |

Figure 9.2   *Reliability does not presuppose validity.*

principal threat to validity, random error is also a problem (Sim and Arnell, 1993).

There is also a difference in the effect of a lack of either validity or reliability. Imagine that targets A and B were not visible, but the shots remained. Because they are reliable, the shots on target A indicate a specific, circumscribed area, which one might take to correspond to the bull's eye. However, the true position of the bull's eye is to the left and upwards. The systematic error associated with these shots gives a *distorted* indication of the true position of the bull's eye. Conversely, in target B the random error associated with these shots provides little indication of where the bull's eye might be; the impression given of its location is an *indistinct* one, rather than a distorted one. Consequently, invalidity may lead the researcher to draw a clear but erroneous conclusion from a set of data, whereas unreliable data often prevent the researcher from drawing any clear conclusions at all (Sim and Arnell, 1993).

As a final point of contrast, it should be noted that whereas data *per se* can be described as reliable, it is not strictly accurate to refer to data as valid. This is because data are only valid for a particular purpose in a particular context (Rothstein, 1993a). For example, temperature readings taken within a room might be a valid indication of the heat of the air within that room, but might not be a valid indication of the comfort felt by its inhabitants. There are other aspects of comfort than how warm one feels, and different people will have different preferences as to how warm a room should be. Hence, it is the inferences drawn from data that are valid or invalid, rather than the data themselves. Carmines and Zeller (1994, p. 4) contend that 'strictly speaking, one does not assess the validity of an indicator but rather the use to which it is being put'.

It follows from this that if the validity of a measure has been established in a particular context or population, this cannot necessarily be transferred to another context or population. For example, the Medical Outcomes Study Short Form 36 (SF-36) quality-of-life questionnaire (Stewart and Ware, 1992) has been translated into a number of languages, and revalidated in each case (e.g. Bullinger, 1995; Sullivan *et al.*, 1995; Aaronson *et al.*, 1998). Streiner and Norman (1995) discuss some of the practical and methodological problems of translating and validating health measurement scales.

The chief differences between validity and reliability are summarized in Table 9.1.

9.2 FORMS OF VALIDITY

There are four main forms of validity; these, with their subtypes, are shown in Figure 9.3.

9.2.1 Face validity

Face validity is concerned with the extent to

Table 9.1 *Points of comparison between validity and reliability*

Validity	Reliability
• Relates to the 'truthfulness' of data	• Relates to the consistency or reproducibility of data
• Is a property of inferences drawn from data	• Is a property of data themselves
• Exists in relation to a specific context and inferential purpose	• Is not related to the context or purpose of data collection (though this may determine the degree of reliability that is considered acceptable)
• Requires independent knowledge of the true nature or magnitude of the entity	• Requires no knowledge of the true nature or magnitude of the entity
• Presupposes at least a moderate degree of reliability	• Does not presuppose validity
• Is undermined chiefly by systematic error	• Is undermined by random error
• When lacking, leads to distorted inferences (bias)	• When lacking, leads to indistinct inferences

125

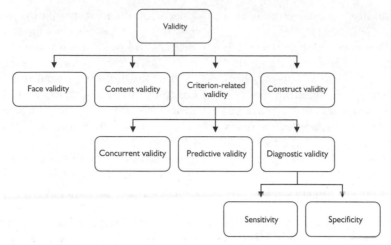

Figure 9.3 *Types of validity.*

which data appear to be valid, in the eyes of either the researcher or the subject (Rothstein, 1985). It is chiefly the latter for whom this is an important issue. For example, respondents should be able to relate the content of a questionnaire to the purpose it is supposed to fulfil. If not, they are liable to be poorly motivated to respond to the questionnaire, or to do so in an incomplete or half-hearted manner. Face validity is therefore a matter of the credibility of the process of data collection, and does not relate to the formal psychometric properties of an instrument (Kazdin, 1992).

9.2.2 Content validity

Content validity is concerned with the scope of a tool: the extent to which it taps the full *domain of content* of a concept or phenomenon. This is particularly important when dealing with multidimensional constructs. To have content validity, any instrument designed to measure such a construct must tap each of its constituent dimensions (Zeller and Carmines, 1980). Thus, to measure the overall experience of pain, it may be necessary to address the sensory, affective, evaluative, cognitive and behavioural dimensions of pain (Sim and Waterfield, 1997).

On occasions, determining the domain of content of a particular construct may be a complex business. Table 9.2 shows how, on one interpretation (Ferrans, 1990), the concept of quality of life can be broken down into four domains, and then into elements within each domain. In principle, any instrument designed to measure quality of life must address each of these domains and each of their constituent elements – or at least all of those relevant to the research question concerned. Determining content validity is thus a question of examining the conceptual and theoretical background against which a research question has been generated. It should be done before an instrument is constructed (Nunnally and Bernstein, 1994).

9.2.3 Criterion-related validity

Three forms of criterion-related validity can be identified: concurrent, predictive and diagnostic.

Concurrent validity

Concurrent validity is established by comparing the performance of a measuring instrument against an independent standard, in respect of the same entity at the same time (Polit and Hungler, 1995; LoBiondo-Wood and Haber, 1994). The independent standard, or criterion, is usually another instrument of accepted validity.

Table 9.2 *The global construct of quality of life, with its major domains and specific aspects, as conceptualized by Ferrans (1990)*

Quality of life			
Health and functioning domain	**Socioeconomic domain**	**Psychological/spiritual domain**	**Family domain**
Usefulness to others	Standard of living	Life satisfaction	Family happiness
Physical independence	Financial independence	Happiness	Children
Responsibilities	Home	Self	Spouse
Own health	Job/unemployment	Goals	Family health
Stress	Neighbourhood	Peace of mind	
Leisure activities	Condition in USA	Personal appearance	
Retirement	Friends	Faith in God	
Travel	Emotional support	Control over life	
Long life	Education		
Sex life	Influence in government		
Health care			
Discomfort/pain			

If the new instrument produces data that agree with those from the criterion measure, when applied to the same entity, it is deemed to be a valid measure. For example, Feldman *et al.* (1990) established the criterion-related validity of the Pediatric Evaluation of Disability Inventory by comparing its scores with those from the previously validated Battelle Developmental Inventory Screening Test, generated from the same sample of children. Similarly, in the Low Back Pain Study, Dr Buckley utilized the Aberdeen Back Pain Scale. This instrument was validated by Ruta *et al.* (1994) by comparing its performance with that of an established measure of health status, the Medical Outcomes Study Short Form-36 (SF-36) (Ware and Sherbourne, 1992).

If the criterion measure is taken to be the best available in terms of validity, and such a measure is available, it might seem strange that a researcher is seeking to introduce an alternative measure that cannot, by definition, be more valid than the criterion measure. However, the new measure will usually have other advantages over existing measures; it may be shorter or easier to use, it may be less hazardous for the subject, it may require less training in its use, or it may involve the use of simpler and more portable equipment (Diers, 1979; Streiner and Norman, 1995).

When dealing with qualitative data, concurrent validity usually takes a rather different form. These data are not measurements, but are usually in narrative or textual form. It is therefore not appropriate to evaluate such data against some type of scale or inventory as the criterion. Instead, use is often made of expert judges. For example, Hinds *et al.* (1990) wished to validate data relating to the cognitive and affective dimensions of the healing process. They achieved this by having their findings reviewed by a panel of experts who were selected for their 'theoretical sensitivity to the studied phenomena' (Hinds *et al.*, 1990, p. 432). This approach does have its problems, however. First, there is the practical problem of making the data available to a third party in a form that is conducive to meaningful analysis. If interviews or observations have been recorded by hand, rather than audiotaped or videotaped (see Sections 10.1.1 and 10.1.2), this may be only partially achievable. A second difficulty is identified by Sandelowski (1998). She asks,

are experts, no matter how impressive their credentials, in any position to certify as valid the findings – descriptions, categories, theories, or meanings – in studies in which they played no part?

(Sandelowski, 1998, p. 467)

An alternative criterion when dealing with qualitative data can be provided by the research participants themselves. They are asked to check the findings to ensure they are accurate and that they have not been misinterpreted, in a process known as *member validation* (Silverman, 1985) or *respondent validation* (Hammersley and Atkinson, 1995). Teresa Ganz employed this technique in the Student Attitudes Study. Once she had completed her interviews and her observations, Dr Ganz talked her findings though with a subsample of the students involved in the study to see if they would endorse them as accurate.

There are a few potential limitations to respondent validation. In the first instance, a decision must be made as to whether its purpose is to check interview transcripts and the like for their accuracy, as Teresa Ganz did, or to pass judgements on the researcher's analytical interpretations; a rather different matter. If the latter is intended, an assumption has to be made that these interpretations are accessible to the participant. If an analytical account is framed principally in researcher-generated concepts, and therefore at a moderately high degree of theoretical abstraction (see Section 11.3), it may not make much sense to the participant. In addition, Morse (1998a) points out that the researcher's analysis is likely to be based on bringing together the perspectives of a number of participants. She argues that it is not necessarily the case that this synthesis of perspectives will – or indeed should – correspond recognizably to that of an individual participant.

Another reason why one might not expect the participant to be able to judge the researcher's analysis is that it may deal with issues of which the participant was unaware. It may, for example, impute certain unconscious motives to the participant or draw inferences from certain non-verbal behaviour of which he or she was unaware. Alternatively, the participant may simply have forgotten what he or she was saying or doing at the time of data collection (Hammersley and Atkinson, 1995). Even if there are no difficulties of recall, there is then a potential problem of retrospective censoring. This is particularly likely to be a problem in a study dealing with potentially sensitive issues, such as those addressed by Teresa Ganz in her study, or in a study where participants may have a vested interest, as might be the case when studying certain managerial issues in health care or those connected with professional politics or professional relationships (Hugman, 1991; Hewison, 1995).

Finally, Burman (1994a) points out that the meaning of apparent confirmation or disconfirmation in the process of respondent validation will depend on the perspective from which the study is being conducted. Within a postmodernist perspective – which emphasizes the diversity, multiplicity and relativity of viewpoints (Grbich, 1999) – the fact that researcher and participant had very different interpretations of an interview would be seen as perfectly normal, whereas it might be problematic from a phenomenological perspective.

Predictive validity

Sometimes, a test or measurement has a predictive function. For example, an aptitude test may be designed to determine who should fulfil certain roles within an institution, a psychological profile may be administered to select patients who would benefit from a particular form of pain management programme, a battery of functional tests may be employed to establish whether a patient is ready for discharge, or a fitness screening protocol may be used to select applicants for a physically demanding job. In cases such as these, the validity of a test can best be determined by seeing whether the future course of events is in line with predictions generated by these tests. Hence, predictive validity will have been achieved if patients who, on the basis of a psychological profile, are classified as highly suitable for a specific pain management programme proceed to achieve good results on this programme, whereas those classified as less suitable fare correspondingly worse. Where predictive validity is used to assign treatment interventions, it is sometimes referred to as *prescriptive validity*. This is said to exist when 'the inferred interpretation of a measurement is the determination of the form of treatment a person is to receive ... [and is] justified based on the successful outcome of the chosen treatment' (Task Force on Standards for Measurement in Physical Therapy, 1991, p. 597).

Diagnostic validity

In epidemiological research, the validity of a diagnostic test is frequently at issue. Here, two specific terms are employed. The *sensitivity* of a test is the extent to which it identifies those patients who do in fact have this disease (i.e. true positives), whereas the *specificity* of a test is the extent to which it fails to pick up those without the disease (i.e. true negatives). These can be calculated according to the following formulae (Farmer and Miller, 1991):

$$\text{sensitivity} = \frac{\text{true positives}}{\text{true positives} + \text{false negatives}}$$

$$\text{specificity} = \frac{\text{true negatives}}{\text{true negatives} + \text{false positives}}$$

A test with high sensitivity serves to rule *out* the diagnosis, whereas one with high specificity rules *in* (i.e. tends to confirm) the diagnosis (Sackett *et al.*, 2000). For example, the Beck Depression Inventory (Beck *et al.*, 1961) is an instrument widely used to screen for depression; i.e. to distinguish patients with depression from those who have another form of psychiatric distress or who are symptomatically normal. If this instrument has high sensitivity when used on a certain population, a *negative* result rules out the diagnosis of depression with a corresponding degree of certainty. If it has high specificity, a *positive* result will establish the presence of depression with a corresponding degree of certainty. With respect to *rival* diagnoses, such as anxiety or neuroticism, it is the specificity of

the test that eliminates these as possibilities (i.e. rules them out).

A test may also be described as having *positive predictive value* or *negative predictive value*. These concepts are related to sensitivity and specificity. However, whereas sensitivity and specificity are constant for any prevalence of a disease, positive predictive value and negative predictive value are a function of prevalence (Box 9.1). Thus, a test with a given sensitivity and specificity will have a higher positive predictive value in a population with a high prevalence than in one with a low prevalence (Gray, 1997; Greenhalgh, 1997). The probability that a person will test positive on the test is therefore conditional upon the prevalence of the disease (Section 13.1.3).

Sensitivity and specificity are usually in an inverse relationship. As attempts are made to increase the sensitivity of a test, this will tend to reduce its specificity, and vice versa (Streiner and Geddes, 1998).

9.2.4 Construct validity

Construct validity is a complex notion that does not lend itself to a straightforward definition (Silva, 1993). Essentially, however, it is a means of validation that relies on the theoretical context in which a test or measure is utilized. Vogt (1999, p. 53) defines it as follows:

> *In practice, construct validity is used to describe a scale, index or other measure of a variable that correlates with measures of other variables in ways that are predicted by, or make sense according to, a theory of how the variables are related.*

Thus, if it is accepted on the basis of theory that a certain relationship should exist between two constructs, data derived from two instruments that purport to measure these constructs should exhibit the same relationship at an empirical level (Zeller and Carmines, 1980). Sim and Arnell (1993) give the example of a questionnaire designed to measure a client's adjustment to physical disability. Certain theoretical relationships might be posited between adjust-

Box 9.1 *Sensitivity, specificity and prevalence*

The role of prevalence in determining the predictive value of a test can be illustrated by considering the formula for positive predictive value (PV+):

$$PV+ = \frac{prevalence \times sensitivity}{(prevalence \times sensitivity) + ([1 - prevalence] \times [1 - specificity])}$$

Assume that in a population of 1000, the prevalence of a disease is 20%, and that a test has a sensitivity of 90% and a specificity of 85%. Under these circumstances, PV+ will be:

$$PV+ = \frac{0.2 \times 0.9}{(0.2 \times 0.9) + ([1 - 0.2] \times [1 - 0.85])} = \frac{0.2 \times 0.9}{(0.2 \times 0.9) + (0.8 \times 0.15)} = 60\%$$

In contrast, for the same sensitivity and specificity, but a population prevalence of 5%,

$$PV+ = \frac{0.05 \times 0.9}{(0.05 \times 0.9) + ([1 - 0.05] \times [1 - 0.85])} = \frac{0.05 \times 0.9}{(0.05 \ 0.9) + (0.95 \times 0.15)} = 24\%$$

The negative predictive value (PV−) of the test is also affected, but a change in prevalence has the opposite effect, and is less dramatic in this case. The formula for PV− is:

$$PV- = \frac{(1 - prevalence) \times specificity}{([1 - prevalence] \times specificity) + (prevalence \times [1 - sensitivity])}$$

From this it can be calculated that a test with 90% sensitivity and 85% specificity would have a PV− of 97% for a prevalence of 20% and a PV− of 99% for a prevalence of 5%.

ment and other constructs. For example, it might be argued that adjustment would be directly related to concepts such as self-efficacy, self-esteem, optimism and an internal locus of control. Conversely, adjustment might be inversely related to social isolation, depressive symptoms, and feelings of catastrophizing (the specific plausibility of these theoretical relationships might be disputed, but can be taken for granted for the purposes of the example).

If adjustment is measured with the questionnaire that is being tested for its validity, and each of these other constructs is measured with existing tools, the relationships between the various sets of scores generated should reflect the theoretical relationships that have been proposed (Figure 9.4). Thus, individuals who score high on the adjustment scale should also score high on self-esteem and optimism, but low on social isolation and depression, and so forth.

If there is a match between these theoretical and empirical relationships, construct validity

has been established. If there is a mismatch, a number of possibilities exist:

- The questionnaire is measuring some concept other than adjustment.
- The questionnaire is indeed measuring adjustment, but one or more of the tools used to measure the other concepts is not measuring the concept it is supposed to measure.
- The questionnaire is indeed measuring adjustment, but one or more of the theoretical relationships between adjustment and the other concepts is mistaken.

The reason(s) for an apparent failure of construct validity must therefore be examined carefully.

Intrinsic to the process of construct validity are the notions of *convergence* and *discrimination* (Campbell and Fiske, 1959). Convergence occurs when positive correlations are obtained between the concept of interest and other

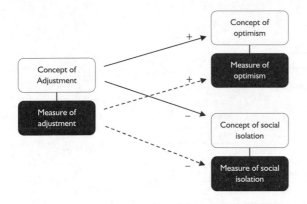

Figure 9.4 *Schematic representation of construct validity. The solid arrows represent theoretical relationships between adjustment and optimism and social isolation, and the broken arrows represent empirical relationships between data produced by measures of these concepts. If the theoretical and the empirical relationships match, construct validity has been demonstrated.*

concepts to which it is in theory positively related (e.g. adjustment and optimism in Figure 9.4). Discrimination occurs when negative correlations are obtained between the original concept and those to which it is considered to be inversely related (e.g. adjustment and social isolation in Figure 9.4), or when near-zero correlations are obtained between the original concept and others to which it has no theoretical relationship (Sim and Arnell, 1993).

The need for construct validity arises when there is no existing criterion measure against which a new measure can be evaluated (this may occur if the construct being measured is theoretically novel), thus ruling out the possibility of concurrent validity. Alternatively, it may be that existing measures of a construct are considered fundamentally flawed in conception or construction, and it is thought necessary to devise a new measure without using existing measures as a yardstick.

9.3 FORMS OF RELIABILITY

The term 'reliability' is used in a broad sense in everyday parlance to refer to the performance of all sorts of living and non-living entities –

friends, colleagues, alarm clocks, vacuum cleaners and the internal combustion engine. In research, the meaning of this term is, or at least should be, more precise. Here too, however, it tends to be used rather loosely. Newell (1996), for example, applies the notion of reliability to samples, in reference to aspects of their representativeness. Also, the findings of a study (i.e. its conclusions, rather than the data on which these are based) are often referred to as being reliable. More often than not, it is unclear whether this is to mean that these findings are ones that can in a general sense be 'relied on', in terms of their having internal and/or external validity, or that they are consistent with those of other studies. To avoid some of this potential confusion, it is preferable to reserve 'reliability' for those contexts in which the consistency or reproducibility of data is at issue.

As defined in this way, there are three broad categories of reliability: equivalence, stability and internal consistency (Figure 9.5). *Equivalence* is a matter of whether an instrument produces consistent measurements, for a given entity, in the hands of two or more investigators, or when utilized in two different forms. *Stability* denotes the extent to which an instrument performs consistently when used to measure the same entity on repeated occasions. Equivalence and stability are sometimes referred to as *reproducibility* and *repeatability*, respectively (Everitt, 1998). *Internal consistency* is a measure of the homogeneity of a multi-item instrument, and will be addressed in Section 15.3.

Central to assessing reliability in any of these forms – and particularly in relation to stability – is an assumption that the entity being measured exhibits, or in the case of stability retains, the same characteristics between measurements. We only expect measurements to be consistent when what is measured has the same value with respect to the relevant variable. If the underlying value of the entity had changed between occasions of its measurement, we would *not* expect an instrument to return the same scores – it would be a matter of concern if it did (Box 9.2). Accordingly, Kline (1993) points out that

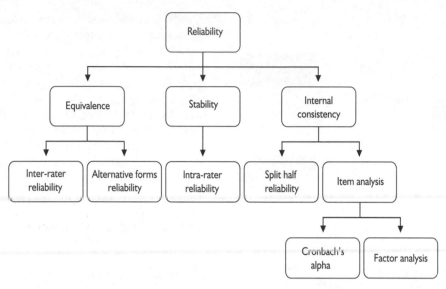

Figure 9.5   *Types of reliability.*

when assessing reliability it is important to take into consideration the nature of the variable concerned and the sample on which it is being measured; each of these will provide some indication as to whether actual change is likely to have occurred between measurements.

Box 9.2   *Analysing reliability*

The statistical methods appropriate for assessing reliability will be considered in detail in Section 18.3. However, it is worth noting at this point that the relationship that needs to be demonstrated between two sets of measurements is usually one of agreement, rather than one of association. In order to show that an instrument returns consistent measurements on two occasions of its use, it must be shown that the two sets of scores are the *same*, not merely that the two sets of scores are *correlated*, and the latter does not imply the former. This said, if two sets of measurements are not on exactly the same scale, correlation is an appropriate form of analysis. This is often the case when assessing internal consistency reliability. As will be seen in Section 15.3, this form of reliability involves assessing the reliability of items within a composite attitude scale. Although all the items may be measuring the same dimension of attitude, they may vary in their strength as indicators; i.e. the same scale point on two items may represent a different intensity of attitude in each case. Correlation, not agreement, should be sought in order to demonstrate reliability. A similar situation may obtain when assessing criterion-related validity. A new measure of functional capacity based on a 1–36 scale might be validated against an existing criterion measure based on a 1–40 scale. Scores on the two measures should correlate in order for the new measure to be validated, but they would not be expected to agree. Whichever index of reliability is used, it is important to realize that reliability may be related to the size of the measurements; i.e. random measurement error may be *heteroscedastic*, varying across the measurement scale (Nevill and Atkinson, 1997). Thus, it is often the case that as the magnitude of measurements increases, their reliability decreases.

For some variables, change over a short period of time can be more or less ruled out a priori. Certain anthropometric measures are, for example, unlikely to change noticeably in the short term. In contrast, certain psychological states may be quite labile. Consequently, it is important to distinguish the reliability of a measurement from the stability of the entity being measured (Knapp *et al.*, 1998). Dunn (1989, p. 50) gives the example of anxiety:

> *The lack of agreement between measures of anxiety taken at two different times could be caused by either changes on* [sic] *the subject's true state or measurement error, or both. In this case stability of the trait or characteristic being measured will be confounded with test reliability.*

Thus, when assessing the reliability of serial measurements, the interval between successive measurements should be sufficiently small to ensure that the construct being measured has not changed. However, the interval should be large enough to ensure that the measures are independent; i.e. that the value recorded on the first occasion has not influenced that recorded on the second occasion, perhaps as a result of observer and/or subject recall of the initial score (Dworkin and Whitney, 1992; Carmines and Zeller, 1994).

9.3.1 Equivalence

Equivalence concerns the reproducibility of measurements. It arises most often when measurements are to be taken by two or more investigators. It concerns consistency *across* raters, and is therefore referred to as *inter-rater reliability*. If data are to be collected on any variable in a study by more than one investigator, inter-rater reliability is an issue that needs to be considered. Tools used in clinical practice almost always require inter-rater reliability, since different practitioners are likely to use them to assess the same individual. The more that active participation is required of the investigator in order to use an instrument, the greater the potential threat to its reliability. A structured observation schedule, in which the researcher has to observe, classify and count specific types of behaviour, normally leaves greater scope for random error on the part of the researcher than a self-completed questionnaire, whose completion requires no direct involvement of the researcher.

It is implicit in the notion of inter-rater reliability that a given method of data collection is likely to perform somewhat differently in the hands of various researchers. It follows from this that levels of reliability that have previously been established for a particular method of data collection cannot always be assumed to apply within a new study. It may be necessary to re-establish reliability within the context of this study. This is not only because the method will be in new hands, but also because the method may have different reliability when used on a different sample. An attitude scale that has a high degree of reliability when used on young adults may be less reliable (and hence less valid also) when used on older people. Thus, Rothstein (1993a, p. 31) argues that if an appeal is to be made to previous work to establish the reliability of a proposed method of data collection, the work in question 'must have examined a similar type of reliability, using similarly trained examiners and similar types of subjects'.

Another situation in which equivalence is important is when it is necessary to use a measuring instrument in a different form on separate occasions. This is normally required on account of testing effects. When measuring knowledge, for example, if the same questions were used on more than one occasion, the second measurements might be biased through subjects' recall of the correct answers following the first measurement occasion. A similar effect might occur when measuring attitudes or personality. Accordingly, the Eysenck Personality Questionnaire (Eysenck and Eysenck, 1975) exists in two equivalent versions. This form of reliability is known as *alternative forms reliability* or *parallel forms reliability*.

It is clearly important that the two (or more) versions of the instrument measure the same concept to the same degree (i.e. that the same, or very similar, scores will be generated by each version in respect of a particular subject). Accordingly, in an attempt to secure such equivalence, test items may be randomly allocated to the various versions of the instrument (Carmines and Zeller, 1994). To verify that the various forms are indeed equivalent, they must be administered one after the other to the same group of individuals. This rests upon an assumption that the concept being measured has not changed in these individuals over this period of time.

9.3.2 Stability

Stability is the extent to which measurements are repeatable. It is usually determined for a single investigator, and is therefore referred to as *intra-rater reliability*. The term *test–retest reliability* is also used, reflecting the fact that serial measurements are involved. Any study in which data are collected from the same individuals or other units on more than one occasion will require intra-rater reliability.

Whereas attempts to secure inter-rater reliability are prone to random error resulting from differences between raters, this source of error is eliminated in intra-rater reliability. This still leaves error that arises from diachronic changes in the investigator's performance. Depending on the period of time between measurements, variability that stems from within-investigator variability is likely to be smaller than that resulting from between-investigator variability. For this reason, it is often reasonable to assume that, if inter-rater reliability has been shown to be at a certain level, intra-rater reliability will be at least as good.

9.3.3 Internal consistency reliability

Internal consistency reliability is assessed in order to determine the homogeneity of a multi-item scale; i.e. the extent to which its constituent items are all measuring the same underlying construct. Techniques such as split-half reliability analysis and item analysis are employed for this purpose. These will be examined in Section 15.3.

9.4 THE VALIDITY AND RELIABILITY OF QUALITATIVE DATA

The idea of validity, as conventionally understood, does not always sit comfortably in research based on qualitative data. For one thing, it suggests that there is a single 'true' account of a phenomenon, whereas exploratory studies are usually premised on the notion of multiple realities among which it is not meaningful to make judgements of relative truthfulness (see Box 15.2). In addition, to talk of 'validation' suggests that there is a highly objective and external process whereby findings can be assessed, which cuts across the essentially interpretive nature of qualitative data. In response to considerations such as these, many researchers prefer to use a term such as *credibility* when examining the 'truth' of findings (Guba and Lincoln, 1981; Sandelowski, 1986; Krefting, 1991; Robson, 1993).

Similar concern is expressed with regard to reliability. It is usually inappropriate to expect that reliability, in its conventional sense, can be achieved in exploratory studies (Schmoll, 1993; Marshall and Rossman, 1999). Many such studies examine somewhat transient phenomena that are not available for reinspection in the same form: we do not expect a person to say precisely the same things or behave in just the same way when interviewed or observed on a second occasion. Accordingly, writers such as those cited above tend to favour the term *auditability* when dealing with qualitative data.

Underlying these contrasting conceptions of validity and reliability is a different idea of the notion of objectivity. In descriptive or explanatory studies based on the collection of quantitative data, researchers usually attempt to secure objectivity by suppressing their own beliefs, expectations, values and emotions at the outset. Many features of the randomized controlled trial are designed to eliminate these subjective, personal influences from the process of data collection and analysis. Similarly, in studies using questionnaires, steps are taken to avoid communicating to the respondent those answers that might be expected or thought desirable (see Section 15.4.2).

In many exploratory studies, however, these options are not available. The sort of environment in which such research often takes place may draw the researcher in psychologically and emotionally, and thus prevent the adoption of a distanced or dispassionate approach to collecting data – it would, for example, be difficult to adopt such a stance if carrying out an observational study of social interaction in a burns unit. Further, as was pointed out in Section 5.5.1, it may not be desirable to take such an approach, even if it were possible to do so. Collecting qualitative data that are meaningful may require a considerable degree of psychological rapport and emotional empathy, qualities that would be lost in an attempt to attain a sense of objective detachment. Indeed, the very idea of objective detachment may be illusory when dealing with qualitative data. Parker (1994, p. 13) argues that objectivity may best be attained

> *through an exploration of the ways in which the subjectivity of the researcher has structured the way it is defined in the first place. Subjectivity is a resource, not a problem, for a theoretically and pragmatically sufficient explanation. When researchers, whether quantitative or qualitative, believe that they are being most objective by keeping a distance between themselves and their objects of study, they are actually themselves producing a* **subjective** *account, for a position of distance is still a position and it is all the more powerful if it refuses to acknowledge itself to be such.*

Accordingly, in exploratory studies, and particularly those conducted from a phenomenological perspective, objectivity is interpreted in a different way. Rather than trying to suppress or eliminate subjective influences from the research process, the researcher discloses and reflects on these factors, both during the process of research (e.g. in a reflective diary; see Section 5.4) and in the written account that is made available to

others. The underlying goal is one of *transparency*:

> *Transparency is simply the notion that researchers' interpretations of the experiential evidence can be checked, examined, critiqued, and used as a basis for convincing others that the research findings are valid.*

(Avis, 1998, p. 144)

Further discussion of the meaning of validity and reliability in different research approaches is provided by Reason and Rowan (1981b), LeComte and Goetz (1982), Kirk and Miller (1986), Avis (1995) and Mays and Pope (1995).

9.5 RESPONSIVENESS

In a longitudinal study involving the collection of quantitative data, the researcher is usually looking for evidence of change in one or more outcome variables. It is important that whatever measuring tool is used for this purpose is able to detect the appropriate magnitude of such change. This is referred to as the *responsiveness* of an instrument (Cole *et al.*, 1994). The term 'sensitivity' is sometimes used in this context – e.g. by Wade (1992) and Gibbon (1995) – in the sense of being 'sensitive to change', but is best avoided so as not to create confusion with the way this term is applied to diagnostic tests (Section 9.2.3).

The degree of responsiveness required of an instrument is determined by the context in which it is to be used. When measuring clinical outcomes, an instrument must be sufficiently responsive to detect the minimum degree of change considered to be clinically important; higher levels of responsiveness are of little value, since they will not add to the clinical usefulness of the data produced.

It was stated earlier that the assessment of stability requires that no change should have occurred in the underlying construct between measurement occasions. Similar considerations apply when assessing responsiveness. For example, if a clinical measure is responsive, it will record a difference in score in those individuals who have changed with respect to the relevant outcome measure between measurement occasions, but will record the same score in those individuals who have not changed over this period of time. The difference in score should, of course, be in the same direction as any underlying change.

Three important practical implications follow. First, the period of time over which responsiveness is tested should be of sufficient length for any change to have occurred. This time will vary from context to context, and is likely to be longer for, say, muscle strength or depression than for muscle spasm or state anxiety. Second, there must be an independent measure of whether or not change has occurred. For example, to determine whether a new measure of neuroticism is responsive, those patients in whom change has or has not occurred must be identified by means of another validated index of neuroticism (Table 9.3). It might be thought that two groups of patients, one treated and one untreated, could be used for such a purpose. On this way of thinking, a responsive measure would be expected to record change in the treated group, but no such change in the untreated group. However, this approach does not provide direct evidence of underlying change, but rests on the possibly dubious assumption that patients who have received treatment have changed while those who have not received treatment are in status quo. Administering treatment is a good means of *eliciting* change, but the fact that treatment has been given is not an indicator that change has in fact occurred.

Third, responsiveness should be tested against an appropriate range of underlying change. To return to the example of neuroticism, let us assume that the patients who exhibited change did so to much the same degree, as judged by the existing validated index of neuroticism. If the new measure of neuroticism recorded change, this would demonstrate responsiveness in relation to this magnitude of change, but it would not indicate whether or not the measure would be responsive to lesser magnitudes of change. Equally, if the new measure failed to record change, this would merely indicate that it is not responsive with respect to this magnitude of change; it would not tell us if it would be responsive to a greater magnitude of change. In contrast, testing against a variety of degrees of change should allow the precise responsiveness of the measure to be identified.

The responsiveness of an instrument is effectively restricted by its test–retest (intra-rater) reliability. Only a difference in score greater than that attributable to random error can be taken to represent true underlying change, and the responsiveness of the instrument cannot therefore be better than its test–retest reliability. In a study of the Roland–Morris Questionnaire (RMQ), a 24-point disability scale (Roland and Morris, 1983), Stratford *et al.* (1996) examined the mean change in scores on the questionnaire on a sample of 60 patients with low back pain undergoing physiotherapy treatment. By examining the reliability of the ratings obtained on the questionnaire both before and following treatment (4 to 6 weeks later), the authors concluded that the magnitude of minimum detectable change lay between 4 and 5 points on the RMQ. They argue that any change of lesser magnitude could not be distinguished from measurement error with 90% confidence.

9.6 THE ROLE OF TRIANGULATION

The use of multiple methods, or *triangulation*, is sometimes proposed as a means of enhancing the

Table 9.3 Use of an independent, validated measure of neuroticism to provide evidence for the responsiveness of a new measure of neuroticism

| | | Validated measure | |
		Change	No change
New measure	Change	Evidence *for* responsiveness	Evidence *against* responsiveness
	No change	Evidence *against* responsiveness	Evidence *for* responsiveness

validity and reliability of research (Brewer and Hunter, 1989; Carr, 1994; Bradley, 1995). Denzin defines triangulation as the use of 'multiple observers, methods, interpretive points of view, and levels and forms of empirical materials in the construction of interpretations' (Denzin, 1989b, p. 270). The rationale for such a strategy is described thus:

> *Triangulation, or the use of multiple methods, is a plan of action that will raise sociologists above the personal biases that stem from single methodologies. By combining methods and investigators in the same study, observers can partially overcome the deficiencies that flow from one investigator or one method.*
>
> (Denzin, 1989b, p. 236)

The various forms of triangulation, as formulated by Denzin (1989b), are described in Table 9.4. In relation to reliability and validity, methodological, investigator and data triangulation are probably most relevant.

9.6.1 Triangulation in relation to reliability

Investigator triangulation is a means of evaluating equivalence in terms of inter-rater relia-

Table 9.4 *Forms of triangulation*

Form	Description
Methodological	The use of more than one method of data collection, either *within* a methodological approach (e.g. two forms of rating scale in a questionnaire) or *between* methodological approaches (e.g. use of both interviews and observation)
Investigator	The use of more than one researcher to collect and/or analyse data
Data	The use of more than one data source within a study (e.g. from more than one time, place, or category of person)
Theory	The use of more than one theoretical perspective to analyse data collected within a study
Multiple	The combination of two or more of the other forms of triangulation

bility. A study may set out to test the equivalence of an outcome measure as a primary objective, or this may be a preliminary requirement when an outcome measure is used to fulfil another primary objective (e.g. to test the relative effectiveness of two or more clinical interventions). Alternatively, if more than one researcher is required for other reasons – the scale of a project, for example, or the fact that cases are geographically dispersed – inter-rater reliability is clearly an important consideration. In either case, the process involved could be described as *investigator triangulation*.

9.6.2 Triangulation in relation to validity

The role of triangulation as a means of securing measurement validity is not straightforward, and requires a clear distinction between different types of validity, and between the roles of methodological and investigator triangulation.

If some form of criterion-related validity is at issue, one of the various methods or approaches must be granted some form of prior, privileged status as a concurrent criterion measure. In terms of investigator triangulation, this might involve identifying expert judges, who may in some cases be the participants from whom the data were collected (see Section 9.2.3).

In terms of methodological triangulation, one method must be viewed as intrinsically more valid than another. This is far from being a straightforward process, as is apparent in the event of discrepant findings. If, for example, a study of patient satisfaction used both interviews and questionnaires, and produced slightly different findings with each, which of the two methods should be seen as invalidating the other? It may be tempting to grant the data from one method some sort of preference – for example, privileging interview data over questionnaire data on the basis that the former are somehow more insightful – but this is liable to be a dubious and arbitrary decision.

Even if the two methods produced similar findings, the question remains. If it is claimed that a form of validation has occurred, at least one of the measures must have the status of a criterion, and, if it is not possible to specify which one, the claim that validation has occurred remains no more than an assertion. There is, moreover, another problem here. If it can be established that one method is indeed a criterion measure, why did we need more than this one method in the first place? If we knew in advance that one method had the status of a criterion measure, why not just use that method alone? The answer to this may be that the alternative method may have advantages over the criterion measure, as described in Section 9.2.3. This, however, is still an argument for using one particular measure in preference to one or more others. The researcher is in something of a cleft stick here:

- The case for criterion-related validity through triangulation fails because there is no satisfactory means of identifying, in advance, a criterion method.
- Or, if such a criterion method can in fact be established, or if one method is superior to others on other grounds, the requirement for more than one method or approach largely evaporates (Sim and Sharp, 1988).

In addition to the impasse just described, the researcher who wishes to use methodological triangulation as a mode of criterion-related validation faces another difficulty. The idea of using multiple methods as a means of validation rests upon the assumption that the individual methods have different patterns of error associated with them – these errors are, in Denzin's (1989b) account, supposed to cancel one another out. However, this overlooks the distinction between random and systematic error. Random error undermines the reliability of measurements, whereas systematic error chiefly undermines their validity. Even if the random error associated with each method differs – which is likely – it is still possible that they share the same type of systematic error (Sim and Sharp, 1998). If so, although the *reliability* of the data produced will tend to improve, there will not necessarily be any increase in their *validity*.

If the focus shifts to content validity, however, the role of methodological triangulation becomes more fruitful. Different methods can be used to capture different components of a multidimensional construct, or different aspects of a complex situation. Hence a number of authors advocate triangulation as a means of securing *completeness* rather than *confirmation* (Fielding and Fielding, 1986; Knafl and Breitmayer, 1991; Redfern and Norman, 1994; DePoy and Gitlin, 1998; Sim and Sharp, 1998). Thus, in the Student Attitudes Study, Teresa Ganz used three different methods so as to gain a broader understanding of the way in which self-inflicted illness is conceptualized within professional health care. She interviewed student nurses and occupational therapists, she conducted non-participant observation of small-group teaching sessions on relevant areas of the curriculum, and she carried out a content analysis of core professional texts. Thus, by using methodological triangulation, Dr Ganz was able to gain a more holistic understanding of the phenomena she was studying. The notion of 'self-inflicted' illness manifests itself on different dimensions and in different contexts in professional health care, and it is unlikely that they could all adequately be accessed by a single methodological approach. However, although the findings that arose from one method shed light on those that arose from another, no attempt was made to validate findings in this way.

9.6.3 Different methods and different objectives

Methodological triangulation is often seen as a means of integrating quantitative and qualitative data and their associated methods (Duffy, 1987; Hinds and Young, 1987; Corner, 1991; Cowman, 1993; Carr, 1994). It is important, however, to examine critically the extent to which different types of data can be reconciled. In seeking to answer this question, it is helpful to decide which research objectives different methods are supposed to address.

If more than one method is used to address

the same research objective, there is a danger that the assumptions of the two methods may be so dissimilar that findings from the two methods cannot be combined. As was demonstrated in Chapters 5 and 6, many of the presuppositions of a study based on unstructured interviews are likely to be incompatible with many of those of a study based on a self-completed questionnaire. For example, there is a very different understanding of what it is for somebody to hold and express an 'attitude' in each of these approaches, and it is hard to see how any kind of common understanding can be gained from an attempt to combine findings from the use of unstructured interviews and self-completed questionnaires within the same study.

If, however, different methods are used in relation to different research objectives, these problems of methodological conflict and incompatibility need not arise. In the Rheumatoid Arthritis Study, Angela Carella conducted two focus groups in order to develop her questionnaire for the main study, following which she carried out unstructured interviews with a subsample of respondents to the questionnaire. Each of these methods fulfilled a separate purpose. The focus groups gathered information that informed the content of the questionnaire, the questionnaire itself served to establish the mode and pattern of practice of therapists working with clients with rheumatoid arthritis, and the interviews sought principally to determine the rationale for some of the practices and procedures described in the questionnaire. Similarly, in the Low Back Pain Study, the randomized controlled trial that constituted the main part of the study was followed by interviews with a subsample of participants from both arms of the trial. Again, the objectives were distinct; the experimental phase of the study was to determine whether or not one intervention was better than the other in general, whereas the interviews were designed to elicit information as to why individual participants did or did not find an intervention helpful, and associated issues to do with patient preferences and treatment acceptability. Although both methods might at first seem to be directed at the notion of treatment effectiveness, this would oversimplify the true situation. The randomized controlled trial was concerned with aggregate, 'objective' effectiveness, whereas the interviews addressed the idea of individual, 'subjective' effectiveness.

These two studies illustrate how methods that produce primarily quantitative data can usefully supplement, and be supplemented by, those that produce primarily qualitative data within a particular study, provided that the methods concerned are linked to distinct research objectives. Neither study would have been so fruitful if just one method had been used.

Further discussion of these and other issues relating to triangulation can be found in Blaikie (1991), Sim and Sharp (1998) and Seale (1999).

9.7 CONCLUSION

This chapter has examined a number of the desirable characteristics of data and the inferences drawn from them. Probably the most important of the characteristics described are validity and reliability. It should be remembered, however, that the way in which these desiderata should be applied will vary between different research approaches. The notion of validity applicable to an exploratory study based on qualitative data is likely to differ from that appropriate to an explanatory study involving quantitative data. Similarly the notion of inter-rater reliability that will be sought when studying physiological variables in a laboratory setting will differ from that sought in the analysis of transcripts of semi-structured interviews.

PART FOUR

PRESENTING AND ANALYSING DATA

10 RECORDING AND ORGANIZING DATA FROM EXPLORATORY STUDIES

SUMMARY

This chapter explores the following topics:

- methods of recording data from interviews
- methods of recording and notating data from observational studies
- the role of reflective notes
- suitable techniques for transcribing interview data

This chapter examines some of the methodological issues that arise when dealing with the data from studies undertaken to answer exploratory research questions. As was explained in Chapter 5, the data concerned will be predominantly qualitative, and are likely to be gathered from interviews, participant or non-participant observation, documentary sources or a mixture of these.

The emphasis will be on the recording and organizing of qualitative data; issues surrounding the analysis of such data will be addressed in Chapter 11. It should be remembered, however, that in practice these processes usually merge, and the division of material in this way is necessarily somewhat artificial.

10.1 RECORDING DATA

Recording data often poses a challenge in exploratory studies. Because these studies tend to take place in natural settings, data usually have to be recorded in as unobtrusive a manner as possible. At the same time, however, the accuracy of the chosen method of data collection is crucial. The data that are gathered in the field during exploratory studies are likely to come from either interviews or observations (or from both).

10.1.1 Recording interview data

Since one of the most consistent challenges to the credibility of qualitative research is the issue of systematic bias through investigator control of data collection and analysis, how interview data are recorded or logged becomes increasingly important.

(K. A. May, 1991, pp. 197–198)

Interview data can be recorded either by handwritten notes or by audiotaping. Each of these methods has its pros and cons. The chief merit of audiotaping is that it provides a full and accurate record of what was said and, moreover, the manner in which it was said (Silverman, 2000). This is vital if the data are to be subjected to linguistic analysis (i.e. an analysis of the *form* of the communication, including its register, syntax, phraseology and vocabulary, as well as its *content*). In addition, some aspects of verbal interaction are effectively unrecordable by hand, e.g. dysphasic or dyspraxic speech. The use of a tape recorder does not, however, obviate the need for careful listening during the interview (Mason, 1996). The chief merit of handwritten notes is that they allow the simultaneous recording of informants' non-verbal behaviour and other aspects of the interaction that takes place during an interview. These observational data can readily be linked to the verbal data being recorded. It is also possible to make a note of who is saying what, which can be very important when more than one informant is being interviewed, such as in a focus group (Sim, 1998). Similarly, comments, questions or ideas for further analysis can readily be inserted in the notes (Lincoln and Guba, 1985). Handwritten notes may also be more natural and acceptable to some informants, who may be suspicious of the idea that their every word is being recorded

(Whyte, 1982; Lincoln and Guba, 1985). Mini-chiello *et al.* (1990, p. 135) note that, for the informant who is being tape-recorded,

> *there is the feeling that once something is on tape it is indelible. There may be a concern that the recorded account may be misinterpreted at a later date when the informant is not present to interject, correct or change an interpretation.*

Rubin and Rubin (1995) and Arksey and Knight (1999) note, on the other hand, that some interviewees may value the use of a tape recorder as a sign that their views are being taken seriously, and as an indication of the researcher's concern to record their views accurately. An assurance that the recorder will be turned off when requested, and even allowing the informant to operate the machine himself or herself, may alleviate anxiety.

A major drawback of handwritten notes, however, is that they inevitably introduce elements of selectivity and interpretation. Because the researcher cannot write down everything, he or she is bound to make choices as to what is or is not important or relevant. This may restrict the scope of subsequent analysis (Sandelowski, 1994). Equally, the fact that paraphrase is often necessary when making notes

by hand means that some degree of interpretation will occur during the process of data recording. Moreover, because this 'pre-interpreted' transcript is the only account available, it is not possible for the researcher to check the validity of the data with a colleague (Section 9.2.3).

On balance, and despite some dissenting voices (e.g. Lincoln and Guba, 1985), audiotaping is usually regarded as the preferable method of data collection for interviews, by virtue of its greater accuracy (Oppenheim, 1992; Fielding, 1993; Maykut and Morehouse, 1994; Holloway and Wheeler, 1996). It should be the method of choice unless there are specific and compelling reasons to favour handwritten notes. Table 10.1 summarizes the principal advantages and disadvantages of the two methods.

10.1.2 Recording observational data

Observational data can be recorded either by means of handwritten notes or through a form of videotaping. Many of the issues that underlie the choice of method for observational data are similar to those outlined for interview data. An important factor is whether the process of observation is to be participant or non-participant, and whether it is to be conducted overtly or covertly (see Section 5.5.3). Videotaping has

Table 10.1 *Advantages and disadvantages of audiotapes and handwritten notes for recording interview data*

	Handwritten notes	Audiotapes
Advantages	• Allow concurrent recording of non-verbal data • Facilitate identification of individual informants • Permit the researcher's comments to be interpolated • Do not require subsequent transcription, and allow immediate review • Encourage the researcher to listen attentively during the interview	• Allow complete, verbatim recording of both the researcher's questions and the informant's responses • Record intonation, inflection, hesitation, pauses, etc. • Unobtrusive, once informants are accustomed to the tape recorder
Disadvantages	• Limit eye contact between researcher and informant • May be obtrusive • Hard to record data verbatim • Prone to effects of inattention or fatigue • Produce selective and 'pre-interpreted' accounts	• May be unacceptable to some informants • Require fairly costly apparatus • Prone to machine failure • Require subsequent transcription • Do not register non-verbal aspects of communication • May encourage inattentiveness during the interview

obvious advantages for some forms of covert observation, whether participant or non-participant. In particular, videotape can be analysed by several researchers but it is often not practicable for multiple investigators to observe a social situation directly. Moreover, videotape can be viewed repeatedly, so that all relevant aspects of behaviour or interaction can be studied. Inter-rater reliability can readily be tested when video-tapes are available (Heacock *et al.*, 1996). A drawback of videotaping, however, is that a single video camera usually has a narrower angle of coverage than the human eye (Carr, 1991). Some aspects of a situation may be obscured from the camera's view, and if the camera is fixed, it cannot move to one side in order to correct this situation in the way that a human observer can. Moreover, it may be hard to capture both the close-in detail of facial expressions and the wider view required to record gross patterns of bodily movement and interaction (Bottorff, 1994). It is difficult to videotape covertly in some situations, such as in small, intimate or dimly lit surroundings, or when those being studied are constantly moving from place to place. In such cases, the researcher is likely to make handwritten notes. If the researcher is acting as a participant observer, this note taking is likely to occur after the interaction of interest has taken place, unless the taking of notes forms a natural or plausible part of the activity in which the researcher is supposed to be participating. Whatever method is adopted, the whole enterprise of covert observation raises fundamental ethical issues (see Section 5.8).

One of the problems facing the observational researcher, particularly when making notes by hand, is that of deciding where to direct his or her attention. It is not possible to record everything that occurs in a social situation, and any attempt to do so would produce a very diffuse and superficial account. Accordingly, some sort of focus needs to be taken. The following are some of the elements within a social situation that may serve as points of focus for the observer:

- the nature of the physical environment in which interaction is taking place
- the identity, role and status of those present
- the orientation and spatial behaviour of participants (i.e. their proximity and degree of physical contact, if any)
- the postures that participants adopt and the actions and activities in which they engage (an 'action' is a form of bodily movement, such as yawning or rising from a chair, whereas an 'activity' is a process or function, such as making a bed or administering medication)
- the duration, frequency and time of occurrence of these actions and activities
- the verbal and non-verbal communication between participants
- the goal or purposes that participants seem to display in their communication or behaviour
- the 'quality' or 'style' of the interaction taking place – whether it is hurried or calm, formal or informal, public or private, expressive or instrumental, and so forth.

Which of these are addressed in a specific study will depend on the research question, which will also determine the extent to which the observation process is structured or unstructured (see Sections 5.5.3 and 6.3.6). It should be remembered that if participant observation is taking place, the researcher should note the way in which participants behave in relation to himself or herself, not just in relation to one another (Silverman, 2000).

Even with certain specific foci in mind, taking full notes is a formidable task. It often helps to use some form of summary or abbreviated note taking. It may be possible to record short pieces of dialogue verbatim, but very often it is necessary to paraphrase. Direct quotation can be identified in the notes by single quotation marks, and paraphrase by double quotation marks. Spatial behaviour can be recorded by means of a series of symbols known as *proxemic notation*

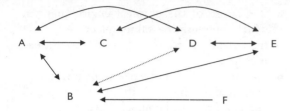

Figure 10.1 *Example of a sociogram of verbal communication.*

(Hall, 1963), and the emotional or communicative relationships between participants can be represented by *sociograms* (Kerlinger, 1986). Figure 10.1 shows a sociogram illustrating the nature and degree of verbal communication between six individuals. The absence of arrows linking C with D, A with E, and B with C indicates that virtually no communication occurs between these dyads, and the dotted line linking D with B illustrates the fact that communication between these two participants is only minimal. It is also evident that F communicates only with B, and the single arrowhead indicates that this is mainly a one-way process.

In many situations, the nature of social processes will change depending on the time of day or day of the week, or in relation to certain key events. The activity that habitually takes place during a Friday afternoon clinic may differ from that of the Tuesday morning clinic, the behaviour of staff on a ward is likely to change depending on whether the senior physician is present, and student nurses are likely to interact in the refectory in a way that they might not when in the lecture room. This suggests that observations should be sampled in some way, so that different situations and time periods are observed. If observation is confined to a single place, key features of the setting may be overlooked and the possibility of new lines of enquiry, not anticipated at the outset of the study, may be lost. This form of sampling can be built into an observation schedule (Bowling, 1997).

It is unlikely that the researcher will be able to make full notes of all that is seen to take place in a setting, particularly if there are concurrent interactions taking place between a number of individuals. It is important, therefore, to supplement written notes from memory as soon as possible after leaving the setting, and certainly not longer than a day later (Bowling, 1997). In some cases of covert observation, *all* notes may have to be constructed from memory, in which case this should be done as frequently as practicable. Temporary absences from the research setting are not only useful to write up field notes while the memory is still fresh; they also provide a means of maintaining the researcher role (Section 5.4). For example, a researcher might return periodically to an academic institution to reaffirm the researcher role, which might otherwise get submerged by the role of participant in the research setting. Furthermore, participant observation is often an exhausting process, and regular breaks are important to minimize the possibility that important issues are not missed due to researcher fatigue.

In many cases, the researcher engaged in a form of participant observation will almost certainly wish to pose questions to those whom he or she is observing. To this extent, interviewing may be part of the process of observational research (Grbich, 1999). However, interviewing normally takes a rather different form in this context. Robson (1993, p. 199) comments that 'in participant observation you are less likely to have "set piece" interviews and much more likely to have opportunistic "on the wing" discussions with individuals'. The smaller quantity of data generated by such 'discussions', and the fact that they are likely to probe the issues concerned in less depth than in an unstructured interview, mean that handwritten notes will usually be sufficient as a means of recording informants' responses. In any case, audiotaping is rarely practicable in such a situation.

Many of the points outlined in this section also apply to the more structured form of observation that may occur in descriptive studies

(Section 6.3.6). However, because the specific actions, events or behaviours to be observed are likely to have been identified in advance, observational data in a descriptive study are normally gathered on a standardized schedule or checklist.

10.1.3 Reflective notes

In addition to making notes of the communication and behaviour that occurs in a social situation, the researcher may wish to make notes on his or her own reactions and reflections during the process of data collection (Box 10.1). These notes are often in the form of a diary or journal, and may include the following topics and issues:

- ideas for subsequent data collection
- strategies or insights relating to data analysis

Box 10.1   *Types of notes*

Burgess (1984) identified three main types of notes that may be made during observational research. *Substantive fieldnotes* are the ongoing record of what the researcher sees and hears in the research setting, and constitute the data for the study. Reflecting the nature of the observation being conducted, these notes may be more or less structured. *Methodological notes* constitute the researcher's contemporaneous reflections on the methodological aspects of a study. They may include notes on methods that are proving to be particularly fruitful, or those that seem to be problematic, and ways in which these can be adapted during subsequent data collection. It is here that the researcher is likely to reflect on the appropriate way to manage the researcher role in the field setting, so as to gather the most insightful data with the least possible disruption to the natural pattern of interaction and behaviour occurring. Finally, *analytic notes* are a record of initial or preliminary analyses carried out in the field setting, and may include new or revised research objectives.

- the researcher's own psychological or emotional reactions to the data
- issues that are unclear and may need further exploration
- thoughts on the researcher's perceived identity and role in the field setting.

One of the values of reflective notes is that they allow the researcher to audit the research process in retrospect and thus separate out – at least partially – his or her psychological and emotional engagement with the research setting and participants (see Section 9.4). In this way, the role of the researcher in the data collection process can be critically evaluated in terms of both methodological and ethical insights (B.A. Smith, 1999). The essence of this process is *reflexivity*:

> *Researchers are reflexive when they refer back and critically examine their own assumptions and actions through being 'self-conscious' and self-aware about the research process.*
>
> (Holloway, 1997, pp. 135–136)

According to Tindall (1994, p. 150), reflexivity 'centralizes, rather than marginalizes or denies, the influence of the researcher's life on the research and the construction of knowledge' (see Box 10.2). The notion of reflexivity acknowledges, therefore, that it is not possible, nor is it necessarily desirable, for the researcher to try to disengage his or her psychological and emotional responses when collecting and analysing data. Indeed, seemingly undesirable elements of subjectivity can be usefully harnessed to enhance the insights drawn from qualitative data (Scott, 1985; Finlay, 1998; see Section 5.5.1).

Reflective notes are not only a resource for the researcher. They can also be used by an independent researcher (Lincoln and Guba, 1985), and by those reading published research (Koch, 1994), to assess the analyses and interpretations made by the primary researcher.

Box 10.2   *Senses of 'reflexivity'*

The term 'reflexivity' is used in rather different ways in different contexts. In Section 6.2, 'reflexivity' was used to describe the way in which an account is not merely something that is said by an informant, but is also a means of accomplishing certain purposes in the course of the interaction with a researcher. Reflexivity here is a notion that applies to the informant and the accounts that he or she provides. In the present section, however, the term pertains more to the researcher's role – the way in which the researcher's subjective self and a consciousness of the social situation in which research occurs should bear upon the way in which an investigation is conducted. Being 'reflective' about one's role as a researcher – such as by keeping reflective notes – is a way in which such reflexivity may be achieved. The 'reflexive' approach to interviewing described in Section 5.5.1 – i.e. one that emphasizes flexibility and responsiveness on the part of the researcher – is broadly in line with this sense of *reflexivity*. See Hammersley and Atkinson (1995) and Seale (1999) for further discussion of this concept.

10.2   TRANSCRIBING INTERVIEW DATA

Audiotaped data from interviews require transcription. Although some advocate direct analysis of the audiotape (e.g. Jones, 1985b), this is not generally to be recommended. It is difficult to juxtapose quotations or sections of data from different parts of the tape, and the need to pause the tape or replay lines of speech can interfere with the sense of flow and progression of the dialogue. The audiotape can, however, be used as a supplementary medium for analysis (see Section 11.2).

The primary purpose of transcription is to record the words used in the interview. However, O'Connell and Kowal (1995) point out that there are other features of the interview that can also be transcribed where appropriate. These are: *prosodic* features (such as the emphasis, timing or rhythm of speech), *paralinguistic* features (non-verbal elements of oral communication, such as laughter) and *extralinguistic* features (such as facial expression, shrugs and other bodily movements).

Transcription is a lengthy process, and an hour's interview is likely to take between 4 and 10 hours to transcribe, depending on one's skill as a typist, the clarity of the recording and the complexity of the data (Maykut and Morehouse, 1994; Holloway and Wheeler, 1996; DePoy and Gitlin, 1998). A specialist recorder, with foot switch operation, is invaluable. Trying to type and operate the rewind, forward and playback switches manually is a slow and frustrating process. It might be tempting to transcribe only those parts of the interview that seem relevant and interesting, and thereby to save a considerable amount of time. This is inadvisable, however, for in order to decide which portions to select for transcription one would need already to have established a fairly well-developed conceptual and thematic framework for the data. Although certain theoretical concepts may need to be identified at the outset, a full theoretical framework should normally emerge from the detailed process of analysis, and should not be developed in detail before this stage (see Section 11.1.1). Fielding (1993) argues that at least the first few interviews should always be transcribed in full.

Views differ as to whether the researcher should transcribe his or her own tapes, or employ somebody to do this. Maykut and Morehouse (1994, p. 101) point out that doing one's own transcribing provides 'an important opportunity to relive the interview and become substantially more familiar with the data'. Whoever does the transcribing, it is important that both the researcher's and the informant's words are reproduced exactly. Any paraphrase at this stage may foreclose certain analytical options.

10.2.1 Transcription techniques

Certain techniques and conventions can be used to facilitate the transcription process. Some of these are illustrated in the following extract from an interview conducted in the Student Attitudes Study. Teresa Ganz is talking to a student nurse about his experience of treating patients who are under the influence of alcohol or drugs:

7   *Teresa: Would you be happy to say*
7   *something about how you felt about treating*
7   *these pts?*
7   James: I didn't have strong feelings about it
7   really, though I wouldn't say they were my
7   favourite pts to treat, compared to all the
7   pts I've had on my clinical placements.
7   *Teresa: In what ways weren't they your ...*
7   James: Well some of them are really abusive
7   and disruptive, and violent sometimes.
7   *Teresa: I can imagine, though it's not all*
7   *of them,* [*presumably.*
7   James: [No, of course not. I don't mean I
7   wasn't happy to look after them, of course I
7   was, it's just that sometimes I felt (pause,
7   sounds uncertain) uneasy, I suppose, about
7   ... because their sort of lifestyle is not one
7   that I'd ever want for myself.
7   *Teresa: What is it about them that you dislike?*
7   James: I didn't say I disliked them (emphati-
7   cally), it's just that I was brought up quite
7   strictly in terms of appropriate ways to
7   behave and I don't like the idea of losing
7   control like that. It's very demeaning and it's
7   also /..?/ and undignified. Anyway, what I
7   think about it isn't really important in the
7   end (pause) if pts need treatment you just
7   get on and do it, 'cause if you don't you
7   know somebody else only has to.

It can be seen that comments interpolated by the researcher have been placed in parentheses so as to distinguish them from the transcript proper. There should be no ambiguity as to which parts of the transcript originate from the researcher's analytical observations rather than from the interview itself (O'Connell and Kowal, 1995). Where the informant has left a sentence incomplete or seems to have changed track, this is marked by a series of three periods (...). An inaudible or indecipherable word or phrase is marked thus: /..?/. Where the speech of the interviewer and the interviewee overlap, this is indicated by a single square parenthesis immediately before the point of overlap. Words that are stressed by the respondent can be underlined. It is important that symbols and notation of this sort are used consistently if their meanings are to be unambiguous when reviewing a transcript at a later stage (Sandelowski, 1994; O'Connell and Kowal, 1995). Silverman (1993) suggests additional symbols that can be used.

There are some parts of the interview that Teresa Ganz has *not* transcribed. These are utterances such as 'right', 'sure', 'uh-huh' and 'I see' that she made while the interviewee was talking. She has omitted these from the transcript, as they will not play a part in the form of thematic analysis that she proposes to carry out. However, had she intended to perform a linguistic analysis on the interview, it would have been important to include such expletives. Even if such an analysis is not anticipated, one should not underestimate the potential analytical importance of apparently trivial aspects of verbal communication (Pope *et al.*, 2000).

A wide margin would have been kept on both sides of the page to allow annotated comments. On the left, a series of 7s have been inserted. This indicates that this is interview number 7, and on a separate card are the details of the informant's identity ('James' is a pseudonym so as to preserve anonymity) and the date and place of the interview. If Dr Ganz decides to cut the transcript up in the process of analysis, each extract will be traceable to its source, since it will have the reference number on it. In order to save time in transcribing, a frequently recurring word like 'patients' has been abbreviated ('pts'). When the transcript is being revised, Dr Ganz will expand this to 'patients' using the word processor's search-and-replace function (Reid, 1992). Finally, the transcript would have double line spacing, to facilitate annotations and the like.

Most of the recommendations outlined above

are applicable, with appropriate modification, to handwritten notes.

10.3 CONCLUSION

This chapter has outlined some of the considerations that underlie the recording and organizing of qualitative data derived from exploratory studies. As issues of design, data collection, and data analysis are closely interrelated in exploratory studies, the material addressed in this chapter should be considered in the light of issues considered in Chapter 5 and those to follow in Chapter 11.

11 ANALYSING DATA FROM EXPLORATORY STUDIES

SUMMARY

This chapter explores the following topics:

- general considerations in the analysis of qualitative data
- principles of grounded theory analysis
- the identification and labelling of categories
- the revision and linking of categories into propositions
- the role of judgement in analysing qualitative data
- the role of quantification in analysing qualitative data

Chapter 10 explored the processes whereby data from exploratory studies are usually recorded and organized. Once these processes have taken place, the data must be analysed so as to extract both their manifest and latent meanings. This chapter presents the principal issues involved in this process, with reference to the Student Attitudes Study.

11.1 APPROACHING QUALITATIVE DATA

It will be recalled from Section 2.4.2 that exploratory studies are usually inductive in their underlying logic. The aim of the study is characteristically one of theory building rather than theory testing. This means that the researcher draws a theoretical framework from the data, rather than seeking to apply a predetermined framework to the data. When applied to the specific process of data analysis, this principle requires that the researcher should not approach the data with a set of definitive conceptual categories already in hand, but should allow these to emerge from the data in the process of analysis.

Of course, the researcher is likely to have some a priori ideas as to what these categories

are likely to be (Locke, 1998); the research question on which the study is based will, at the very least, suggest some broad potential categories. Miles and Huberman (1994) recommend drawing up a provisional 'start list' of codes before analysis. However, it is probably preferable to set such expectancies aside as far as possible; there is always a danger of finding what you are looking for, whether or not it is really there. This process of suspending prior expectations is often referred to as *epoché* or *bracketing*, and is an important element in phenomenology. Beech (1999, p. 36) describes it as 'a process by which the researcher resolves to hold all preconceptions in abeyance in order to reach experiences before they are made sense of, before they are ordered into concepts that relate to previous knowledge and experience'. An important part of bracketing is an avowal on the part of the researcher of exactly what his or her prior expectations were. This allows the consumers of a study to evaluate possible sources of bias (Liehr and Marcus, 1994).

To say that prior expectations should be put to one side is not to say that they should be discarded irrevocably, since they may be usefully invoked at certain stages of the analysis (see Section 11.2.1). Nor should it be assumed that bracketing is easily achieved. It may be cognitively problematic to attempt to set aside certain subjective expectations and at the same time retain a sense of intuitive responsiveness:

> [T]he qualitative researcher's perspective is perhaps a paradoxical one: it is to be acutely tuned-in to the experiences and meaning systems of others – to indwell – and at the same time to be aware of how one's own biases and preconceptions may be influencing what one is trying to understand.
>
> (Maykut and Morehouse, 1994, p. 123)

Ahern (1999) provides practical guidance on how to manage the process of bracketing and maintain an appropriate balance between these two requirements.

It should be noted that the possibility of bracketing is not universally acknowledged. A key tenet of the philosophy of hermeneutics (see Box 5.1) is that the observer is inseparable from that which he or she is observing, and cannot set aside past experience in the way required if bracketing is to occur. The observer is set within a particular culture and cannot step outside it in order to attain some sort of 'neutral' stance – indeed, this culture is an essential element within the process of understanding (Hughes, 1990).

Figure 11.1 shows the steps involved in the analysis of qualitative data. It can be seen that the analysis moves upwards from the specific and concrete (pieces of raw data) to the general and abstract (theory). It will also be noticed that this has not been represented as a wholly unidirectional process. It is usually argued that one should also work back through the stages, reviewing and where appropriate revising prior decisions. In particular, the analyst is encouraged to return frequently to the data, to ensure that

the whole process of analysis is firmly grounded in the actual data.

11.1.1 Grounded theory

A particular inductive approach to qualitative data analysis that has recently gained considerable popularity in health care research – and within nursing research especially (Benoliel, 1996) – is 'grounded theory'. Barney Glaser and Anselm Strauss first proposed this approach in the 1960s (Glaser and Strauss, 1967). Further accounts of the method have followed (Glaser, 1978, 1992; Strauss, 1987; Strauss and Corbin, 1998), together with a book of readings (Strauss and Corbin, 1997). The fundamental principles of grounded theory analysis can be summarized as follows:

- All inferences should be firmly 'grounded' in the data.
- Prior theoretical expectations are avoided as far as possible, and for this reason it is considered undesirable to conduct a full literature review at the outset of a study (Box 3.2).
- Data collection and data analysis are iterative (i.e. the researcher moves back and forth between the two, rather than collecting and analysing data in sequence).
- In a similar way, sampling proceeds in parallel with data collection and analysis – insights derived from analysis of the data prompt the choice of sources of further sources of data.
- All categories identified within the data should be regarded as provisional, and are subject to revision or modification on further examination of the raw data (a process referred to as the *constant comparative method*).
- The researcher should take a sceptical view of any conclusions reached and consciously seek disconfirming instances in the data.
- The ultimate purpose of analysis is to construct a coherent theory from the data that is rooted in the reality of human experience and interaction.

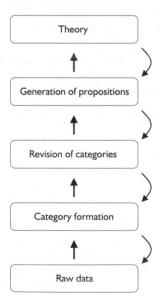

Figure 11.1 *Steps in the analysis of qualitative data.*

A significant achievement of grounded theory was to systematize and make explicit the process of qualitative data analysis, which had hitherto been somewhat unclear, lacking guidelines, and open to charges of arbitrariness. There are, however, differences in emphasis and interpretation within the grounded theory approach, and not all proponents of grounded theory would endorse the above principles equally. Indeed, there has lately been something of a schism between its originators, with Glaser (1992) vehemently criticizing a recent account of the method by Strauss and Corbin (1990). In essence, Glaser maintains that Strauss and Corbin have described a method of conceptual description rather than one of theory construction, which he sees as the true purpose of grounded theory. Melia (1996) provides an interesting commentary on this dispute.

It has also been argued that many studies that purport to be based on grounded theory depart from some of its basic canons (Bryman, 1988). A particular point of debate centres on the place of theory. Although grounded theory suggests that theory should emerge exclusively from the data gathered in a study, it may not be possible or even desirable to suspend all theorizing in the initial stages of a study (Bulmer, 1979). Indeed, the researcher will need some sort of preliminary or provisional theoretical framework in order to decide which of the numerous potential sources of data are worthy of attention. Furthermore, the methods to be used in a study will make certain theoretical assumptions about the nature of the object of study and the way in which it can be apprehended (Section 2.3). In other words, methods must be theoretically informed from the outset. The role of the literature in this respect is addressed in Box 3.2.

The account of qualitative data analysis in this chapter will be framed to a considerable extent, but not wholly, in terms of the principles of grounded theory. Because there are a variety of approaches to qualitative data analysis, and no clear set of agreed rules to guide the process, we shall try to avoid being prescriptive in our recommendations. It is in any case unlikely that many analysts follow a single model of analysis, such as grounded theory, in its entirety (Bryman and Burgess, 1994). We would endorse the following comments on the analysis of qualitative data:

> *There is no need to search for an orthodoxy here: the format chosen is likely to be one which fits both the investigator and the kind of problem under scrutiny.*
>
> (Turner, 1994, p. 200)

11.1.2 Illustrative extracts from the Student Attitudes Study

To illustrate the practical steps in qualitative data analysis, three extracts from the interviews conducted by Dr Teresa Ganz in the Student Attitudes Study will be used. These are taken from one-to-one interviews with health care students on their experiences of dealing with patients whose conditions might in some sense be deemed 'self-inflicted'. The principles that will be illustrated are, however, applicable to the analysis of other forms of textual data, such as documentary sources. See Section 10.2.1 for an explanation of the transcription symbols and conventions used.

Extract from interview with student nurse, Emma

5   *Teresa: You must have encountered some*
5   *patients who'd committed suicide – or tried*
5   *to, perhaps I should say – when you were*
5   *working in the emergency unit. Am I right?*
5   <u>Emma</u>: Yes, there were a few, though I
5   wasn't directly involved with many of them.
5   It's not always clear, though, whether
5   someone's tried to kill themself or not.
5   <u>*Teresa: How would you describe the general*</u>
5   *reaction when these patients are brought in?*
5   <u>Emma</u>: It's hardly something you think
5   about really (pause) well, not at the time.
5   There's so much going on, and if there's
5   someone needing their stomach pumped you
5   just get on with it. I have to say, though,
5   you do get rather snide comments being
5   made sort of off the cuff . . . you know,

things like 'as if we didn't have enough to do without him putting himself in here', and I sort of see their point sometimes. But when you think about it, it's not really as if they had a real choice. You don't just decide to swallow a bottle of pills just like you'd decide to take a bath or watch the TV (laughs). Mind you, I think one reason why the staff's got mixed feelings about the suicides is because it's so hard to understand. You can't imagine why someone would want to do away with themselves. When someone comes in from a road accident or something like that, you often think to yourself 'that could have been me', but you don't think like that with a suicide. It's really hard to relate to, and that makes it hard to be very sympathetic sometimes, although I know we shouldn't really think like that.

Teresa: So do you think that the suicidal patients that you get in are perceived differently from the accident [victims?

Emma: [Yes, I do. Although they obviously look after them when they come in, same as they would for anyone else, there's a sort of feeling that this isn't really what they're there for.

Teresa: When you say 'they' ...?

Emma: I mean the staff. Some of them think that their job's really to deal with the heart attacks and the appendicitises and the broken legs, and things like that. I probably feel a bit like that myself, and I'm sure some of the other students do too.

Teresa: Is the treatment that they receive the same, then, – the suicides, I mean – the same as for other patients who'd have the same medical problems? I mean, somebody who'd had the same sort of injury, but not in the course of a suicide attempt.

Emma: Yes, I think so. It's just not always so (pause) enthusiastic.

Teresa: In what sense do you mean?

Emma: Well, I think we sometimes just go through the motions. I don't mean we're not trying, because we are, don't get me wrong.

It's just that some of the staff don't seem to put their heart into it. It's funny, though, I say that, but I have seen one of the qualified nurses who was really over-enthusiastic with a young girl who'd swallowed pills when her boyfriend broke up with her all of a sudden. She was quite rough with her, really, especially when she was putting the tube down her stomach.

Teresa: Why do you suppose that was?

Emma: I think to teach her a lesson, so she wouldn't try it again. There was one of the staff – not the same one – that said that this sort of patient should only be given so many chances, and they should be told that if they kept on swallowing pills or slicing away at their wrists or whatever, there'd come a point where they wouldn't get any more treatment. I don't know how serious he was, though (laughs uneasily). Seriously though, I don't think you could really have a policy like that, because it would mean turning somebody away at the door.

Extract from interview with occupational therapy student, Martine

Teresa: You mentioned that some of the clients on the psychiatric unit had tried to commit suicide. What are your feelings about suicide?

Martine: I know some people say that suicide, or at least attempted suicide, is an act of total selfishness ... as though, when it comes down to it, the person's just thinking of himself. Because you've also got to think of the family that's left behind, and they really do feel awful. We've lots of relatives coming in to the unit where I was before Easter, and the qualified staff always say that the relatives nearly all feel really, really guilty, as though it's their fault, and they should have done something or other to prevent it. (pause) And I think also it seems to be a rejection to them – you know, like 'I've got to the stage where nobody can be of any help to me, not even my family', that sort of thing.

9 *Teresa: Is that what you think, yourself?*
9 Martine: I don't know, really. It can't
9 always be like that, because some people try
9 to kill themselves because they don't want to
9 be a burden on /.. ?/ people, and you can
9 hardly call that selfish. Anyway, I don't
9 know that one can ever really say what's in
9 the mind of someone who's trying to kill
9 themselves, seeing as how ... It's not
9 something that one can really visualize, is it?
9 I think some of the clients that we think of
9 as killing themselves aren't really thinking
9 that way at all. It's like that with some of
9 the anorexics. On the surface, it seems as
9 though they're deliberately starving
9 themselves to death, but I don't think that's
9 what's in their mind at all. It may be the
9 result of what they're doing by not eating,
9 sure, but I'm sure it's not what they're
9 aiming at. When we did anorexia in class, it
9 was always stressed that their perception of
9 their body image is completely different
9 from what you or me would see – what we'd
9 regard as really thin, they see as overweight.
9 So I don't think they see themselves as
9 starving themselves as we might think they
9 are.
9 *Teresa: So how would that sort of thing*
9 *affect your work as* [*an OT?*
9 Martine: [I don't know
9 really, because I've never had any contact
9 with anorexic clients who've reached that
9 stage. I've been at case conferences though
9 on one of my placements where they
9 were dealing with these clients, and
9 they were always talking about trying to
9 reinforce good eating habits and sanction
9 the bad ones, so that the client would
9 change their behaviour during their stay.
9 This was very much an across-the-team
9 approach, and involved the OTs as well as
9 the nurses and the psychologist.
9 *Teresa: Is that an appropriate strategy, do*
9 *you think?*
9 Martine: Well it must work on some clients,
9 otherwise I don't suppose they'd be using it.
9 I always suspect that it will work as long as

9 they're in the unit, but as soon as they're
9 out, where you can't apply all the rewards
9 and sanctions, they're going to do as they
9 please. Anyway, I heard that some of the
9 clients find ways round the system, and hide
9 their food, or get rid of it without anyone
9 knowing how. ... And some of them really
9 couldn't care about some of the sanctions.
9 Like the withdrawn ones don't care if they
9 can't take part in the social activities in the
9 unit – hardly surprising, really (laughs).
9 There's only so much you can do. After all,
9 they've really got to want to get better,
9 haven't they, and ultimately it's down to
9 them. We can only support them in the
9 process, and if they're not prepared to take
9 part in the first place, you're probably on a
9 bit of a loser.

Extract from interview with student nurse, Joanna

10 *Teresa: Do you think there are some illnesses*
10 *or conditions that one could describe as 'self-*
10 *inflicted'?*
10 Joanna: Oh yes, of course there are. Things
10 like drug overdoses. And also, people who
10 do really risky things like motorbike racing
10 and mountaineering and hang-gliding, or
10 boxing, or ...
10 *Teresa: How would you describe your*
10 *reaction to patients like these? I mean your*
10 *psychological reaction, not what you*
10 *actually do in the way of treatment and such*
10 *like.*
10 Joanna: Well, I sometimes think to myself
10 something like 'If you hadn't been tearing
10 about the streets, this wouldn't have
10 happened'. I certainly don't understand why
10 people want to take these drugs, certainly
10 not the amount some of them do, because
10 they must know how bad it is for them.
10 Mind you, I'm not sure that's always in their
10 mind at the time. It's one thing knowing you
10 shouldn't take too many drugs, but you
10 probably blot that out of your mind when
10 you get the urge for a fix, or whatever. I
10 suppose that if a mountain climber was

10 always thinking of how dangerous it was,
10 they'd never get off the ground! Also,
10 sometimes you don't really have any choice.
10 I've seen a professional footballer who
10 ruptured two of the ligaments in his knee. It
10 was his job, so I don't suppose he could
10 really decide to do something else instead on
10 the spur of the moment.
10 *Teresa: Are there any other conditions that*
10 *you can think of that you might describe as*
10 *'self-inflicted'?*
10 Joanna: Well, heavy drinkers sometimes get
10 serious liver problems, and you'd certainly
10 call that self-inflicted. (pause) I suppose you
10 could also say that people who get ill
10 because of eating the wrong sort of diet or
10 not taking any exercise at all are bringing
10 their illness on themselves. That's rather
10 different, though.
10 *Teresa: How is it different?*
10 Joanna: Well, you can never be sure exactly
10 why someone's had a heart attack. It could
10 be because they've eaten a bad diet or never
10 done any exercise, or it could be because
10 they've chosen the wrong set of genes
10 (laughs). You can't know for sure, but if
10 someone breaks a leg coming off a
10 motorbike, it's pretty clear what the cause of
10 that was.
10 *Teresa: Do you think the fact that some*
10 *patients are seen as having 'self-inflicted'*
10 *illnesses affects the sort of care they get?*
10 Joanna: I daresay it does sometimes, though
10 I don't think it really ought to.
10 *Teresa: Can you say a bit more about why*
10 *you don't think it should?*
10 Joanna: I think it's because their needs
10 aren't any different. I remember reading
10 about this famous person in the last century
10 – I forget who it was – who drank some
10 carbolic, because he mistook it for his
10 sleeping medicine. I think he died actually,
10 but suppose he came into hospital at the
10 same time as someone who'd taken an
10 overdose of pills. They'd both need their
10 stomachs pumped just as much as ... The
10 fact that one took it by accident and the

10 other on purpose isn't really relevant, I
10 don't think. As a nurse, just like anyone else,
10 we like some patients more than others, and
10 some of them we really disapprove of their
10 lifestyle and such like ... and I won't say
10 that staff are reluctant to look after these
10 patients, but they don't really do any extra
10 for them, if you see what I mean. At least ...
10 But really, what you think of a patient ought
10 really to be kept apart from the treatment
10 we give them, because it's all too subjective.
10 *Teresa: I see what you're saying there, but*
10 *what if the person who'd taken the pills was*
10 *coming in not for the first time, but let's say*
10 *for the fourth [or fifth?*
10 Joanna: [What, you mean like 'three
10 strikes and you're out'? I think that's a
10 difficult one (pause) but I suppose what you
10 have to say is that if he keeps on coming
10 back like that, in that sort of state, things
10 are probably out of his control, and that's
10 not going to be helped by threatening that
10 there's going to be no more treatment.

11.2 CATEGORY FORMATION

In common with other aspects of data analysis, the computer can do much of the work involved in identifying analytical categories (see Box 11.1). In what follows, however, we will explain how the steps in the process might be undertaken by hand, since this probably illustrates the underlying logic of the process more effectively. The steps described are purely illustrative and by no means prescriptive – there are other, equally legitimate strategies that can be applied to this task.

In analysing interviews, the basic materials with which the analyst works are the transcripts. These are likely to be read through a number of times during the process of analysis. It may also be beneficial to return to the audiotapes, so as to get a first-hand impression of paralinguistic features of the data, such as mood, intonation, fluency and hesitation (Jones, 1985b); it is hard to represent these fully through annotations or symbols in the transcript. A further resource is

Box 11.1 *Computer-based analysis*

Virtually all of the procedures that are performed in the analysis of qualitative data can be performed on a computer. Specialist software programs have been developed – e.g. NUD.IST, Ethnograph, Hypersoft, WinMax – and there are now at least 20 such programs available (Dohan and Sánchez-Jankowski, 1998). The computer can search for and identify categories and store all of the associated databits. In a similar way, links between categories can be identified and stored. Hence, virtually at the press of a button, the analyst can call up all the data that relate to a particular category, or all data that are common to two or more specified categories. Even if quotations are extracted and examined in new combinations, the software program maintains the links with the appropriate parts of the parent transcripts. Some programs are adept at creating diagrams of the relationship between categories. If frequency counts are required, these are readily available (see Section 11.6). The computer can also keep a record of all the decisions taken and processes performed during analysis, thus facilitating a retrospective 'audit' of

the analysis process (Dey, 1993). Setting aside the time required to become acquainted with the software, the larger the dataset being analysed, the greater the economies of time and effort provided by computer analysis (Holloway and Wheeler, 1996). There is, however, a danger that the computer can handle more data than the analyst can (Dey, 1993). Perhaps the major drawback of computer-based analysis is that the process of analysis may be determined more by the facilities and procedures offered by the program concerned, than by the theoretical sensitivity of the analyst (Reid, 1992; Tak et al, 1999). On the other hand, Dohan and Sánchez-Jankowski (1998) suggest that the computer may prevent the researcher from being overwhelmed by his or her data, and thereby may make the process of analysis more manageable. Further discussion of the role of computer analysis can be found in a number of texts (e.g. Fielding and Lee, 1991, 1998; Reid, 1992; Dey, 1993; Miles and Huberman, 1994; Richards and Richards, 1994; Weitzman and Miles, 1995; Holloway and Wheeler, 1996; Gahan and Hannibal, 1998).

any reflective notes made during the process of data collection (see Section 10.1.3).

The process whereby textual data are analysed is often referred to as *content analysis*. This term was originally employed in reference to documentary data, but tends also to be used in relation to any form of textual data, including interview transcripts. Content analysis was originally quantitative, involving an analysis of the frequency of occurrence of certain elements in a text (Holsti, 1969; Weber, 1994). More recently, however, the term has been extended to denote qualitative forms of analysis (Holloway, 1997; Schwandt, 1997), as is the case in the present example.

The first stage in the process of analysis involves reading though the transcript and assigning sections of data to analytical *categories*. These sections of data, which Dey (1993) refers to as *databits*, may be a word or two, a phrase,

or one or more sentences. This process of category formation is referred to by some writers as *coding* (Strauss and Corbin, 1998; see Box 11.2), and the categories themselves are sometimes referred to as *themes* (Schmoll, 1993). The term 'theme' can, however, also be applied to levels of analysis above that of the individual category, such as a relationship between two or more categories (Section 11.4) or a taxonomy of categories (De Santis and Ugarizza, 2000).

At its simplest, category formation is a process of summarizing the data by identifying similarities and differences within them. An interview transcript represents a multitude of words, phrases, concepts and ideas. In their raw form, these would be impossible to analyse effectively. By searching for commonalities and contrasts within the data, while also preserving the individuality of informants' perspectives, more manageable elements are created for the process of analysis. The need for this is apparent if one considers the two extremes – either treating each piece of data as a wholly unique idea or, on the other hand, regarding each piece of data as part of a single overall notion. Each of these extremes would be an analytical dead end.

Box 11.2   *Open coding and axial coding*

In grounded theory, steps in the analysis process are given specific labels, and these are often encountered in accounts of research analysed according to this method. The process of category formation is known as *open coding*. This is defined as 'the process of breaking down, examining, comparing, conceptualizing, and contextualizing data' (Strauss and Corbin, 1990, p. 61). The process of linking categories to identify relationships between them is known as *axial coding*, and is defined as '[a] set of procedures whereby data are put back together in new ways after open coding, by making connections between categories' (Strauss and Corbin, 1990, p. 96).

The categories arrived at may represent fairly concrete ideas (e.g. 'overdose', 'diet', 'injury') or more abstract concepts (e.g. 'guilt', 'disapproval', 'ambivalence'). Miles and Huberman (1994) refer to the first type of category as *descriptive* and the second type as *interpretive*. A third type of category, which expresses how other categories relate to one another and may feature particularly in the later stages of analysis, could be described as *relational* (see Section 11.4).

Turning to the practicalities of category formation, an index card can be created for each category identified in this way. The title of the category, or the 'code', is written on the top of the card and is cross-referenced to the transcript. Thus, the number and page of the transcript on which the relevant databit occurs are entered on the index card. Similarly, the transcript is cross-referenced (in pencil) with the index card. However, it is advisable to mark the transcript

with a letter for the category, rather than the category itself, since there may be a number of changes in the label attached to the category. Notes can be made on the card as to the criteria used to assign databits to the category (*coding criteria*). These too may change. As new categories are identified, new cards are created, and when further examples of existing categories are encountered, additional cross-references are entered on the existing cards corresponding to these categories.

To illustrate, Emma's observation that 'it's not always clear ... whether someone's tried to kill themself or not' might be placed in a category labelled 'ambiguity'. Later, she comments that it is hard to understand 'why someone would wish to do away with themselves' and, in the second extract, Martine suggests that it hard to know what is really in the mind of a suicide. It might be felt that these databits also express a similar idea, and if so they would be added to the card labelled 'ambiguity' (Figure 11.2).

Emma also comments that the staff have 'mixed feelings' about suicides. This expresses a slightly different idea. The uncertainty here is not so much one relating to the staff's understanding of the motive for an act of suicide as to their feelings towards the individual. This databit probably belongs in a fresh category labelled 'ambivalence'. To take another example, when Dr Ganz reaches the transcript of the interview with Joanna, she encounters her comment 'you can never be sure exactly why someone's had a heart attack'. This seems to be another example of ambiguity, but the context is very different: it concerns myocardial infarction not suicide, and it is ambiguity as to aetiology rather than motivation. Here, Dr Ganz might have chosen to include this databit in the 'ambiguity' category. In the event, she decided to create a new category to reflect the rather different nature of this databit, with the label 'aetiology and diagnosis'. Notice, however, that Dr Ganz has cross-referenced the two cards to remind herself that there is a potential analytical link between them (Figure 11.3).

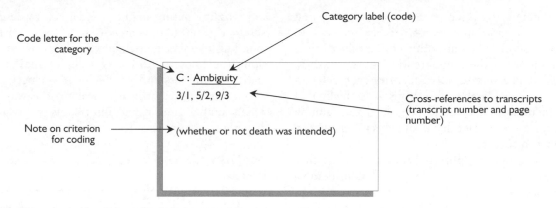

Figure 11.2 *An example of an index card.*

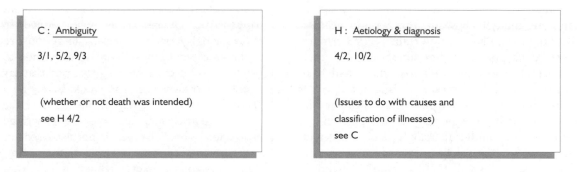

Figure 11.3 *Cross-referencing of index cards.*

Often, a particular databit may appropriately be subsumed under more than one category. For example, Emma's statement 'I think one reason why the staff's got mixed feelings about the suicides is because it's so hard to understand' could be categorized under the 'ambivalence' category and also under a category such as 'incomprehensibility', which expresses the idea that suicide is hard for others to understand.

11.2.1 Desirable features of an analytical category

What, then, are the attributes of a 'good' analytical category? Above all, it should be faithful to the data – Dey (1993) refers to this as the *internal* aspect of a category, and it is one of the core principles of grounded theory. In addition, it should be meaningful to other categories –

which Dey (1993) calls its *external aspect*. It should be possible to construct theoretically relevant relationships between categories. This may depend upon striking the appropriate balance between generality and specificity (Skelton, 1997). A very broad category, such as 'self-inflicted illness', is unlikely to permit many interesting theoretical relationships to be generated, since it does not reflect the variety of such illnesses and the theoretically relevant distinctions that might be drawn among them. In contrast, a category such as 'hang-gliding' refers to just one example of a broader category of 'hazardous leisure activity', and as such is probably too specific to play a part in a theoretical relationship.

A category should also strike the right balance between inclusivity and exclusivity in relation to the databits to which it refers. A category that refers to a large number of databits may fail to discern subtle but important conceptual distinctions between these apparently similar databits. Equally, if a number of categories each refer to just a single databit, this leads to a feeling of fragmentation and may suggest that common themes in the data have not been adequately identified (Glaser, 1992).

It is important not to be dogmatic on this, however. Sometimes ideas of considerable interest and theoretical significance may be expressed only once, and by the same token, on occasions a specific idea may genuinely be represented by numerous databits. That which occurs repeatedly is not necessarily theoretically significant, and that which occurs rarely is not necessarily theoretically unimportant. Furthermore, some concepts may be significant by their absence. For example, suppose there had been no mention of the notion of blame in any of Dr Ganz's interview transcripts. This is a theme that would have been expected to arise, given the topic of the study. It may not be sufficient, therefore, to rely solely on the data to identify categories, as this will exclude 'empty' categories that are theoretically important even though not represented in the data. The researcher's own expectations – which should generally be bracketed (see Section 11.1) – can be called up to form a comparison with categories that have emerged from the data.

11.3 LABELLING AND REVISING CATEGORIES

Choosing a label for a category is not a straightforward process. According to Lofland (1976) a distinction can be drawn between *member-generated* and *observer-generated* categories. A member-generated category is one that is expressed in the phraseology and concepts of the informants, whereas an observer-generated category is one generated by the researcher (Box 11.3). The use of the label 'ambiguity' when describing the uncertainty surrounding the would-be suicide's intentions, and the use of 'incomprehensibility' to refer to the unfamiliar

and puzzling nature of the suicidal act, represent observer-generated categories. The corresponding member-generated categories might be along the lines of 'did they want to die?' and 'hard to understand', which are closer to (though not necessarily identical to) the way in which Emma and other informants expressed their thoughts or attitudes on this issue.

Box 11.3 *Member-generated and observer-generated categories*

Qualitative data analysts differ in their views on the relative appropriateness of these two kinds of categories. Much will depend upon the sort of theoretical account that the researcher seeks to construct. A researcher who wished to understand lay decision making in relation to health care would most likely be concerned to produce an account of the processes that lay people themselves use. This would largely be a *first-order* account, framed in the terms of the research participants, and member-generated categories would be an important element within this. In contrast, a study of the professional ideologies expressed in health care textbooks might seek to generate a *second-order* account, expressed in more abstract theoretical terms at a remove from the actual words used in the raw data. Observer-generated categories would have an important part to play here.

In general, however, there is a tendency to use member-generated categories in the early stages of analysis, and to substitute observer-generated categories as analysis proceeds (Hammersley and Atkinson, 1995). This reflects the way in which categories are provisional and subject to ongoing reappraisal and revision. It also accords with the process depicted in Figure 11.1, in which the process of analysis moves from raw data towards more abstract theory. It follows, therefore, that the researcher needs to attain both closeness to and distance from the data, moving back and forth between these two standpoints. A process of 'immersion' in the data is important in order to grasp the often subtle meanings that lie within them. At the same time, identifying theoretical concepts and relationships requires the researcher to stand back from the data and the specific context from which they were gathered (Bryman, 1988). Richards (1998, p. 324) describes the process thus:

> *Qualitative research requires an in-out process; researchers have to achieve and manage both ways of zooming in and ways of achieving a wide-angle view.*

11.3.1 Joining and dividing categories

When analytical categories are reviewed, three things may become apparent. Sometimes, new data may suggest that existing categories need a degree of adjustment. Thus, Joanna suggests on more than one occasion that it is often unclear what is in the minds of people who incur apparently self-inflicted illnesses or injuries. This idea seems to belong to the 'ambiguity' category created from data in the interviews with Emma and Martine. However, this category does not relate to suicide, and the coding criterion therefore needs to be changed from 'whether or not death was intended' to something broader, such as 'the intention or motivation of an action'.

Alternatively, the researcher may decide that what is at present a single category should be divided into two or more categories. For example, Dr Ganz might notice that the category 'moral censure' represents two separate phenomena. Sometimes staff *express* their moral censure, such as in the 'snide comments' that Emma describes, whereas on other occasions they *enact* their criticism, as in Emma's later description of the apparently punitive manner in which a nurse passes a gastric tube on an overdose patient. This category would therefore

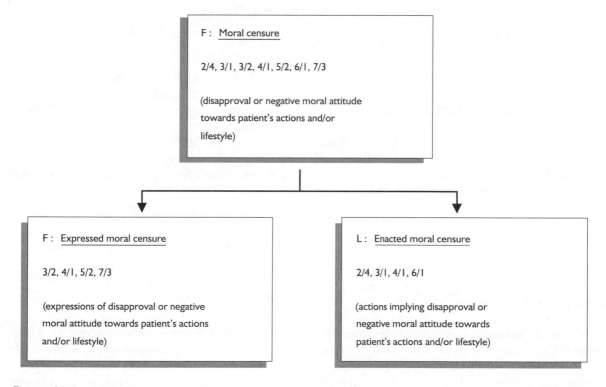

Figure 11.4 *Splitting categories.*

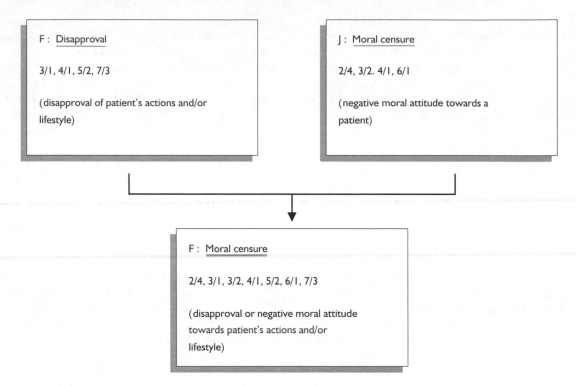

Figure 11.5   *Splicing categories.*

be divided into two (Figure 11.4).

The third possibility is that some categories that were initially regarded as separate may seem not to be distinct after all. For example, in analysing her interview transcripts, Dr Ganz might have identified two categories relating to the students' reaction to patients with self-inflicted conditions: 'disapproval' and 'moral censure'. On re-examining the databits associated with these categories, she might well decide that they are all expressing the same idea and decide to merge the two categories (Figure 11.5). If one category has been subsumed by another, as in this example, the newly formed category may bear the same label as one of the original categories. Sometimes, however, the new category may express a somewhat different meaning from that of either of the original categories, in which case a new label is likely to be required. As categories are joined, the resulting category

is likely to be at a higher level of abstraction than those from which it has developed, and thus merged categories tend to be observer-generated categories.

Dey (1993) refers to these processes of merging and dividing categories as *splicing* and *splitting*, respectively. He summarizes their purposes as follows:

> *We split categories in a search for greater resolution and detail and splice them in a search for greater integration and scope. The fewer and more powerful our categories, the more intelligible and coherent our analysis*
>
> (Dey, 1993, p. 139)

It can be seen from Figures 11.4 and 11.5 that when categories are either split or spliced, the index cards are amended accordingly. The transcript cross-references are either amalgamated or split, the category labels and code letters are changed as appropriate, and the coding criteria are revised. Additionally, the cross-references to the code letters that appear on the transcripts themselves should be updated. Note that, in the case of splitting (Figure 11.4), although most databits will probably relate to one or other of the new categories, some may relate to both of the new categories.

11.3.2 Creating definitive categories

Sometimes it is necessary to establish fairly definitive coding criteria for a set of categories. This may be required when more than one analyst is working on a project and it is desirable that the data are categorized in an agreed, consistent manner. In a situation such as this, analysis probably needs to take place in two stages. After the researchers involved have analysed a certain amount of data independently, they can meet and compare their categories and the criteria whereby data have been assigned to them. Through discussion and negotiation, a single set of categories and criteria can be generated, and used to analyse the remaining data. In this way, the problems associated with creating a set of categories prior to analysis are avoided, since categories are finalized only when they have emerged from the data. In fact, 'definitive' and 'finalized' may not be the right words, since even agreed categories and criteria should be modified if necessary.

11.4 DEVELOPING THEORETICAL PROPOSITIONS

In Section 2.4 it was pointed out that a theory will contain within it a number of theoretical propositions, which state relationships between certain theoretical concepts. It follows that if a theory is to be constructed in the process of data analysis, the categories (i.e. the concepts) identified need to be linked to form relationships between them (i.e. theoretical propositions). The use of index cards facilitates the exploration of these relationships, since they can be laid out in various ways to represent possible groupings or links between them. A copy of the transcripts

themselves can also be cut up, so that the relationships between key quotations can be compared in a similar way.

There are a number of possible relationships that may exist between categories (and thereby between concepts). It is worth noting that some of these relationships between concepts can themselves be regarded as categories (relational categories); they may also be referred to as themes (Section 11.2). The relationships that may be discerned include:

- juxtaposition: some categories may occur together
- non-juxtaposition: some categories may tend *not* to occur in proximity to one another
- similarity: one category may be likened, explicitly or implicitly, to another
- contrast: one category may be contrasted, explicitly or implicitly, with another
- means-end: two or more categories may be linked in terms of purposes and intended results
- causation: two or more categories may be linked in a cause-effect relationship (see Box 11.4)
- explanation: one category may be used in an explanatory role with respect to another category.

If we turn to the transcripts, we can see some examples of these relationships. The concepts of choice and suicide appear together on a number of occasions ('juxtaposition'). Joanna suggests that drug overdoses and motorcycling injuries are comparable in terms of being self-inflicted ('similarity'), but draws a distinction between taking a drug overdose and mistakenly drinking carbolic ('contrast'). As an example of the 'causation' relationship, Joanna proposes diet and alcohol as potential causes of heart disease and cirrhosis of the liver. Meanwhile, Martine contends that a desire not to be a burden may result in some people's suicide attempts, and Emma expresses the view that staff's ambivalent feelings towards suicides may arise from the incomprehensible nature of the suicidal act. A

Box 11.4   *The notion of causation in qualitative analysis*

When qualitative data are analysed, relationships of cause and effect will often emerge from the data. These are *subjective* notions of causation. They represent informants' perceptions of the factors they regard as having generated or influenced actions or events in their lives. This view of causation is a very different matter from trying to establish *objective* cause-effect relationships by means of isolating certain potentially causative factors and testing their effect on an outcome, such as occurs in a controlled experiment. It is unlikely that studies based purely on the analysis of qualitative data will establish the existence of such objective causal relationships, though they may do much to elucidate the precise way in which such relationships operate, once they have been identified through other methods.

'means-end' relationship can be discerned in several of Martine's comments about the intentions of would-be suicides, or in Emma's account of the apparently punitive intentions of the 'over-enthusiastic' nurse.

A relationship of 'explanation' is often rather more complex. Figure 11.6 depicts the contrast drawn by Joanna between the high-risk activities of a professional footballer and those of a mountaineer. This relationship of contrast is in turn explained by the concept of 'choice'. Similarly,

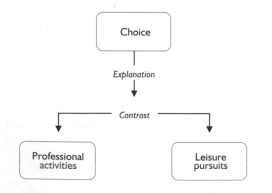

Figure 11.6   *An example of an 'explanation' relationship.*

Martine suggests that there is a contrast between the *result* of an anorexic patient's failure to eat, and the *motive* for this; this may be explained by the concept of 'body image' to which she then refers.

Some relationships between categories will emerge readily from the data. Sometimes, however, the researcher may find it hard to interpret the data in other than a very literal way. Theoretically important insights may simply not strike the analyst, possibly because of the familiarity of the subject matter and his or her common-sense assumptions. At such times, some form of lateral thinking is required, such as what might be called *counterfactual analysis*. This involves focusing on what is *not* present in the data – events that did not occur, views that were not expressed, situations that did not obtain, and so forth. A technique of this sort advocated by Strauss and Corbin (1998) is the *flip-flop*. Here, the researcher seeks insights by imagining that the data were expressing the opposite of what they actually are, or by conceptualizing a situation very different from the one under consideration (a counterfactual case). By way of example, Strauss and Corbin (1998) suggest that a greater understanding of the world of teenage drug use may be gained by imagining that access to drugs was a complex and difficult process, rather than the relatively straightforward and easy process that it is. In the current example, Dr Ganz might find it helpful to explore the meanings attached to self-inflicted illness by imagining a situation in which a patient's condition could *not* conceivably be seen as self-inflicted, for example victims of natural disasters or terrorism. This may suggest new ways to explore her data in an imaginative way.

The relationships that have been outlined are, of course, based on just three extracts from interviews. However, we can see how they might form the basis of certain theoretical propositions relating to patients with putatively self-inflicted illness. For example, the students' attitudes to self-inflicted illness appear to be conditioned by their perception of the degree of choice or autonomy that patients were able to exercise over their actions or the factors that may have led to their condition. Moreover, the care received by these patients would seem on occasions to be influenced by the moral acceptability of their lifestyles.

11.4.1 Saturation

Ultimately, a point will be reached in the process of analysis when examining further data does not add to the insights already gained, in terms of either the identification of new categories or the discovery of new relationships between existing categories. At this point, the analytical framework is said to be *saturated*, and further analysis is not strictly necessary. If, as is often the case, fresh data are being gathered in parallel with the process of analysis, this means that, for example, further interviews need not be conducted. Similarly, if there are interviews still to be transcribed, this may not be necessary after all. However, one can never be certain what unexamined data may reveal, and if there are a manageable number of already-transcribed interviews remaining, it may be advisable to analyse these even though saturation appears to have been achieved. It is always possible that one or more of these interviews will add an unexpected, one-off insight.

The achievement of saturation is not determined by the *amount* of data gathered, as is the case when sampling for statistical purposes (Morse, 1995). The determinant of saturation is the *nature* of the relationships that have been revealed between categories. If these are rich and theoretically informative, and if they are not significantly modified by the analysis of further data, saturation has occurred, irrespective of the amount of data that has hitherto been analysed.

11.4.2 Keeping notes

Throughout the process of analysis, it is helpful to keep a record of the theoretical and methodological decisions made (Wainwright, 1994). Not only does this clarify the process of analysis at the time, but it also facilitates a retrospective audit of this process. Strauss and Corbin (1998,

p. 217) refer to such notes as *memos*, which they define as 'written records ... that contain the products of analysis or directions for the analyst'. They also advocate the use of *diagrams*, to depict visually the relationships among concepts.

Memos are similar in purpose to the reflective notes made during the process of data collection (Section 10.1.3). They may include the coding criteria used to assign databits to categories, observations on possible relationships between categories, plans for further data collection, and various forms of more abstract theorizing. Orona (1997) provides an interesting account of her use of memos in the study of Alzheimer's disease. She highlights three key purposes that they fulfilled.

First, they allowed a speculative form of 'free association' when reading her interview transcripts:

> *I allowed myself the freedom to say whatever I wanted, in whatever form seemed to flow. I did not attempt to be grammatically correct or to find sociological terms to describe what I was thinking ... I went with an idea without monitoring or making judgments about it.*
>
> (Orona, 1997, p. 180)

Second, the memos allowed Orona to 'unblock' her thought processes when she found it hard to clarify her thinking when analysing her data. The memos were written as though to another analyst, and new insights and clarification often resulted from this 'dialogue'. Third, memos served to document the process of conceptual and theoretical thinking:

> *I used memos to document the beginnings of a conceptualization which had emerged from the data, 'tracking' its levels from the raw data (words used by the respondents) to my notes in the coding and finally, to the concept.*
>
> (Orona, 1997, p. 180)

Charmaz (1995) recommends that memos should be written spontaneously and without editing, so as to preserve the researcher's own voice in the memo and thereby to capture more accurately the thought processes occurring in his or her mind at the time. Memos should be dated, so that they can be re-examined in the context of a particular stage of a study (Corbin, 1986).

11.5 THE ROLE OF JUDGEMENT IN QUALITATIVE ANALYSIS

The basis for the assignment of datahits to categories and the subsequent formation of relationships between categories is the researcher's own judgement. This involves the researcher in responding personally to the data (Jones, 1985b) – using his or her intuition, imagination and, at times, empathy. The criteria whereby data are categorized emerge from a reading of the data themselves and are not predetermined in the way that is usual when coding a questionnaire. The researcher therefore has considerable scope for creativity, which is an important element in the process of analysis (Strauss and Corbin, 1998). The challenge for the researcher, however, is to ensure that the process of interpretation is used to understand the meanings expressed by the informants, rather than to project his or her own meanings on to the data. The interpretation of the data should be imaginative without being fanciful, personal without being idiosyncratic, and creative without losing an analytical perspective.

One way to try to strike the correct balance is to stay in close contact with the data. This is in accordance with the principles of the constant comparative method in grounded theory. By returning frequently to the actual words used by informants, the researcher can check that insights and inferences are substantiated by the data. Thus, the grounded theory approach advocates that any insights or hypotheses that suggest themselves to the analyst should immediately be tested by turning back to the raw data.

Similarly, it is often recommended that the researcher should, as far as possible, use *low-inference descriptors* when analysing data. A low-inference description is one that is expressed largely in terms of the words and concepts of research informants and participants, with the minimum of higher-level interpretation. The use of member-generated categories, described in Section 11.3, is in keeping with this principle.

An important part of returning to the data is the search for what are known as *negative cases*. Insights that are developed from the data are regarded as tentative hypotheses, and an attempt is made to disconfirm them by re-examining the data for datahits that seem to disconfirm these hypotheses. This reinforces the way in which the emerging theory is grounded in the data (see Box 11.5). The characteristics of negative cases may also shed important light on those cases that do fit the general pattern. Bailey (1997) gives the example of a rehabilitation programme that most participants complete successfully, subsequently returning to work. An analysis of the few patients who drop out of the programme may provide insights about the reasons why the majority see it through (compare the discussion of counterfactual analysis in Section 11.4).

Box 11.5 *'Hypotheses' in qualitative analysis*

Although researchers may talk of developing hypotheses during the analysis of qualitative data from exploratory studies, this is a very different notion of 'hypothesis' from that used in explanatory studies. An exploratory study does not stem from a hypothesis but from a fairly broad research question, and its purpose remains one of theory building, not theory testing as in an explanatory study. The fact that the analyst may develop tentative hypotheses as part of the analysis process in an exploratory study does not mean that such a study should be described as a hypothesis-testing study.

There is, therefore, a crucial balance to be struck. On the one hand, the analyst should move from the concrete reality of the data to higher levels of abstraction, so as to generate imaginative theoretical prepositions. On the other hand, the analyst must not move too far from the data, so that these propositions are firmly substantiated by what has actually been said or taken place.

It should not be inferred from this, however, that there is a single 'correct' interpretation of a particular text or account. Any account will be susceptible of a number of readings (Burman, 1994a), reflecting the fact that different analysts will bring different types of response to the data. One reading may well be more plausible than others, particularly in terms of its relationship to the data, but that is not to say that it has attained some sort of final truth.

11.6 TO QUANTIFY OR NOT?

Strictly, qualitative analysis is, by definition, a process that does not seek to quantify data. Many qualitative analysts are therefore wholly opposed to the use of numbers or other quantities when describing or analysing qualitative data. There is, nonetheless, justification for a limited use of quantification in the analysis of qualitative data (Silverman, 1985, 1993).

It is quite difficult to conduct any form of qualitative analysis without at some point making statements such as 'many respondents suggested that ...', 'this theme recurred frequently in the transcripts', 'occasionally, respondents reacted defensively to any suggestion that ...'. Indeed, it is not easy for someone reading a report of an exploratory study based on qualitative data to get a feeling of these data without some such indication of the prevalence of a certain concept or theme. Hence, it may be appropriate to quantify the *frequency* with which certain themes occur in the data. Furthermore, the identification or construction of theoretical propositions from categories may sometimes depend on some form of basic quantification. Hence, Dey (1993, pp. 179–180) argues that

it is difficult to see how, in practice, it is possible to identify associations between categories or to assess the strength of relationships without recourse to a numerical evaluation. If we are looking for substantive connections between categories which are 'contingent' (i.e. not true by definition), then we should be concerned to make an empirical (and numerical) assessment of our evidence. If we want to claim that transposition of temperament results in infliction of suffering on patients, we want to know whether and how far the evidence supports this connection.

Silverman (1985, p. 147) provides an example of how simple frequency counts may elucidate relationships between concepts. Reporting the findings of a study of the management of children with Down's syndrome, he notes that in a random sample of ten consultations with affected children, the doctor made reference to the child's 'wellness' on only one occasion (10%) while initiating the consultation. In contrast, 'wellness' was referred to in the initiation of 13 out of 22 cases (59%) involving unaffected children.

It would seem, therefore, that some forms of frequency count may be an appropriate part of qualitative analysis. There are, however, some caveats to be considered here. First, it has already been suggested that the frequency with which a category or a relationship occurs is not necessarily a direct index of its importance, either to respondents or to the analyst. Although issues that are significant may often be mentioned more often than those that are less important, this may not always be the case.

Second, it is particularly important to be wary of judging the *relative* significance of two or more categories by such means (e.g. to suggest that informants found a certain issue more important than another simply because they referred to it more frequently). There are many other factors that may influence the frequency with which an issue is referred to, such as its perceived social acceptability, the emotional associations it may hold for the informant, or certain interpersonal aspects of the interview process.

Third, although it may be appropriate to

comment on the strength or intensity with which an attitude or an emotion may be expressed by a particular informant, it can be unwise to attempt to make comparisons of magnitude *between* informants' accounts. The way in which an informant expresses his or her feelings and perceptions has an individuality that markedly limits the extent to which this account can be compared with another, in quantitative terms, on a common scale of measurement. In other words, these accounts are at least partially *incommensurable*. Hence, if Dr Ganz wished to compare her informants in terms of their acceptance of patients with deviant or morally questionable ways of life, it would be difficult on the basis of the interview transcripts to generate an accurate ranking of informants on this dimension. At best, some tentative and fairly crude judgements of degrees of acceptance could be made.

Finally, the researcher should not allow the uniqueness of specific databits to be lost in the desire to produce tallies within themes; as Britten and Fisher (1993, p. 271) point out, '[i]t is inappropriate to force complex responses into simple categories in order to count them'.

11.7 CONCLUSION

This chapter has examined some of the principles and procedures of analysing qualitative data generated from exploratory studies. It is important to remember that there is no single correct way in which to approach the analysis of such data. Moreover, many researchers tend not to follow a single set of precepts when analysing qualitative data, but follow a more eclectic approach, geared to their particular theoretical and empirical concerns. Whatever strategy is adopted, the general issues explored in this chapter – such as the development of theoretical propositions and the use of intuition and judgement – will need to be considered. Moreover, as with all forms of data, the methods by which data are collected – as outlined in Chapter 5 – should be compatible with the way in which they will be analysed.

12 PRESENTING DATA FROM DESCRIPTIVE AND EXPLANATORY STUDIES

SUMMARY

This chapter explores the following topics:

- the role of descriptive statistics
- the levels of measurement associated with numerical data
- appropriate summaries for data at each level of measurement
- presentation of summaries of quantitative data

Earlier chapters have discussed the interrelationships between the research question, methodology, design and data collection in a study. In general, descriptive and explanatory research questions lead to the collection of data in the form of numbers (Chapter 4). To many researchers, these numbers (often referred to as *raw data*) appear to be a frightening maelstrom of information without order or meaning. If they are to be used to inform health care practice, these raw data must be organized, summarized and presented in a form that succinctly communicates their important features and their underlying meaning. This chapter introduces the methodological and technical issues underlying this process. Since most researchers will use a statistical computing package to organize the data and to perform all the calculations, we will not present details on how to perform calculations manually.

12.1 THE ROLE OF DESCRIPTIVE STATISTICS

The word 'statistics' has several meanings. In everyday use, it stands for numerical facts; e.g. number of births, number of deaths, tax rates. Many numerical facts that are compiled routinely are published as official statistics (for example,

unemployment trends) and used as a basis for decision making. Statistics is also a discipline that helps the researcher to make sense of numerical data collected from groups of units or cases, where these might be people, items, objects, institutions or geographical regions. It is a tool and, in common with all tools, its usefulness depends upon the researchers knowing when, why and how to use it. Further distinctions can be made within the discipline of statistics. *Descriptive statistics* are methods for collecting, organizing, summarizing and presenting numerical data (Gissane, 1998). When the data comprise all relevant information from the population of interest (a rare situation in practice), the raw data can be condensed to a few quantities called *parameters*. These parameters convey the important features of the population (for example, mean, standard deviation and skewness) and also enable comparisons to be made across different populations. When the data comprise a sample of relevant information from the population of interest (the more likely situation in reality), the descriptive summaries calculated from the sample are called *statistics*. *Inferential statistics* are used to generalize from samples to populations and will be dealt with in later chapters (Chapters 13, 14 and 18).

Descriptive statistics serve two main purposes. The first is to organize and summarize numerical data so that their important features are presented clearly and succinctly in tables and visual displays (also referred to as *diagrams*, *charts* or *graphs*). This might be the extent of the analysis for some fairly straightforward descriptive research questions. The second purpose is to aid the more detailed statistical analysis associated with more complex descriptive research questions and explanatory research questions. In this case, the diagrams might provide an insight into the structure of the data or a check on assumptions necessary to perform a particular analysis. In such a situation, the permissible methods of analysis are dependent upon the levels at which variables are measured. Although this is a very basic concept within statistics, it is central to almost all decisions regarding statistical analysis. Hence, it will be considered in some detail in the following section.

12.2 LEVELS OF MEASUREMENT

Numbers result from the measurement of variables within a study. The nature of the characteristic being measured determines the rules for assigning these numbers, and these rules then determine the methods that are appropriate to organize and summarize the numbers. A commonly used typology for the rules was proposed by Stevens (1946) and categorizes measurements according to four major classes or levels of measurement: nominal, ordinal, interval and ratio (see Box 12.1). These levels reflect the quantity of information conveyed by the measurements, from the simplest to the highest, respectively.

Box 12.1   *Controversy over levels of measurement*

There is controversy over the conventional approach to levels of measurement developed by Stevens. The debate has been going on since about 1951, when Stevens first published work on the transformations and statistics permissible at each level (Stevens, 1951). A convention establishes the scale properties of a measure, with the implication that different conventions lead to different permissible statistical methods on the same data. A method valid under one convention might be invalid under another. Nunnally and Bernstein (1994) summarize the argument. We follow Stevens' approach in this text, but common practices are discussed.

The main characteristics of the four levels of measurement are given in Table 12.1; allowable

mathematical operations and transformations can be found in Nunnally and Bernstein (1994).

12.2.1 Nominal level of measurement

Nominal is the lowest level of measurement. Two of the questions used in the Rheumatoid Arthritis Study – 'What is your profession?' and 'In the past 12 months, have you seen patients/clients with a confirmed diagnosis of rheumatoid arthritis?' – are examples of questions associated with variables on a nominal level of measurement. In the first example, each therapist who responds is categorized as either an 'occupational therapist' or a 'physiotherapist' according to which response option is ticked. These two categories cover all possibilities in this study, since the questionnaire is sent only to members of these two professions. No therapist should tick both response options. Hence, it is an easy task to count how many occupational therapists and how many physiotherapists responded. The professions could be presented in any order; an alphabetical order is used here. This information is simplified for entry into a computing package by using a number (e.g. 1) for every occupational therapist and a different number (e.g. 2) for every physiotherapist. These numbers are labels or codes and have no quantitative meaning: any numbers could be used. Similar comments apply to the second example in which the response ('yes' or 'no') is used to categorize each respondent according to whether or not, within the past 12 months, the therapist has seen patients/clients with a confirmed diagnosis of rheumatoid arthritis.

Thus, at a nominal level of measurement, numbers represent labels for unique categories into which persons or items can be classified. The numbers have no intrinsic quantitative meaning and can be chosen arbitrarily without affecting the information. They are used as codes for entering the data into a computing package. The categories can be presented in any order. They must be defined so that:

- all cases with the same characteristics are assigned the same number

Table 12.1 Main characteristics of the four levels of measurement

Level	Examples	Zero point	Relationship of scale points	Permissible arithmetic operations	Continuity	Hierarchy	Categorization
Ratio	Duration (hours), distance (cm), weight (kg), angle (degrees), temperature (K)	Zero on the scale represents a true zero point	Equal differences between scale points have equal meaning	Multiplication, division, addition, subtraction, counts	Continuous or discrete	Represent a rank order among cases	Classify cases into mutually exclusive and collectively exhaustive categories
Interval	Intelligence (IQ), temperature (°C, °F).	Zero on the scale represents an arbitrary zero point		Addition, subtraction, counts			
Ordinal	Agreement (Likert scale), pain (verbal rating scale), occupational grade, social class, duration/distance, etc. (measured on adjectival ranking scale)		Equal differences between scale points do not necessarily have equal meaning	Counts	Discrete		
Nominal	Sex, ethnicity, profession, diagnostic category	Zero on the scale has no quantitative meaning	Differences are not calculable, since scale has no quantitative meaning			No rank order between categories	

- cases with different characteristics are assigned different numbers
- every case can be assigned only one such number (i.e. the categories are *mutually exclusive*)
- all plausible characteristics are associated with a number (i.e. the categories are *collectively exhaustive*).

12.2.2 Ordinal level of measurement

Ordinal is the next level of measurement in the hierarchy. Here, numbers convey unique categories of membership, as in the case of the nominal level of measurement, but also a rank order for the categories. Higher numbers indicate progressively more of some characteristic (or less of some characteristic, depending upon the selected coding), but the numbers have no meaning in a mathematical sense and it is not possible to quantify the increments. For example, the measurement of attitudes is frequently performed at an ordinal level using a Likert scale with categories 'strongly agree', 'agree', 'neither', 'disagree' and 'strongly disagree', which might be coded as 5, 4, 3, 2 and 1, respectively (see section 15.2.1). The numbers 1 to 5 reflect progressively stronger levels of agreement with a statement. A person responding 'agree' (coded as 4) does not necessarily have twice as much agreement as another person who responds 'disagree' (coded as 2). In fact, two individuals who 'agree' with the statement will have selected that option based on their own individual perception of that level in relation to the other choices of response. Therefore, although both responses would be coded as 4, the true strengths of agreement might differ. A change in attitude following an intervention might be from 1 to 2 for one person and from 4 to 5 for another person – seemingly equal shifts. However, a change in attitude from 'strongly disagree' to 'disagree' cannot be assumed to equate with a change from 'agree' to 'strongly agree'. Satisfaction (rated as 'highly satisfied' through to 'highly dissatisfied'), balance (rated as 'good', 'fair', 'poor') and ability to perform activities of daily living (rated as 'with no difficulty', 'with some difficulty', 'with great difficulty' and 'unable to do') are further examples using an ordinal level of measurement (see Box 12.2).

12.2.3 Interval level of measurement

Numbers on an interval level of measurement define distinct categories of information, are ordered according to rank, and also possess the property of known and equidistant intervals between the units of measurement. Temperature in degrees Celsius or Fahrenheit and many educational tests are measured at an interval level. A temperature of 10°C is lower than 15°C, which is lower than 20°C. The temperatures convey more information than just this rank ordering. A temperature of 15°C is 5° higher than 10°C (i.e. the intervals are known). Further, the difference between 10°C and 15°C is equal in some sense to the difference between 15°C and 20°C (i.e. the intervals are equidistant). However, zero on the Celsius scale is not an absolute or true zero indicating no molecular motion. Therefore, 20°C is not twice as hot as 10°C.

Summative rating scales (see Section 15.2.1) comprise many individual items usually at an ordinal level of measurement. Summing the responses (or numbers) across the individual items forms a scale score. It is common practice to assume that this score is at an interval level of measurement (Spector, 1992; Pett, 1997).

12.2.4 Ratio level of measurement

Ratio is the highest level of measurement. The numbers possess all the properties of those at an interval level, with the addition of a true or absolute zero (representing total absence of the characteristic being measured). Many physical variables are measured at a ratio level, for example, height (m), weight (kg), blood pressure (mm Hg), lung capacity (cc), range of joint movement (degrees) and temperature (K or kelvin). A weight of 60 kg is twice as heavy as a weight of 30 kg. A temperature of 200 K is twice as hot as 100 K, since 0 K is an absolute zero representing no molecular motion. Time, distance and force are usually measured on a ratio scale.

Box 12.2 *Data at nominal or ordinal levels and 'qualitative' data*

Some writers, such as Haber and Runyon (1977) and Last (1988), explicitly refer to the nominal and ordinal levels of measurement as 'qualitative'. Others, such as Coggon (1995), do so implicitly by excluding these levels of measurement from the description 'quantitative'. There is, admittedly, some justification for this terminology, but it is misleading in two ways. First, data at an ordinal level of measurement are hierarchical. Although it is true to say that data at this level denote 'position in an ordered series' (Haber and Runyon, 1977, p. 23), in many cases they also express a sense of degree or magnitude, and to that extent are performing a quantitative function. Thus, a five-point scale running from 'strongly agree' to 'strongly disagree' conveys the respondent's degree of agreement, and a scale of occupational grades denotes the degree of seniority of each practitioner. Similarly, pain intensity expressed on a verbal rating scale indicates how much pain the patient is experiencing. Second, to describe nominal level data as 'qualitative' invites confusion with the way in which this term is used in much exploratory research (see Chapter 10). Essentially, data at a nominal level only represent a process of categorization (with, perhaps, frequency counts based on such categorization). In exploratory approaches, the data usually have a far richer descriptive meaning that that of simply expressing differences in category, and frequency counts are not usually a central element within their analysis. Moreover, the epistemological assumptions that underlie the collection and analysis of data in these studies are radically different from those underlying the statistical analysis of nominal-level data. For example, in the latter approach, cases placed in the same nominal category are taken to be equivalent. In contrast, data from an exploratory study that are placed in a single category are considered to retain an essential individuality of meaning derived from the informant's own unique framework of perceptions, and to that extent cannot sensibly be regarded as equivalent. Hence, referring to data at the nominal or ordinal level of measurement as 'qualitative' is best avoided. In other texts (e.g. Altman, 1991a; Daniel, 1991; Bland, 1995), data at a nominal level of measurement are also referred to as 'categorical' as distinct from 'numerical'. This terminology is also best avoided, since there is a sense in which *all* numerical data are categorical. For example, all persons aged between 80 and 89 years are octogenarians. In fact, each level of measurement has all the properties of the weaker (or lower) levels.

In many (though not all) statistical analyses, the distinction between interval and ratio levels of measurement is not a crucial one.

12.2.5 Deciding upon the level of measurement

The optimal level of measurement for each variable in a study will depend upon the nature of the variable, the research question (or hypothesis), resources such as time, money and the skills of the researcher, and the availability of existing standard measurement tools. The implications of a chosen level of measurement for permissible statistical methods and generalizability of findings need to be pursued at the design stage. Other things being equal, the higher levels of measurement contain more information, support a greater choice of permissible statistical methods and can be collapsed to lower levels (if necessary) at the summary or analysis stage. It should be noted that we cannot raise measurements to a higher level than that at which the data were collected.

12.2.6 Discrete and continuous variables

Variables that can be assigned numerical values can be classified as either discrete or *continuous*. *Discrete* variables are those for which there are a countable number of distinct and separate possible values. They are usually counts, some function of counts (e.g. percentages or ratios of counts), or numbers reflecting some system of artificial grading (Armitage and Berry, 1994). Examples in the data from the Rheumatoid Arthritis Study include: the number of clients seen in the last 12 months who have a confirmed diagnosis of rheumatoid arthritis, the proportion of weekly clinics that are usually attended by clients with rheumatoid arthritis, and the assessment of pain on an 11-point scale from 0 ('no pain'), 1, 2 . . . up to 10 ('pain as bad as can be imagined'). *Continuous* variables are those for which, in theory, there is an infinite number of possible values within a specified range. Examples include weight, joint range and body temperature. In reality, the resolution of a measuring instrument limits the precision with which continuous variables can be measured – for example, whether the scales are graduated in kilograms, grams or milligrams. Similarly, a decision may be made to measure a respondent's age only to the nearest year (e.g. age last birthday).

Hence, although an underlying *variable* may be continuous, the *scale* on which it is measured may be discrete. A discrete variable can, of course, only be measured on a discrete scale. Nonetheless, Nunnally and Bernstein (1994) suggest that, based on experience, if a discrete variable is measured on a scale with 11 or more distinct values, such a variable can be treated in the way that we would a continuous variable. Thus, when a continuous variable is measured on a discrete scale, or when a discrete variable can take on many distinct values, it is important to distinguish carefully between the intrinsic measurement properties of the variable and those of the scale on which it may be measured.

12.3 SUMMARIZING DATA MEASURED AT A NOMINAL OR ORDINAL LEVEL

The first step in any analysis of data is to examine each variable separately (Munro, 1997). This creates an overall picture of the sample and, through this, the researcher begins to understand the data. Later, two or more variables might be considered jointly, especially when this is necessary to address a research question.

12.3.1 Counts and percentages

Data at a nominal or ordinal level of measurement can be summarized in a table that contains the categories, the number of units (or cases) in each category, and the corresponding percentage of the total number of units in the study. That is, the summary describes how many units are associated with a specific response to a question or possess a specific attribute. The individual response from every unit is apparent in this summary.

In the simplest situation there are two responses at a nominal level of measurement, for example, responses to the following question from the Rheumatoid Arthritis Study:

Profession   Occupational therapist   ☐ 1
             Physiotherapist   ☐ 2

An appropriate summary is given in Table 12.2. Categorizing respondents according to profession creates a simple variable for which the main features are obvious from the table, and a graph would not provide any further insight. In this study, 41% (61) of the respondents were occupational therapists and 59% (89) were physiotherapists.

The percentage figures have enabled comparisons to be made that might be useful in later discussions, but the number of cases has been clearly reported. This is particularly important when the sample size is small, since a percentage can convey a very different impression from that conveyed by the same percentage in a larger sample. For example, if one case in a sample of four were to change between two categories, this

Table 12.2   *Number and percentage of respondents according to profession*

Profession	Number of respondents (%)
Occupational therapy	61 (41)
Physiotherapy	89 (59)
All respondents	150 (100)

would be a shift of 25%. It would require 20 cases to change category to produce the same percentage shift in a sample of 80.

12.3.2 Pie charts and bar charts

When the number of categories is greater than two, a pie chart or bar chart might aid the understanding and, hence, interpretation by providing a visual display of the tabular information. A pie chart is a circle that is divided into segments. The area of each segment is proportional to the number of cases (or frequency) of the respective category, with the total area representing the total number of cases in the sample. The largest segment will represent the *mode* (i.e. the category with the highest number of cases).

Other than for the comparison of frequencies across a few categories, pie charts are not recommended by graphics experts, since they present more perceptual difficulties than alternative forms of display (Henry, 1995). Bar charts are easier to assimilate and far more flexible. Empirical studies have provided evidence of a smaller absolute error when comparing differences across two bars than across two slices in a pie chart (Cleveland and McGill, 1984). Essentially, a simple bar chart comprises a series of bars of equal width, separated by equal gaps, where each category is represented by one bar whose height (and therefore area, given that the bar width is equal) is proportional to the number of cases in that category. The axis representing the frequency (or number of cases) must begin at zero, or the visual comparison across categories is distorted. More generally, bar charts can be used to portray:

- the number (or percentage) of cases against the different categories of one item across the whole sample
- the number (or percentage) of cases against different categories of one item according to specified subgroups within the sample
- the number (or percentage) of cases against the different categories for a series of items on a common response scale.

There are several formats in which the same information can be presented and it is worthwhile experimenting at the preliminary stage so that a graph conveys the important pattern or association on which the researcher wishes to focus the viewer's attention. Some examples are given below. The interested reader is referred to Kosslyn (1985) and Henry (1995) for more detail on such multiple component and multiple stacked bar charts.

The following question (from the Rheumatoid Arthritis Study) requires the respondents to endorse one or more options from a checklist:

By what means do you assess the *intensity* of the rheumatoid arthritis patient's pain (please tick all that apply)?

Numerical rating scale (e.g. 1–10)	☐ 1
Verbal rating scale (e.g. 'severe, moderate …')	☐ 2
Visual analogue scale	☐ 3
McGill Pain Questionnaire (long or short form)	☐ 4
Other (please state below)	☐ 5
None of the above because I do not routinely assess pain intensity	☐ 6

An appropriate summary of the responses is presented in Table 12.3 and visually displayed in a bar chart in Figure 12.1. The order of the tools has been rearranged in both the table and the graph so that the pattern of usage is easier to discern visually. No meaning of the data has been distorted by this reordering, as would be the case with ordinal or higher levels of measurement. The researcher should articulate the main features of the data. At this initial stage in the analysis, the objective is to describe the data, not to discuss findings or try to generalize from the findings. For example, it is obvious that the majority of therapists (81%) in this study assessed pain intensity for rheumatoid arthritis patients, and only 12% (13) assessed pain intensity through the McGill Pain Questionnaire. No one tool in the list dominated the assessment of pain intensity for rheumatoid arthritis patients, although the visual analogue scale was

175

Table 12.3 *Tools used by therapists to assess the intensity of rheumatoid arthritis patients' pain*

Method	Number of therapists (%)
Tool:	
McGill Pain Questionnaire	13 (12)
Numerical rating scale	19 (17)
Verbal rating scale	21 (19)
Visual analogue scale	25 (22)
Other tool to assess pain intensity	28 (25)
Do not routinely assess intensity	21 (19)
Any assessment tool	92 (81)

Note: Numbers of therapists are out of a total of 113; a therapist might use more than one tool.

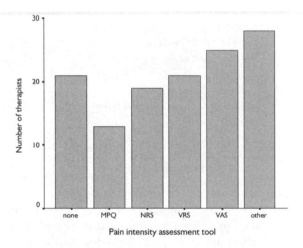

Figure 12.1 *Tools used by the therapists to assess the intensity of rheumatoid arthritis patients' pain. A therapist might use more than one tool. MPQ = McGill Pain Questionnaire; NRS = numerical rating scale; VRS = verbal rating scale; VAS = visual analogue scale.*

chosen by 22% of therapists (25) compared with 19% (21) and 17% (19) for the verbal and numerical rating scales, respectively. Tools other than those specified in the list were used by 25% of therapists (28).

As is typical with questions involving checklists, respondents were allowed to tick as many options as were applicable. Accordingly, useful information might be afforded by calculating the number of tools that each therapist routinely used to assess intensity. Such information is discrete, at a ratio level of measurement and is summarized in a frequency table (Table 12.4) and might also be depicted in a frequency diagram (Figure 12.2). Although really the domain of the next section, these are included here to complete the preliminary inspection of responses from the above question. In this sample, 19% of therapists (21) did not routinely assess the pain intensity of rheumatoid arthritis patients, 69% (78) used one tool and 12% (14) used two tools to assess intensity.

12.3.3 Two-way tables or cross-tabulations

The following question (from the Rheumatoid Arthritis Study) comprises a series of items on a common adverbial rating scale.

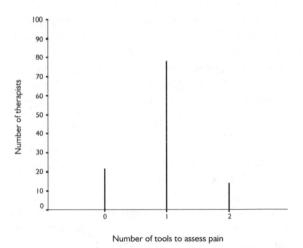

Figure 12.2 *Number of tools used by therapists to assess the intensity of rheumatoid arthritis patients' pain. Numbers of therapists are out of a total of 113.*

Table 12.4 *Number of tools used by therapists to assess the intensity of rheumatoid arthritis patients' pain*

Number of tools used	Number of therapists (%)
0	21 (19)
1	78 (69)
2	14 (12)

Note: Numbers of therapists are out of a total of 113.

Please indicate the frequency with which patients with rheumatoid arthritis are referred to you from each of the following sources:

	Very often	Often	Sometimes	Seldom	Never or almost never
	5	4	3	2	1
Rheumatologist	☐	☐	☐	☐	☐
Orthopaedic surgeon	☐	☐	☐	☐	☐
Other therapist	☐	☐	☐	☐	☐
General practitioner	☐	☐	☐	☐	☐
Self-referral by patient	☐	☐	☐	☐	☐
Other (please state below)	☐	☐	☐	☐	☐

The summary table (Table 12.5) uses the columns to show the frequency with which patients with rheumatoid arthritis are referred to therapists, and the rows to identify the different sources of referral. The rows have been re-arranged from the most common to the least frequent source of referral to highlight this pattern of referrals across all participating therapists. The columns denote information at an ordinal level of measurement and as such have a natural order, which has been preserved. A separate table might be created to show the corresponding percentage figures.

12.3.4 Component and stacked bar charts

Several formats are possible when depicting these data in a bar chart. The choice is based on what aspects of the pattern of referral the researcher wishes to emphasize. Figure 12.3(a) is a *multiple component* bar chart that encourages comparisons to be made across the frequencies of referral (represented by the neighbouring bars) *within* each source of referral (represented by each group of bars). In this example, the same number of therapists responded against every source; therefore, it is possible also to visually compare the patterns of referral *across* the sources. In general, however, differing numbers of responses against each source would confound such a comparison. A *multiple stacked* bar chart, with the vertical axis changed to a percentage scale, encourages comparisons across the sources of referral, as in Figure 12.3(b).

These summaries, along with the other tables and graphs discussed in this section, have retained the individual responses from the therapists. There are many situations in which this strategy produces too much information, making it difficult to discern a general pattern or trend, or to perform comparisons across subgroups of cases. A typical example is the use of an ordinal measure comprising more than ten scale points.

Table 12.5 *Frequency of referrals from various sources of patients with rheumatoid arthritis to therapists*

Source of referral	Never or almost never	Seldom	Frequency of referral			Total number of therapists
			Sometimes	Often	Very often	
Rheumatologist	0	0	6	40	71	117
General practitioner	21	25	32	24	15	117
Other therapist	0	32	48	26	11	117
Orthopaedic surgeon	0	31	52	34	0	117
Patient self-referral	20	53	29	15	0	117
Other	0	0	0	0	0	0

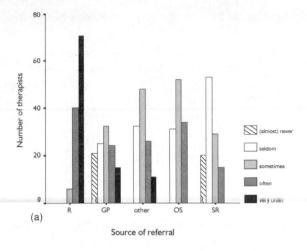

(a)

Source of referral

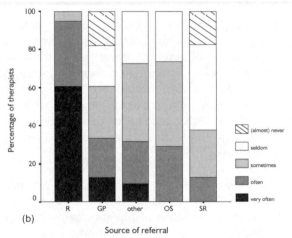

(b)

Source of referral

Figure 12.3 *(a) Referral of patients with rheumatoid arthritis with respect to source and frequency: multiple component bar chart. (b) Referral of patients with rheumatoid arthritis with respect to source and frequency: multiple stacked bar chart. R = rheumatologist; GP = general practitioner; other = other therapist; OS = orthopaedic surgeon; SR = self-referral.*

Responses from such a measure might be summarized through boxplots and six-figure summaries; these are described in the next section.

12.4 SUMMARIZING DATA MEASURED AT AN INTERVAL OR RATIO LEVEL

In general, variables that are measured at an interval or ratio level are capable of taking on

many distinct values, for example age, weight, distance walked and angular movement. The values that are recorded in a study contain information about the characteristics and features of each variable, subject to the conditions under which the data were collected. The important features can be encapsulated in graphical and/or numerical summaries.

Graphs are particularly helpful in the preliminary stages of data analysis. They depict the pattern or distribution of values and make obvious any values that are atypical. This might guide the researcher towards appropriate numerical summaries or analyses to be performed at a later stage. Common graphs include frequency diagrams, frequency polygons, histograms, stem-and-leaf plots, boxplots, time-series graphs and scatter plots (Altman, 1991a; French and Sim, 1993; Munro, 1997). Numerical summaries provide the essential characteristics of the distribution of values and can be compared across samples or subgroups. Data at an interval or ratio level of measurement possess the property that equal differences between scale points have equal meaning. This permits mathematical operations such as addition and subtraction to be performed and, hence, the calculation of numerical summaries such as the mean and standard deviation. Other summaries include frequency distributions, medians, quartiles, modes and ranges. The appropriate summaries depend upon the manner in which the values were measured, the size of the dataset, and the inherent pattern of values. Ages of patients or participants are reported in many studies and will be used to illustrate some of the commonly used graphs and summary statistics.

12.4.1 Frequency distributions and histograms

Age is inherently a continuous variable which is often measured using a category list comprising specified age bands (which are mutually exclusive and collectively exhaustive). It is also frequently measured on a discrete scale to the nearest hour (for neonates), day (for babies), month (for young children) or year (for adolescents and adults). Table 12.6 shows the ages of 130 patients who participated in the Low Back Pain Study. These ages could be presented in a frequency distribution comprising a listing of the possible distinct ages and the associated observed number of participants at each age. This would preserve all the individual responses, but would produce a table that had 48 rows, from which it would be difficult to identify a pattern or particular shape for the distribution of ages. A frequency distribution for a discrete variable with only three distinct values is exemplified by the number of tools used by therapists ᵗᵒ ᵃˢˢᵉˢˢ ᵗʰᵉ ᵖᵃⁱⁿ ⁱⁿᵗᵉⁿˢⁱᵗʸ ᵒᶠ rheumatoid arthritis patients. This information was presented in Table 12.4 and depicted in Figure 12.2. When there are more than ten distinct values, it is usual to summarize the data in a grouped frequency distribution (Table 12.7). This can be displayed in a histogram (Figure 12.4), which is basically a series of adjacent rectangles, one per interval in the grouped frequency distribution. Individual responses are not identifiable in such summaries.

There are many rules for the specification of interval limits, the optimum number of intervals, and the recommended ratio of the height to the width of the rectangles in a histogram (Altman, 1991a; Munro, 1997). In this illustration, the lower and upper limits represent the youngest and oldest ages, respectively, in each interval. The number of intervals and the graphical dimensions affect the visual pattern that is portrayed by the histogram. Ten to 15 intervals are commonly used, and the

Table 12.6 *Ages in years of 130 patients participating in the Low Back Pain Study*

57 63 34 32 41 38 35 20 27 28 34 50 42 38 57 50 49 47 53 18
47 34 48 25 36 29 46 53 64 28 35 43 28 56 31 45 32 47 42 38
48 43 28 65 32 38 29 34 39 32 62 40 41 53 36 62 60 41 38 51
44 27 48 60 51 52 62 35 33 58 45 56 36 51 38 45 27 28 38 24
53 39 47 34 60 42 34 44 33 48 60 29 54 60 57 32 52 41 41 43
45 35 35 31 20 49 42 47 63 33 49 46 61 31 55 34 43 60 49 61
36 56 45 31 32 21 26 43 65 50

Table 12.7 *Distribution of ages of patients who participated in the Low Back Pain Study (n = 130)*

Age (years)	Number of patients	% of patients
18–22	4	3.1
23–27	6	4.6
28–32	18	13.8
33–37	19	14.6
38–42	19	14.6
43–47	19	14.6
48–52	16	12.3
53–57	12	9.2
58–62	12	9.2
63–67	5	3.8

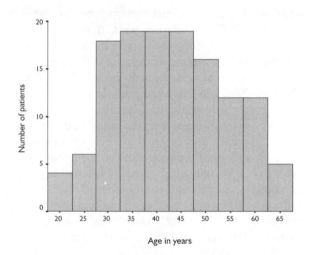

Figure 12.4 *Histogram of ages of patients participating in the Low Back Pain Study. The horizontal axis has been labelled with the midpoint of each class interval.*

graph is normally drawn so that the tallest rectangle is two-thirds of the width of the whole graph. The underlying principle is that the area of each rectangle represents the number (or percentage) of cases in the associated interval, and the total area represents the total number of cases (or 100%).

It is worth noting that the strict mathematical limits extend outside the limits that are customarily ascribed to an interval. The mathematical limits are usually assumed to be one half a unit below the lower limit and one half a unit above the upper limit. Thus, in a distribution of body weights, an interval described as '70–79 kg' strictly includes weights equal to or greater than 69.5 kg and less than 79.5 kg. The presentation of mathematical limits can, however, confuse non-mathematical readers and is for this reason mostly avoided.

12.4.2 Common shapes of frequency distributions

Some commonly used descriptions for the shape of a distribution include skewed, symmetrical, uniform, unimodal and bimodal. A unimodal distribution has one clearly identified peak or modal interval (that is, the interval associated with the highest frequency) and a bimodal distribution has two. When the peak is towards the right of a histogram, the distribution is said to exhibit a negative skew, compared with a positive skew when the peak is towards the left. A symmetrical distribution has symmetry in terms of its shape either side of the middle interval. Uniform distributions possess the feature that every interval contains approximately the same number of cases, such that the rectangles of the histogram are of approximately equal height. Some idealized shapes are shown in Figure 12.5.

In real situations, measurement and sampling errors (Section 13.2.2) contribute towards a more rugged outline. Therefore, the shape of the distribution should be judged against a smoothed profile. For example, the histogram in Figure 12.4 exhibits a slight positive skew, but could be said to be fairly symmetrical. It might be prudent to query the underlying situation when bimodality is apparent. For example, a sample of households encompassing both one and two wage earners might exhibit a bimodal distribution on household income as a direct consequence of the two distinct subgroups in the sample. Further analyses might be performed on the separate subgroups.

12.4.3 Mean and standard deviation

The mean and standard deviation are appropriate numerical summaries when the grouped

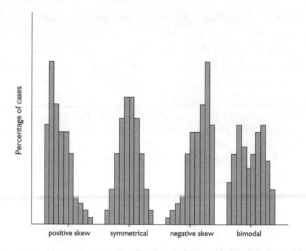

Figure 12.5 *Common shapes of histograms.*

frequency distribution observed in the sample is consistent with a unimodal, symmetrical population distribution and the data satisfy the conditions of an interval or ratio level of measurement. These two statistics convey information about the central location and the spread of values, respectively.

Mean

The mean (or, more precisely, the 'arithmetic mean') is the common 'average'. It is the sum of the data values (across all cases) divided by the number of cases. It is usual to use $\bar{x}$ to represent the mean from a sample and x_i to represent the ith individual value in the sample. The formula for the sample mean is given by:

$$\bar{x} = \frac{\sum x_i}{n}$$

where Σ stands for 'take the sum of', and n = number of cases.

It is obvious from this definition that the mean is calculated from every value in the sample and, consequently, is affected by atypical values, especially when the sample size is small. Hence, the addition of a single extreme value will exert considerable leverage on the mean (see Box 12.5).

As a measure of central tendency, the mean is a 'typical' value, but might not be equal to any value in the sample. The mean age of patients in the Low Back Pain Study was 42.7 years, yet individual ages were measured in whole years (Table 12.6). The mean is unsuitable when some values are *censored*. Censored values are those for which incomplete information is available; for example, when it is known only that they are above or below a certain value. These are referred to as *right-censored* and *left-censored* values, respectively, on the basis of the direction in which the true value lies on the horizontal axis of a frequency distribution (Bland, 1995). Thus, in a study on the clinical course and recurrence of neck pain, the time to recurrence would be absent for those participants whose neck pain did not recur during the duration of the study, and thus would be a right-censored value.

However, the mean possesses many important mathematical properties that make it a useful statistic. These properties will become apparent in later chapters and underlie the use of transformations. Many sets of data exhibit skewed distributions; for example, duration of a chronic illness, survival following a stroke. The mean is influenced by the direction of the skew and is not a representative value. Sometimes, a mathematical operation (such as the square root or logarithm) can be applied to the data to transform them to a scale that exhibits a symmetrical pattern (Altman, 1991a; Bland, 1995). There is often a theoretical rationale for the appropriate mathematical operation or transformation.

Range

The mean represents a central value in a symmetrical distribution. It conveys no information about the variability of the individual sample values around this central position; that is, whether the data are closely clustered (low variability) or highly dispersed (high variability). Two or more samples with precisely the same mean may exhibit very different variability. The span from the minimum value to the maximum value is called the *range* and is one measure of variability. However, although the range represents the extent of the recorded data, it is an unstable measure of variability, since it is greatly affected by an atypical value at one or other end of the distribution.

Standard deviation

The most widely used measure of variability is the *standard deviation*. The standard deviation is a measure of the scatter of individual values around the mean and therefore is suitable for symmetrical distributions only. The sample standard deviation is defined by the following formula.

$$\text{Standard deviation} = \sqrt{\frac{\sum (x_i - \bar{x})^2}{n - 1}}$$

This statistic is calculated on the basis of the distances between the sample mean and every individual value in the sample $(x_i - \bar{x})$. Hence, a small standard deviation indicates that the individual values are clustered around the mean, whereas a large standard deviation indicates that the individual values are spread out around the mean (demonstrating high variability between the individual values). In this context, small and large are judged by comparison with the mean value (Box 12.3).

It is difficult to put a precise interpretation on the standard deviation unless it can be associated with a specific distribution, in particular a theoretical or statistical distribution such as the normal distribution (Section 13.2.1). At this stage, the standard deviation might be taken to represent a 'typical' distance between an individual value and the sample mean. Its role in inferential statistics is discussed in Chapter 13. The standard deviation is usually quoted to three significant figures and the sample mean value to the corresponding precision. For example, the 130 patients in the study on the management of low back pain had a mean age of 42.7 years with a standard deviation of 11.5 years, indicating a fair spread of ages (the units of measurement should always be specified).

Box 12.3   *Coefficient of variation*

The standard deviation provides a measure of dispersion of individual values in a set of data with a symmetrical distribution. When we wish to compare the dispersion in two sets of data measured on a ratio scale, we use values of a statistic called the coefficient of variation (CV), which is given by:

$$CV = \frac{\text{standard deviation}}{\text{mean}} \times 100$$

The coefficient of variation is a dimensionless quantity that provides a measure of dispersion of values relative to the mean value in a distribution. It can be used, therefore, when comparing measures on different scales as well as on scales with the same units. For example, data on age (years) and physical ability (on a scale from 0 to 10 units) were recorded for a random sample of 200 people with rheumatoid arthritis. The physical function score is a mean value derived from 12 items, for each of which 0 denotes no limitation of performance and 10 denotes inability to perform the activity in question. The corresponding mean values, standard deviations and coefficients of variation are given below:

Measure	Mean	Standard deviation	CV
Age (years)	54.9	13.8	25.1
Physical ability (scale 0 to 10)	5.07	2.14	42.2

Using the standard deviation, it would appear that ages have far more variability than values on physical ability. However, when the magnitude of the mean is accounted for, the CVs show that values on physical ability demonstrate far more variability than ages.

Standard deviation and variance

All statistical packages, spreadsheets and most hand calculators will compute the mean and standard deviation, and a statistic called *variance*. The variance is the square of the standard deviation and is the basic measure of variability, as will be seen when we discuss analysis of variance (Chapter 18). When the data comprise a random sample from a population, the sample mean provides an unbiased estimate of the population mean, and the sample variance provides an unbiased estimate of the variance in the population. The standard deviation is the preferable measure of variability in descriptive studies, since it possesses the same units as the sample mean, whereas the variance is associated with squared units.

Error charts

When it is necessary to display means and standard deviations from a number of samples, or from subgroups within a sample, an error chart is an appropriate graphical format to employ (see Box 12.4). Figure 12.6 shows an

Box 12.4   *Misuse of bar charts*

Bar charts are commonly used to display mean values. As the purpose of the chart in such a situation is to display a single summary measure of location for each subgroup, rather than a frequency count, a bar chart is strictly inappropriate. If a bar chart were used to display the mean age of the male and female subjects in the Low Back Pain Study, the bars would pass through all age values below the mean, whereas there are no subjects in the study aged less than 18: this is potentially misleading. Similarly, one would gain the impression that values above the top of the bar are not represented in the subgroup. However, unless the value of every case is precisely the same, there is always at least one value in the dataset greater than the mean value. Indeed, in this respect it would make just as much (or as little) sense for the bars to extend from the top of the vertical axis. Bar charts should be reserved for frequency data (Swinscow and Campbell, 1996).

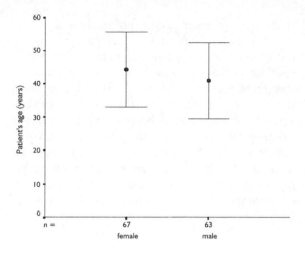

Figure 12.6   *Error chart of patients' age in years (mean and one standard deviation bars).*

error chart for the ages of male and female participants in the Low Back Pain Study. The solid circular marker indicates the mean value and the error bars above and below it denote one standard deviation above and below the mean.

Other statistics that are often computed at the preliminary stage are measures of 'skewness' and 'kurtosis'. The former denotes the extent of asymmetry in a distribution and the latter the flatness or peakedness of the pattern. These statistics are also used to assess whether the distribution of sample values is consistent with a random sample drawn from a normal distribution (Section 13.2.1), an assumption that is made in many inferential testing procedures (Chapters 14 and 18).

12.4.4 Medians and percentiles

It has been emphasized that the mean and standard deviation are appropriate summary statistics for data that are measured on at least an interval scale and that exhibit a symmetrical distribution with one mode. There are many occasions on which these conditions are not satisfied. Percentiles (also known as 'centiles') provide a summary for distributions that might be skewed and for data that are measured on at

least a ten-point ordinal scale. They can also be used for symmetrical distributions.

The data are rearranged from the lowest value through to the highest value and five statistics are calculated – the minimum value, the lower quartile, the median, the upper quartile and the maximum value. There are three quartiles in a dataset and they can be defined as follows:

- 25% of values are smaller than or equal to the lower quartile (25th percentile)
- 50% of values are smaller than or equal to the median value (50th percentile)
- 75% of values are smaller than or equal to the upper quartile (75th percentile).

Boxplots and five-figure summaries

These five statistics are called a five-figure summary and can be displayed in a boxplot (often also called a box-and-whisker plot). The number of cases in the sample is also a valuable piece of information, and when this is reported together with the five-figure summary, a 'six-figure summary' is produced. Most statistical packages have options that enable these summaries to be computed and will draw boxplots. These graphs are particularly useful for making comparisons across subgroups. Table 12.8 shows the six-figure summaries for the age of patients participating in the Low Back Pain Study, Figure 12.7 is a boxplot of ages for all participants and Figure 12.8 compares ages across the two treatment approaches.

Table 12.8   *Age in years of patients participating in the Low Back Pain Study (according to treatment approach)*

Statistic	Treatment approach		All patients
	Individual	Group	
Ages:			
Youngest	20.0	18.0	18.0
Lower quartile	34.0	33.5	34.0
Median	42.0	43.0	42.0
Upper quartile	49.0	51.5	51.0
Oldest	65.0	65.0	65.0
Number of patients	62	68	130

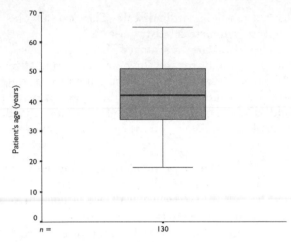

Figure 12.7 *Boxplot of ages of patients participating in the Low Back Pain Study.*

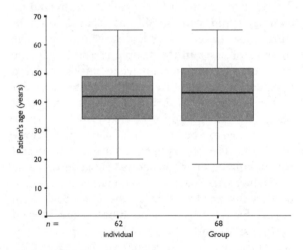

Figure 12.8 *Comparison of patients' ages across the individual and group approaches in the Low Back Pain Study.*

In Figure 12.7, the bottom and top of the box denote, respectively, the lower and upper quartile ages for the 130 patients. The length of the box (17 years) is the distance between the lower and upper quartiles (34 to 51), the middle 50% of ages. This is called the *interquartile range* and is a measure of variability of age; the longer the box, the higher the variability. The width of the box has no meaning. The horizontal line within the box denotes the median age. Fifty per cent of patients in this

study are younger than the median age, 42 years. This is a typical or representative age in the sample. It is a point estimate of the corresponding typical value in the population (assuming that the patients constitute a random sample). However, when the values are very variable, it might be debatable in what sense a single value can be typical. The distance from the lower to the upper quartile presents an interval of values that can be expected to be representative of the population. Fifty per cent of patients who participated in the Low Back Pain Study were between 34 and 51 years of age.

Vertical lines (or 'whiskers') usually extend from the top and bottom of the box to the maximum and minimum values, respectively (Figure 12.7). Some statistical packages separately identify outliers and extreme values (Figure 12.9), and in this case the vertical lines extend to the limit for 'typical' values as defined by the package – generally, any values that lie within 1.5 box lengths from the upper or lower limit of the box (Norušis, 1997). No outliers or extreme values are identified on Figures 12.7 or 12.8. The boxplot is analogous to the error chart shown in Figure 12.6, but displays a median rather than a mean value, and the interquartile range rather than the standard deviation. It also provides information on the range of values, which is not present in an error chart.

The boxplot of ages with respect to the treatment modalities (Figure 12.8) shows no major differences in the two distributions of age (which is to be welcomed in a randomized controlled trial). The maximum and minimum ages are similar (as indicated by the ends of the vertical lines). The box length for the 'group' modality is slightly larger than for the 'individual' modality, indicating slightly higher variability in the middle 50% of ages. The median values (the horizontal lines inside the two boxes) are similar. These observations can be confirmed by considering the summaries in Table 12.8, from which it can be seen, for example, that responses were received at baseline from 130

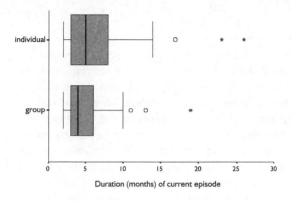

Figure 12.9 *Boxplot of duration of current episode of low back pain (in months), for individual and group approaches, demonstrating a positive skew of distribution. The circles represent outliers and the asterisks represent extreme values. In this graph, the boxplot has been drawn in a horizontal, rather than a vertical, orientation; the minimum value, lower quartile, median, upper quartile and maximum value are therefore located from left to right.*

patients, whose ages ranged from 18 to 65 years, with a median age of 42 years and typical ages between 34 and 51 years (lower to upper quartile).

The boxplot also displays the shape of a distribution. A symmetrical distribution has the same shape either side of the median; that is, the distance between the median and the lower quartile is the same as that between the median and the upper quartile, and the two whiskers are approximately the same length. With a negative skew, the median will shift towards the upper quartile, and towards the lower quartile in the case of a positive skew (Box 12.5), as illustrated in Figure 12.9 and Table 12.9.

12.5 PRESENTING SUMMARIES

The final report for a study will rarely contain all the graphical, tabular and statistical summaries that were produced during the preliminary stage in the data analysis. A judicious process of selection, summarizing and editing is needed and the level of detail that is finally reproduced depends upon the purpose of the report and its expected readership.

The presentation of substantive data from a study should normally be preceded by a summary of demographic and other background data (e.g. the age, sex, ethnicity and occupation of respondents to a questionnaire). This places the findings of the study within a particular context, and enables their potential relevance to be judged.

Some basic principles are that tables and graphs should enhance the reader's understanding without distorting the facts, provide clear and simplified summaries of the data, complement the text by containing more detail or by focusing on specific aspects, and be capable of standing alone without the need for recourse to the text (Chapman and Mahon, 1986; French and Sim, 1993; Price, 1996a, 1996b). Hence, unambiguous titles, clearly labelled axes (including a marked origin), legends and footnotes are important features for tables and graphs. Graphs that appear too complex or too busy are unhelpful; the information might be better presented across a series of graphs. Further, charts that use a projection technique to achieve the illusion of a third dimension (e.g. 3-D pie charts) can distort comprehension of the data and should be avoided (French and Sim, 1993; Daly *et al.*, 1995; Henry, 1995).

As a final point, the tables and graphs that are presented in a report form part of the evidence on which a reader bases his or her judgement about the validity of the stated conclusions and, as such, they must be a truthful representation of the data collected in the study.

12.6 DATA INPUT AND AUDITING

A statistical package (or, perhaps, a spreadsheet) performs the tasks of organizing the data, creating the tables, drawing the graphs and calculating the summary statistics. However, more often than not, the task of entering the data into a worksheet accessible to the package is a tedious, manual process. The integrity of a soundly designed and executed study is sacrificed if errors exist in this worksheet. It is prudent,

Box 12.5   *Means, medians and modes*

Influence of extreme values and shape of distribution

Every value in a dataset contributes towards the calculation of the mean, which is therefore affected by extreme values. The value of the median, in contrast, is determined by the rank order of the values in the dataset, and is therefore unaffected by extreme values. Consequently, the shape of the distribution of a dataset (Figures 12.5 and 12.9) will influence the relationship between the mean and the median. In a symmetrical distribution, the mean and the median will have the same value. In a negatively skewed distribution, however, the mean will be lower than the median. The extreme low values associated with the cases in the tail of the distribution will tend to draw the mean value downwards but will not affect the value of the median. Conversely, in a positively skewed distribution the mean will be higher than the median (Table 12.9). In this case, the high values associated with the cases in the tail of the distribution exert an upward leverage on the mean; again, this does not influence the median value.

Different averages and level of measurement

The mathematical properties of the sample mean make it more useful than the median for performing comparisons across subgroups (Bland, 1995). However, it is applicable only to variables measured on interval or ratio scales. The median is a useful summary for symmetrical and for skewed distributions, and is applicable to variables measured on at least an ordinal scale. If there are identifiable cases at the extremes of a distribution whose exact values cannot be ascertained (perhaps because they lie beyond the range of a measuring instrument), the mean is not calculable, but the median is (Altman and Bland, 1994). Both the mean and the median are fairly insensitive to small changes in a sample of data (Bowers, 1996). The mode is the value that occurs most frequently in a dataset. It is a useful statistic for discrete data that can take on a small number of values. In particular, it represents a typical attribute for variables measured at a nominal level of measurement.

Other measures of average

Other measures of average that are sometimes used include a *trimmed mean* (the mean value calculated after excluding, for example, the lowest 5% and highest 5% of values, hence eliminating the influence of extreme values), the *geometric mean* (based on the multiplication rather than the summing of individual values, and used to represent average rates of growth over time, which usually exhibit a positive skew), and the *harmonic mean* (used in calculations of sample size and in multiple comparison tests).

Table 12.9   *Comparison of mean and median duration of current episode of back pain (months) for a distribution with a positive skew*

Statistic	Approach	
	Individual	Group
Mean (standard deviation)	6.44 (4.65)	5.31 (3.42)
Median	5.00	4.00
Lower, upper quartiles	3.00, 8.00	3.00, 6.00

therefore, to build preventive strategies into the process of data collection, to develop a procedure for handling the data input process and to perform an audit of the data worksheet.

The process of coding a questionnaire (i.e. converting responses from closed-ended questions into a numerical value for entry into a computer worksheet) is simplified if the questionnaire is *precoded*; i.e. numerical scores are printed in a small font above or alongside the response options (see Section 15.5.3).

Each step in this process should be audited. In small studies (about 50 questionnaires or cases), the coding and data entry of every questionnaire should be verified. In larger studies, random samples of 10% at the coding and at the data entry stages should detect the presence of any major problems. Once the computer worksheet is completed, then one further data check is useful. Computing the minimum and maximum scores against every item will identify values that lie outside permissible ranges; for example, a '77' instead of '7' against a ten-point scale. Additional procedures, such as cross-tabulations, can also be performed to detect other implausible features in the data which would raise suspicions of erroneous input (Dijkers and Creighton, 1994).

When the data comprise clinical or physical measurements rather than responses to questions, a clear, unambiguous data collection sheet is necessary. Each sheet should contain data from one case only, to prevent the possibility of entering information against the wrong case.

A few further points are worth a mention. The data need to be entered into the worksheet in a format that allows the desired statistical analyses to be performed. In many packages, data from each case (or unit) occupy a row in the worksheet and every variable occupies a column that is identified by a unique name. One variable, usually in the first column, represents a unique identification number for each case; this allows a crosscheck to be made against the questionnaires or data collection sheets and can be used to locate atypical values (it is unwise to rely on the row number provided by the package, since this may change if an earlier row is moved or deleted). Before inputting any data, it is prudent to gain a working knowledge of the

chosen package, to plan the content of the computer worksheet and to decide upon suitable names for every variable. Whenever possible, data from individual items or variables should be input and any necessary mathematical operations (such as summing the scores across several items to form a total score for a summated rating scale) should be performed through the functions available within the package. This method is less prone to undetectable mathematical errors. Missing values should be identified as such. They might occur through two routes: no response was recorded but one was expected; or no response was expected, since the question was inapplicable. These can be distinguished if information is represented through the use of two different missing value codes.

12.7 CONCLUSION

Quantitative data result, in the main, from studies that address descriptive or explanatory research questions. The data are collected, organized, summarized and presented in textual, tabular and graphical forms using descriptive statistics. These serve to depict the important features in the data and can be an aid to more detailed analyses. The appropriate methods for any analysis are dependent upon the level at which variables are measured. Hence, permissible analyses need to be identified at the design stage in a study. A computing package will perform *any* analysis requested of it as long as the data are inputted in the appropriate format. The researcher must accept the responsibility for performing appropriate analyses to support meaningful conclusions.

13 ANALYSING DATA FROM DESCRIPTIVE AND EXPLANATORY STUDIES: PRINCIPLES

SUMMARY

This chapter explores the following topics:

- the role of inferential statistics
- basic principles of probability
- statistical distributions
- the use of statistical interval estimation, and its limitations
- the use of statistical hypothesis testing, and its limitations
- the concept of statistical significance
- the principal characteristics of parametric and of nonparametric statistical methods

The preceding chapter has stressed the importance of communicating numerical information in a manner that is comprehensible and appropriate to the nature of the data concerned. Many descriptive and explanatory studies involve the investigation of associations between attributes, or the differences between characteristics of subgroups, or change in such characteristics over time. In these situations, the statistical analyses entail more than graphical and numerical summaries, and the published reports of such studies necessarily contain some rather more technical statistical terminology (for example, Tables 14.7 and 14.8). To judge the usefulness of such research findings to health care practice, and to make a judicious choice of analyses within his or her own research, the practitioner needs to have a clear understanding of the principles underlying statistical methods and the associated terminology. This chapter aims to provide the foundation for this understanding and for the specific inferential procedures to be presented in Chapters 14 and 18.

13.1 BASIC CONCEPTS FOR INFERENTIAL STATISTICS

13.1.1 Samples and populations

Much empirical research involves collecting information about a sample of cases that has been selected from the accessible population. The rationale for sampling in relation to statistical representativeness, and some common sampling strategies were discussed in detail in Chapter 8. The use of inferential statistics enables the characteristics of the accessible population (parameters) to be inferred from the known characteristics in a sample (statistics), through an objective process based on probability theory and sampling error. Further inference from the accessible population to the target population (all the cases of interest to the researcher) is generally based on non-statistical considerations (Daniel, 1991). It rests on the assumption that the accessible population is similar to the target population, at least with respect to the characteristics under investigation. For example, in the Low Back Pain Study, Dr Buckley might assume that the accessible population that formed his sampling frame – the patients in the three hospitals and in the caseloads of primary care physicians – was representative of such patients in general. In this chapter, the accessible population will be referred to simply as the 'population'.

At its most basic, statistical inference is concerned with two types of procedures:

1. estimation of the values of population parameters;
2. testing of hypotheses concerning stated values for population parameters.

These processes will be considered in detail in Sections 13.3 and 13.4, respectively. However,

Box 13.1   *Objective and subjective probabilities*

There are two approaches to probability: (1) *objective*, which is further categorized into classical probability and the relative frequency concept of probability, and (2) *subjective* (Daniel, 1991). Classical probability theory originated in the seventeenth century when two mathematicians, Pascal and Fermat, investigated the outcomes of games of chance, such as the rolling of dice and the drawing of a particular hand from an ordinary pack of cards. In these situations, the probability of any particular event (for example, a 6 uppermost when rolling a fair six-sided die) can be calculated through abstract, logical reasoning. In the given example, there are six possible outcomes (1, 2 ... 6 uppermost), which are mutually exclusive and equally likely. One of the outcomes represents the desired event, a 6 uppermost, leading to a probability of 1 out of 6, or 1/6, for the occurrence of this event. In most practical situations, this approach is not possible. There is no logical rationale on which to base the relative rate of occurrence for the possible outcomes. The relative frequency approach, in contrast, is based on empirical observation and defines probability as the proportion of occasions, under certain circumstances, on which some specified event occurs in the long term. This definition requires the occasions to be repeatable and countable, and the event of interest to be clearly identifiable and countable. For example, low back pain is reported to affect 14% of the UK population at any one point in time (Rose *et al.*, 1997). Hence, the probability that a randomly selected member of the UK population has low back pain is estimated as .14, based on relative frequency. In contrast, subjective probability is not based on theory or observation, but on a particular individual's personal belief that a specified event will occur. This concept can be used to provide a probability for some future, one-off event, such as the discovery of a cure for all cancers within the next 10 years (Daniel, 1991).

in order to make sense of these procedures, it is necessary to understand some basic elements of probability (Sections 13.1.2 and 13.1.3) and the notion of a sampling distribution (Section 13.2).

13.1.2 Probability

Probability is concerned with uncertainty, and statistical inference is based on the theory of probability. It follows, then, that an understanding of the basic principles of probability will contribute to an understanding of statistical inference. Probability theory is an unfamiliar field to many, and grasping the way in which it works might therefore be a rather daunting prospect. In reality, however, all those involved in health care routinely encounter the concepts of probability in the care of patients. This is exemplified by remarks such as 'there is a 50% chance that a particular antibiotic therapy will be successful', 'the likelihood of regaining full mobility is about 90%', or 'a complete recovery of cognitive function is highly unlikely'. These comments imply an uncertainty in clinical outcome. The stated percentage in the first two quotations reflects the proportion of occasions on which the specified event has occurred over many past cases. This is a *relative frequency* approach to probability (Box 13.1). That is, data recorded on many past cases show that 90% regained full mobility. Hence, for future patients with a similar condition, medical history and personal attributes, there is support for the proposition that 90% will regain full mobility, and 10% will not.

13.1.3 Properties of probability

There are three features of probability that are crucial to an understanding of inferential statistical analysis:

- the numerical representation of probability
- the probability of independent events
- the idea of conditional probability.

When speaking of probability, an 'event' is an occurrence or an existing state of affairs.

Numerical representation

Mathematically, the probability of occurrence of some event is represented by a number between zero and one (Hodges and Lehmann, 1964). The less likely the occurrence of an event, the closer the probability is to zero, and the more likely the occurrence of an event, the closer the probability is to one. Strictly speaking, the end points do not represent uncertainty, since the number zero would be assigned to an event that can never occur and the number one to an event that is certain to occur. For example, it is impossible for a baby to be born (at least from a physical point of view) more than once and it is a certainty that a person will die at some point in time.

A percentage occurrence can be converted to a probability through division by 100 (e.g. 90% is equivalent to a probability of .9) and a probability to a percentage occurrence through multiplication by 100 (e.g. a probability of .5 is equivalent to an occurrence of 50% of cases). A number representing probability cannot, of course, be negative. Our practice with regard to placing a zero before the decimal point is explained in Box 13.2.

Box 13.2 *When to place a zero before the decimal point*

Throughout this text we have followed the practice advocated by the American Psychological Association (APA, 1994) of not placing a zero before the decimal point when the quantity in question cannot exceed unity. This also applies to correlation coefficients (Section 14.1.2), which always lie between −1 and 1. Quantities that can exceed unity should, however, take a zero before the decimal point; 'half a per cent' would be written as '0.5%', not '.5%'.

Independent events

Two events are independent when the occur-rence of one event provides no information about the occurrence or non-occurrence of the other event (Hodges and Lehmann, 1964). The events 'a patient contracts a urinary tract infection' and 'the retail price index falls' are independent (except in the most bizarre and far-fetched of scenarios). The probability of two independent events occurring is given by the product of the probabilities of individual occur-rence; for example, if two such independent events each have a probability of .5, the prob-ability of their both occurring is .25.

Hence, 'statistical independence' is a very precise concept that is defined through prob-ability. It is an important consideration in many statistical procedures and is a basic feature of the chi-square test of independence or association (see Section 14.1.1).

Dependent (or conditional) events

Two events are dependent when the occurrence of one event provides some information about the occurrence or non-occurrence of the other event. That is, the probability of occurrence of one event is *conditional* upon the situation with respect to the other event. Howell (1997) gives the example of the probability of a person contracting AIDS being conditional on whether or not he or she is an intravenous drug user. Similarly, the probability of a person having ankylosing spondylitis will be condi-tional upon whether that person is male or female, and the probability that a person will have blue eyes will be conditional upon whether or not he or she has blond hair. In each of these cases, knowledge of one event (being an intravenous drug user, being female, etc.) causes a different level of probability to be assigned to the other event (having AIDS, having ankylosing spondylitis, etc.) than if the first event were unknown.

The idea of conditional probability will later be seen to be important in relation to the prob-ability value obtained through a hypothesis test (Section 13.4.6). It is also relevant when calcu-lating positive or negative predictive values for diagnostic tests (Section 9.2.3).

13.2 STATISTICAL DISTRIBUTIONS

13.2.1 The normal distribution

A statistical distribution may be likened to a histogram (Section 12.4.1) drawn from all data in a population, with the histogram scaled to have a total area of one. The normal (or Gaussian) curve is an important statistical distribution that:

- has well-defined properties
- approximates the distribution of the population of values taken by many biological, psychological, socioeconomic and physical phenomena
- has a special connection with the mean values from large random samples; this enables us to make generalizations about the population from which the samples were drawn.

Many standard tools used by health care professionals are developed so that the values follow a normal distribution; for example, Draw A Person (used to assess the graphic skills of children with learning or motor coordination difficulties) and the Wechsler Intelligence Scale for Children (Wechsler, 1974; Naglieri, 1988; Beery, 1989).

Properties of the normal distribution

A normal distribution possesses the following properties:

- It is bell shaped.
- It requires two parameters for complete definition of the curve, viz.:
  - its mean, which determines its location along the horizontal axis (Figure 13.1)
  - its standard deviation, which determines its 'width' (Figure 13.2).
- It is symmetrical around the mean.
- Its mean, median and mode values coincide.
- The area under the distribution curve represents probability, such that:
  - 68.3% of values are within one standard deviation of the mean

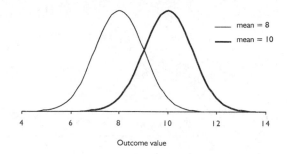

Figure 13.1 *Two normal distributions. Population means = 8 and 10; standard deviations = 1.*

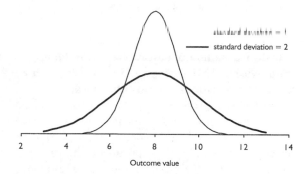

Figure 13.2 *Two normal distributions. Population means = 8; standard deviations = 1 and 2.*

  - 95.4% of values are within two standard deviations of the mean
  - 99.7% of values are within three standard deviations of the mean (Figure 13.3).
- It follows from the preceding point that there is a decreasing chance of values occurring at increasing distance from the mean, such that:
  - 31.7% of values are more than one standard deviation from the mean
  - 4.6% of values are more than two standard deviations from the mean
  - 0.3% of values are more than three standard deviations from the mean (Figure 13.3).

Tables of scores for Draw A Person (DAP) and the Wechsler Intelligence Scale for

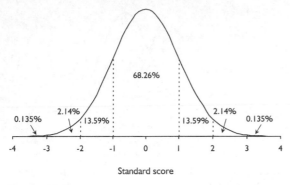

Figure 13.3   *The normal distribution, indicating the percentage of values in the population within one, two and three standard deviations of the population mean.*

$$\text{standardized score} = \frac{\text{variate score} - \text{population mean score}}{\text{population standard deviation}}$$

or in symbols,

$$z = \frac{X - \mu}{\sigma}$$

where: z is the standardized score;
 X is the score of the outcome variable, or variate score;
 μ is the population mean;
 σ is the population standard deviation.

The relationship between standardized scores and percentage of cases with more extreme values in the population is tabulated in statistical tables (e.g. Murdoch and Barnes, 1974) and in an appendix of many textbooks (e.g. Portney and Watkins, 1993; Munro, 1997). It is provided, also, in statistical packages and spreadsheet packages. Standardized scores form the basis of many inferential tests.

13.2.2 Sampling distributions

In statistical inference, the objective is to draw inferences about a population's characteristics from the information contained in a random sample that is representative of that population (Section 8.2). This is achieved if we can specify the relationship between the parameters (such as the population mean) and the statistics (such as the sample mean). Parameters are constants; that is, once the population has been defined it is assumed that its characteristics are fixed quantities (albeit unknown). Statistics, however, are random variables whose values depend on the actual sample selected – the value of a statistic is known only when the data in a particular sample have been collected and analysed. For example, the sample mean is the arithmetic mean of all the data in a sample; hence different data produce different sample mean values. For a given random sample, the value of the statistic might or might not equal the value of the parameter.

Children have been published with a mean of 100 and a standard deviation of 15. Hence, a child with a DAP score of 55 (which is three standard deviations below the mean) and a Wechsler score of 70 (which is two standard deviations below the mean) would have performed as well as or better than 0.14% of children in his or her age group on the drawing test and 2.28% of children on the intelligence test (the percentages here are given to two decimal places). With such extreme scores, this child might be considered to have learning or motor control difficulties.

Because these two tools are published with the same mean and standard deviation, it is easy to see that the child in our example has scored relatively better on the intelligence test than on the drawing test. If the tools had been published with different means or standard deviations, the comparison would have been more difficult to make. Standardized scores are useful for making comparisons in these situations, and many assessment tools are based on such scores (Davies and Gavin, 1999).

Standardized scores

The last two properties of the normal distribution were worded in terms of the number of standard deviations between a specific value of an outcome variable (*variate score*) and the mean. This quantity is called the *standardized score* and can be expressed as:

Sampling error

The difference between the value of a statistic and that of the parameter is known as sampling error. Some random samples will produce positive sampling errors (e.g. sample means higher than the population mean) and others negative sampling errors (e.g. sample means lower than the population mean). The nature of random sampling does not allow this direction to be predicted for a given sample, since it is due to chance, but the mean error will be zero when calculated on many random samples (i.e. positive and negative sampling errors will tend to cancel one another out). When the pattern of the sampling errors can be described by a statistical distribution, the properties of that distribution enable us to answer questions such as:

- What is the likely difference between the value of a statistic and that of the corresponding parameter, based on chance?
- How extreme is the value of the statistic relative to an assumed value of the parameter, based on chance?

The second question is equivalent to:

- What is the chance of selecting a random sample (from a population with an assumed parameter value) for which the value of the statistic is as extreme as, or more extreme than, that of the obtained statistic?

These questions are central to inferential testing procedures. The problem lies in the choice of an appropriate distribution to model the sampling errors or statistics. This could be found empirically by graphing the distribution of the values of the statistic that would arise from all possible random samples (of a fixed size) selected from a population. Such a curve is called the *sampling distribution* of the statistic. Of course, this approach is not feasible in practice. An alternative is to derive the sampling distributions mathematically (Hoel, 1962). Fortunately, we can avoid this mathematical exercise by referring to standard statistical texts for those sampling distributions in common use.

Sampling distribution of means

One important sampling distribution will be discussed in more detail here – the distribution of the sample means, called the sampling distribution of means. This underlies the data analyses in many studies that set out to do one or more of the following:

- investigate change in the mean value of an outcome variable over time (such as change in mean pain intensity for patients following attendance at a programme for the management of low back pain)
- compare mean values of an outcome variable across subgroups of cases (for example, change in mean pain intensity for patients who have and those who have not received previous therapy)
- investigate change in the number of cases exhibiting some attribute following an intervention (for example, a change in the number of clinically anxious patients following relaxation sessions)
- compare proportions of cases responding to different treatments (for example, the proportion of patients who are discharged home within 10 days from each of two surgical wards).

Some general properties apply to the sampling distribution of means:

- It has a mean equal to the mean of the population from which the samples were drawn.
- It has variance equal to the variance of the original population divided by the sample size (n).
- When random samples of size n are drawn from a normally distributed population, the distribution of sample means is normal.
- When random samples of size n are drawn from a population with unknown distribution, the distribution of sample means is

approximately normally distributed when the sample size is large.

This last point is referred to as the *central limit theorem* and applies to sample means, proportions and totals of a set of values in a sample (Altman, 1991a). The implication of the theorem is that as long as the sample is large, approximately the same results can be expected when sampling from non-normally distributed populations as would be obtained if the populations were normally distributed (Wilkes, 1993). In such situations, the normal distribution might be used for inferential purposes. What constitutes 'large' is open to debate. Daniel (1991, p. 110) contends that in most practical situations a sample size of 30 is a satisfactory rule of thumb, the actual number depending upon the extent of non-normality present in the population. One should consider not only the total sample size, but also the size of separate subgroups when these are examined in the analyses (Pett, 1997).

Standard error of the mean

In section 13.2.1, a standardized score was used to find the percentage of cases with as extreme or more extreme values than a given variate score. When the distribution of sample means is normal, the standardized score for a sample mean is given by:

$$\text{standardized score} = \frac{\text{sample mean} - \text{population mean score}}{\text{standard error of the mean}}$$

The standard error of the mean is the square root of the variance of the sample means and, as such, is a standard deviation of sample mean values. It is calculated by taking the standard deviation of the distribution of individual values divided by the square root of the sample size (or $\sigma/\sqrt{n}$ in terms of the symbols used in Section 13.2.1).

The standard error of the mean reflects the likely distance between the population mean and a sample mean – the sampling error. High variability across individual values in the population

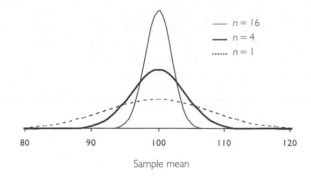

Figure 13.4   *The effect of increasing sample size; larger sample sizes produce smaller standard errors. Sample means are more precise estimates of the population mean for larger sample sizes.*

produces a larger standard deviation and, hence, a larger standard error for a fixed sample size. As the sample size increases, the standard error decreases and the sample mean becomes more precise as an estimate of the population mean, as depicted by the curves in Figure 13.4 (see Box 13.3 for a fuller explanation).

Box 13.3   *Standard error of the mean*

With reference to Figure 13.4, values in the population (which can be thought of as samples of size 1) are normally distributed with a mean of 100 and a standard deviation of 15, so that 68.3% of values are between 85 and 115. When samples of size 4 are drawn from this population, the mean of the sampling distribution is 100, and the standard error of the mean is 7.5 (15 divided by the square root of 4), so that 68.3% of sample means from samples of size 4 are between 92.5 and 107.5. When samples of size 16 are drawn from this population, the mean of the sampling distribution is 100 and the standard error of the mean is 3.75, so that 68.3% of sample means from samples of size 16 are between 96.25 and 103.75. Smaller standard errors give rise to smaller sampling errors.

13.3 ESTIMATION AND CONFIDENCE INTERVALS

Estimation of population parameters is an important aspect of inferential statistics. Its purpose is to aid practitioners in inferring the properties of a population by analysing the information contained in a sample from that population. It provides answers to questions such as: 'What is the difference in the effectiveness of individual-based and group-based cognitive-behavioural approaches to the management of low back pain?' (Low Back Pain Study); 'What proportion of therapists routinely measure pain intensity for patients with rheumatoid arthritis?' (Rheumatoid Arthritis Study).

Interval estimates

The value of a population parameter is estimated by the value of a statistic calculated from a random sample drawn from that population. This provides a *point estimate* – one numerical value that conveys no information about how far or how close it might be to the value of the parameter. The sampling error is quantified by the standard error of the sampling distribution of the statistic (Section 13.2.2). Combining the information in the statistic and the standard error enables an *interval estimate* to be constructed for the value of the parameter. When the form of the sampling distribution is known, this interval can be associated with a level of confidence that it contains the value of the parameter. Such an interval is called a *confidence interval*.

Confidence interval for the population mean

For example, the mean from a random sample of size n is a point estimate of the mean in the population from which the sampling was performed. When the sample size is sufficiently large to invoke the central limit theorem (greater than 30, say), then using the properties of the normal distribution we know that 95% of sample means are within 1.96 standard errors of the population mean. This interval might (with probability .95) or might not (with probability .05) contain the population mean. This cannot be determined conclusively without knowledge of the population mean value. A confidence interval for the unknown population mean value is constructed by taking a certain number of standard errors (in this case 1.96) below and above the known sample mean value. The end points are called *confidence limits*. If the mean value from the collected sample were within 1.96 standard errors of the population mean, then this confidence interval would contain the population mean value. An interval based on 1.96 standard errors is called a '95% confidence interval'. Phrasing this in a different way, 95% of all intervals constructed in this way would contain the population mean value, hence one can be 95% confident that the interval in question contains the population mean.

Similar procedures are used to construct confidence intervals for parameters (e.g. population variance) when the statistic follows other known shapes of sampling distributions. The interested reader is referred to Gardner and Altman (1989a), Altman (1991a) or Daniel (1991) for further details. The conventional levels used for confidence intervals are 90%, 95% and 99%. The higher confidence levels are associated with wider intervals – to increase the confidence that the interval contains the population parameter. However, wider intervals reflect lower precision in the estimate of the parameter. The width of the interval is also determined by the size of the standard error, which is affected by the variability in the population from which a sample is taken and by the sample size. Quadrupling the sample size reduces the width of an interval by one half (assuming the population standard deviation is known).

In terms of symbols, a 95% confidence interval for the population mean (μ) is given by:

$$\bar{x} - 1.96\left(\frac{\sigma}{\sqrt{n}}\right) \text{ to } \bar{x} + 1.96\left(\frac{\sigma}{\sqrt{n}}\right)$$

where: $\bar{x}$ is the mean of a random sample;

σ is the standard deviation of the individual values in the sampled population;

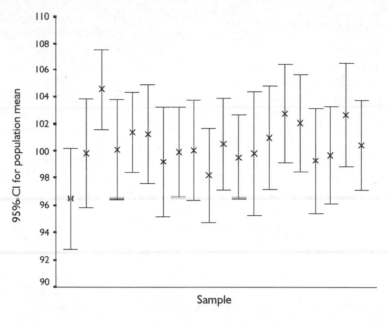

Figure 13.5 *Twenty 95% confidence intervals for the population mean from 20 random samples of size 64. Actual population mean = 100; population standard deviation = 15.*

n is the size of the random sample drawn from the sampled population;

1.96 is a standardized score and is related to the level of confidence associated with the interval (in this example, 95% of sample means are within 1.96 standard errors of the population mean).

Figure 13.5 shows 95% confidence intervals for a population mean, constructed from 20 random samples of size 64. In this example, the population mean value was actually known (100) and the standard deviation was 15. Nineteen of the intervals contain the population mean. In practice, it is likely that values of both the population mean and standard deviation would be unknown. The sample standard deviation is used as the population standard deviation when the sample size is large. In this situation, quadrupling the sample size can reduce the width of an interval, but only by approximately one half – larger samples produce diminishing returns in terms of the precision of the

estimates obtained. The application of confidence intervals is discussed in Section 13.5.

13.4 HYPOTHESIS TESTING PROCEDURE

Hypothesis testing is the form of statistical inference that has received most attention within the health care literature. Its role is to address questions such as: 'Is there a difference in effectiveness between individual-based and group-based cognitive-behavioural approaches to the management of low back pain?' (Low Back Pain Study), or 'Do differences exist in the routine practices and attitudes of occupational therapists and physiotherapists with respect to the management of rheumatoid arthritis?' (Rheumatoid Arthritis Study). Ignoring questions of operationalization (covered in Section 7.2.3), the first question involves a comparison of the mean measures of functional ability for patients randomized to the two different approaches. Even if no differential effect on mean functional ability exists between the two approaches, the observed mean measures relating to the approaches will differ as a result of chance between-group differences in patients' characteristics arising through the randomization process, and in events occurring during the data collection period. Hypothesis testing provides a procedure whereby, under certain assumptions, chance differences in the effects can be distinguished with some degree of confidence from 'real' differences. In general, it is a process of inferring from a sample whether or not to retain a certain statement (i.e. a hypothesis) about the population from which the sample was drawn.

Both estimation and hypothesis testing draw conclusions about population parameters from the information obtained from a random sample. Estimation is a means of assigning a value (or a range of values) to certain population parameters, on the basis of the corresponding statistics observed in the sample. Hypothesis testing is a method of deciding whether or not a difference between a sample statistic and the assumed population parameter represents some form of sampling error.

13.4.1 A simple hypothesis test

A simple hypothetical example may illustrate the basic rationale of hypothesis testing. Imagine a ratio-level variable that is normally distributed within a population, such that it has a mean of 100 and a standard deviation of 28. A sample of 64 units, which are claimed to have been randomly selected from this population, are examined and found to have a mean of 110.5 on this variable. Is this sample statistic consistent with the stated population mean of 100? In other words, is it credible that this sample did indeed come from this population?

This question is answered by calculating the standardized score:

- From the properties of the distribution of sample means (Section 13.2.2), the standard error of the mean is 3.5 (28 divided by the square root of 64).
- The difference between the sample mean and the population mean (110.5 minus 100) is 10.5.

- The reported sample mean is, therefore, three standard errors above the stated population mean (10.5 divided by 3.5 is 3).
- Only 0.3% of random samples from the stated normally distributed population would have more extreme mean values (Section 13.2.1).

This represents an unlikely situation. There are two possible explanations:

1. The sample is indeed derived from the population in question, and the difference between the population mean of 100 and the reported sample mean of 110.5 is due to sampling error; i.e. a 3-in-1000 chance event has occurred.
2. The sample is in fact derived from another population whose mean value of the variable in question is closer to the sample mean of 110.5.

Faced with this choice, most researchers would reject the first explanation in favour of the second, with a probability of .003 that the decision to do so is erroneous. A conclusion might be that, based on these data, there is evidence that the mean score for the variable is greater than that of the population from which it was supposedly drawn, such that it is more credible that the sample derives from a different population. A confidence interval would provide an estimate of the actual mean of the sampled population (Section 13.3).

The hypothesis testing procedure described above is based on a *frequentist* model and is discussed in more detail in the rest of this section. Other approaches exist (Box 13.4) but, for many researchers, their use is limited by the lack of readily available computing packages to perform the data analyses.

13.4.2 Goodness-of-fit tests

Goodness-of-fit tests are those that assess the extent to which the statistical properties of a sample (e.g. central tendency, dispersion, distribution) match those of a known population, or some specified model. Goodness-of-fit tests are

Box 13.4   *Approaches to statistical inference*

The approach to statistical inference adopted in this book is predicated on a *frequentist* model. In this model, the underlying principle of statistical inference is based on a relative frequency interpretation of probability, and the starting point for statistical decision making is the null hypothesis. It is important to realize, however, that there are different interpretations of this approach, and an alternative approach that rejects this underlying model of inference (Howson and Urbach, 1989). Within the frequentist approach, two schools of thought can be identified: one based on the writings of Ronald Fisher and one based on those of Jerzy Neyman and Egon Pearson. The points of difference between these perspectives are complex and detailed, but are principally concerned with different approaches to setting a level of statistical significance. At the risk of oversimplifying the matter, Fisher tended to advocate a standard cut-off for statistical significance, whereas Neyman and Pearson suggested that this should be adjusted according to the context of inference, and in relation to the relative likelihood of a Type I and a Type II error. Gigerenzer argues that contemporary frequentist statistical inference is a hybrid of these approaches: 'the offspring of the shotgun marriage between Fisher and Newman and Pearson' (Gigerenzer, 1993, p. 322). The

Bayesian approach – named after the eighteenth-century cleric and mathematician Thomas Bayes – is based on a subjective interpretation of probability (Bland and Altman, 1998). In this approach, before conducting an experiment a scientist will estimate the probability of an outcome or effect (the *prior probability*), based on what he or she already knows on the subject. The results of the study will then be used to modify this subjective probability (which then becomes the *posterior probability*). Rather than starting each experiment in an area of study with a null hypothesis and effectively ignoring prior knowledge, as is advocated by the frequentist, the Bayesian uses each experiment to update knowledge from the previous experiment. Thus, the Bayesian revises the probability of a hypothesis, given the evidence, whereas the frequentist examines the probability of the evidence, given the (null) hypothesis. Bayesian and frequentist methods have differing implications for certain specific aspects of statistical analysis, such as the presentation of results, interim analyses, and the analysis of subsets of data (Spiegelhalter *et al.*, 1999). Further discussion of these issues can be found in Oakes (1986), Howson and Urbach (1989), O'Hear (1989), Gigerenzer (1993), Winkler (1993) and Chow (1996).

often used when testing whether the assumptions of a particular statistical test hold in relation to data in a sample. They are also referred to as *one-sample* tests, since only one set of sample data is utilized. In a *two-sample* test, two sets of sample data (which may be either related or unrelated) are used to perform the statistical test. Although one-sample tests are referred to from time to time in this book, they are not covered in detail.

13.4.3 Outline procedure for hypothesis tests

The decision to include statistical tests in a

research project is taken at the design stage, when one also considers what test might be most applicable. The procedure for this process is discussed in the following sections. An outline procedure for the process and the ensuing analyses is given in Figure 13.6. Steps 2 through to 5 might be considered conjointly or repeatedly until a practical and realistic compromise is reached; they are considered before beginning data collection. Throughout the process, we assume that a statistical package would be used to perform the analyses.

Stage 6 is often preceded by a pilot study

1. A research hypothesis is specified

2. Outcome variables are operationalized *A decision is made about what data to collect and under what conditions (Section 7.2.3). Other aspects of design are addressed as appropriate.*

3. Statistical hypotheses are identified *Both the null hypothesis and its alternative hypothesis are specified. The levels of measurement implied in the hypotheses and those anticipated in the collected data should be consistent. (Section 13.4.4)*

4. A statistical test is selected *The chosen test should be appropriate for: the given research design; the selected sampling method and conditions; the anticipated level(s) of measurement of the data; the specified null and alternative hypotheses; the nature of the population(s) from which the sample is to be selected; a plausible maximum sample size. (Section 13.4.5)*

5. A significance level and the required power of the test are specified *The required sample size is calculated using this information together with the chosen statistical test. An allowance is made for attrition or non-response. (Sections 13.4.7 & 13.4.8)*

6. Data are collected and entered into a computer file *The data file should be checked for accuracy (Section 12.6). A standard procedure is followed to minimize the amount of missing or erroneous data.*

7. The assumptions required by the statistical test specified at Stage 4 are checked *These assumptions are checked against: the actual sampling method and conditions appertaining to the study; the achieved level(s) of measurement; the achieved sample size. A different statistical test or analysis is selected if necessary. (Section 13.4.5)*

8. A check is made for outliers and for violations of the assumptions underlying the selected statistical test *If the assumptions are violated to an extent that is not tolerated by robustness of the test, then a different statistical test or analysis is selected, or data transformations might be considered. Statistical summaries are produced and considered at this stage. (Sections 13.4.5 & 13.4.11)*

9. The statistical test is performed on the data *For many tests, a test statistic and a p value are obtained; for exact tests, only a p value is obtained. It is important to remember that the p value is a conditional probability; it assumes the truth of the null hypothesis (Section 13.4.6).*

10. A decision is made either to reject or not to reject the null hypothesis *This is done using the significance level specified at Stage 5 and the computed p value from the test. If the p value is smaller than or equal to the significance level, the null hypothesis is rejected; if the p value is larger than the significance level, the null hypothesis is not rejected (Section 13.4.7).*

11. Further analyses are performed as appropriate *Whenever possible, the computation of confidence intervals should be considered (Section 13.3). Other analyses might include comparisons across groups (Sections 18.1.3 & 18.1.4).*

12. The results are interpreted *(Sections 13.4.9 & 13.4.10)*

13. Clinical or practical implications of the findings are discussed *Limitations of the study and data analyses should be acknowledged. (Section 13.4.10)*

Figure 13.6 *Steps in statistical hypothesis testing.*

(Section 6.1). This provides an opportunity to test the study protocol and the appropriateness and practicality of measurement tools. It might be feasible to go through the proposed analysis, but usually there is insufficient data to check any assumptions at the pilot stage.

13.4.4 Research and statistical hypotheses

A distinction should be drawn between the research hypothesis and the statistical hypotheses within a study (Stages 1 and 3 in Figure 13.6).

Research hypothesis
The research hypothesis provides a focus and direction for a study. It often relates to a generic outcome, such as 'effectiveness' of therapy, that the researcher operationalizes in terms of one or more outcome variables for which valid and reliable measurement tools exist. For example, in the Low Back Pain Study, effectiveness was evaluated through values of pain intensity, pain affect and the Aberdeen Back Pain Scale.

Statistical hypotheses
Statistical hypotheses corresponding to each outcome variable are formulated from the

research hypothesis. The null hypothesis (written as H_0) is a statement of no effect (e.g. no difference, no change, no association) and the corresponding alternative hypothesis (written as H_1) is a statement of effect, covering all other possible situations. The null and alternative hypotheses are thus *collectively exhaustive* and *mutually exclusive* with respect to possible outcomes of a study (i.e. all possible outcomes should be ascribable to one or other of the null and the alternative hypotheses, and no outcome should be ascribable to both hypotheses). Table 13.1 shows some examples of statistical hypotheses and Table 13.2 displays some of their properties.

Issues concerning statistical hypothesis tests
There are two issues here that need further discussion. The first concerns the use of the null hypothesis as the basis for the statistical testing procedure when, usually, the researcher is performing the study because some difference is expected. A formal condition for a hypothesis is that it must be formulated in such a way that its corroboration, or lack of it, can be achieved through data collected on an outcome variable. This condition can be satisfied when the null

Table 13.1 *Examples of research and statistical hypotheses*

Hypothesis	Example statement
Research	There is a difference in effectiveness between individual-based and group-based cognitive-behavioural approaches to the management of low back pain.
Null	There is no difference in the mean changes in pain intensity scores following an individual-based and a group-based approach to the management of low back pain.
Alternative	The mean change in pain intensity scores is different following an individual-based compared with a group-based approach to the management of low back pain.
Research	There is a difference in how occupational therapists and physiotherapists perceive the responsiveness to therapy of patients with rheumatoid arthritis.
Null	There is no association between profession and perception of responsiveness to therapy of patients with rheumatoid arthritis.
Alternative	There is an association between profession and perception of responsiveness to therapy of patients with rheumatoid arthritis.
Research	Deaf children are more likely to have impaired vision than are children with normal hearing.
Null	The proportion of deaf children who have impaired vision is the same as the proportion of children with normal hearing who have impaired vision.
Alternative	There is a difference between the proportions of deaf children and those with normal hearing who have impaired vision.

Table 13.2   *Properties of null and alternative hypotheses*

Null hypothesis (H$_0$)	Alternative hypothesis (H$_1$)
The tested hypothesis	The complement of H$_0$
States a 'null' situation – no difference, no change, no effect or no association	States all possibilities not covered under H$_0$ – there is some difference, change or effect of an unknown magnitude; there is some association but of an unstated relational form
States assumed value(s) for specific characteristic(s) of the population	Does not state specific values or relational form
Reflects the situation that the researcher believes is false (usually)	Reflects the situation that the researcher believes is true: the research hypothesis (usually)
Data that are inconsistent with H$_0$ can be used as evidence to reject it, in favour of H$_1$	Data that are consistent with the alternative hypothesis cannot be used to establish its truth

hypothesis is tested, but *not* if an attempt were made to test the alternative hypothesis.

A decision to reject or not to reject the null hypothesis can be based on the probability that the data are a random sample from the population that is specified by the null hypothesis. A large probability provides evidence that the data are consistent with the null hypothesis and a small probability that the data are inconsistent; that is, the data are unlikely to be a random sample from the assumed population. A large probability provides no reason to doubt the null hypothesis, whereas a small probability provides evidence to reject the null hypothesis in favour of the alternative hypothesis. The alternative hypothesis is the complement of the null hypothesis and as such does not specify a single value for the population parameter against which to perform the testing. For example, when considering a possible difference in outcome between two intervention groups, the null hypothesis specifies a single value for this difference – zero. The alternative hypothesis, on the other hand, does not specify any specific value for this difference; it states only that the difference will be other than zero. All values greater than or less than zero are covered by the alternative hypothesis. As the statistical hypothesis test operates on a specific value of the population parameter, it can do this only in relation to the null hypothesis.

The second issue concerns the wording of the alternative hypothesis. Irrespective of the expected direction of any difference or change implied in the *research* hypothesis, we have worded the *alternative* hypothesis as non-directional. This non-directional alternative hypothesis (also referred to as 'two-sided' or 'two-tailed') is in contrast to a directional ('one-sided' or 'one-tailed') alternative hypothesis such as 'medication A is more effective than medication B'. In this book, we follow the position advocated by Armitage and Berry (1994), Bland and Altman (1994a) and Greenhalgh (1997). Armitage and Berry (1994, p. 97) argue that

> one should decide to use a one-sided test only if it is quite certain that departures in one direction will always be ascribed to chance, and therefore regarded as non-significant however large they are. This situation rarely arises in practice, and it will be safe to assume that significance tests should almost always be two-sided.

In other words, in order to use a directional alternative hypothesis, the researcher would have to believe that only a change in a specified direction would make sense within the theoretical framework of the study. Any observed change in the other direction would be theoretically implausible, and would therefore be ascribed to chance (Box 13.5).

Box 13.5 *Unidirectional effects*

It is not easy to think of effects that could work in only one direction. It might seem likely that a certain painkiller will either reduce or leave untouched a person's level of pain, but it may still be theoretically conceivable that in some circumstances it could increase the level of pain. Equally, it is perhaps reasonable to suppose that if there is any correlation between a person's level of occupational achievement and their level of self-esteem, this will be a positive correlation; but can a negative relationship between these variables really be ruled out categorically? We would argue, therefore, that a directional hypothesis should not be used on the basis of what the researcher may hope or expect to find (as might be expressed in the research hypothesis), and should be reserved for those occasions when an effect in the opposite direction can be excluded on theoretical grounds.

Whatever the researcher's belief, the choice between directional and non-directional hypotheses should never be made after viewing the data. To do so would allow statistical sleight of hand. If a change is observed to lie in a certain direction, the magnitude of such change required to reject the null hypothesis is smaller with a one-tailed than with a two-tailed test (Gravetter and Wallnau, 1988). Hence, switching from a two-tailed to a one-tailed test on the basis of having examined the data would be an improper means of ensuring that a null hypothesis is rejected. One further word of caution concerns the use of the term 'experimental hypothesis' instead of 'alternative hypothesis'. This practice should be avoided on the basis that such a hypothesis might exist within a study that does not employ an experimental design.

13.4.5 Selecting a statistical test

Experimental designs are constructed to answer an explanatory question of cause and effect, and will lead to the use of inferential statistics. It is common practice to perform different tests according to the number of groups of patients involved in the design (one, two or more) and according to the employed methods of randomization (Section 13.6) and control. A further distinction is drawn between designs in which data are collected repeatedly over time on the same group of cases or on individually matched cases (*repeated* or *related* measures, respectively) and designs in which data are collected on independent groups of cases (*unrelated* measures).

Survey designs are often employed to test associations between variables or to test for differences between specified subgroups of cases, in the absence of the manipulation of an intervention variable. The appropriate statistical hypothesis tests will depend upon the research question to be answered and upon the sampling method employed.

Levels of measurement for the outcome variable

The level of measurement chosen for each outcome variable is, perhaps, the most controversial determinant of what test is and is not appropriate in a situation. Controversy arises through different perspectives in measurement theory with respect to ordinal scales (Labovitz, 1970; Knapp, 1990). There are two key issues here: determining whether a scale is ordinal or not, and deciding what mathematical operations are valid on an ordinal scale. We shall follow Stevens' (1946) typology, given in Section 12.2.2; that is, there is a meaningful ordering of values on an ordinal scale, but the numbers have no meaning in a mathematical sense and it is not possible to quantify differences. On this premise, tests that have been established for the analysis of data measured at an interval or ratio level involve statistics such as means and standard deviations, and these tests should not, therefore, be applied to ordinal scales – nor, of course, to nominal scales. However, tests established for the analysis of data measured at a nominal or ordinal level involve statistics such as counts and (for ordinal scales) medians, and can be applied to data at an interval or ratio level of measurement (sometimes following a suitable grouping of values). Many authors believe that the real issue in practice is whether the results from an analysis have a meaningful interpretation (Knapp, 1990), which may very well not be the case if tests are applied to data at an inappropriate level of measurement.

Assumptions of normality and homogeneity of variance

Many tests involving continuous data (as defined in Section 12.2.6) require additional assumptions concerning the distribution of values in the population. These tests can be performed if the collected data are consistent with the assumptions. The most common assumptions are that the data from the study groups constitute random samples from normally distributed populations having equal variances (Altman, 1991a; Daniel, 1991). When the groups have equal sample sizes, investigations have shown that these tests are *robust*, in that they are approximately valid for distributions that are moderately non-normal or have small departures from equal variance (Domholdt, 1993; Howell, 1997; Conover, 1999). Here, 'moderately' and 'small' are difficult to define (Bland, 1995). The situation is more uncertain when the groups have unequal sample sizes (Myers and Well, 1995). Statistical tests exist to check the assumption of normality, and to check whether variances are equal (*homogeneity of variance* or *homoscedasticity*) or unequal (*heterogeneity of variance* or *heteroscedasticity*). Examples of such tests are given in Box 14.3. It is difficult to test these assumptions with any real power (Section 13.4.8) when the sample size is small. Furthermore, and rather paradoxically, if the sample is large enough for the test for normality to have acceptable power, it is quite likely that the central limit theorem can be invoked, making the test redundant.

In many instances the data can be *transformed* to a scale on which the assumption of normality is satisfied and statistical tests are then performed on the transformed data (Ferketich and Verran, 1994). A transformation is a mathematical operation applied to the data, such as taking the reciprocal, square root or logarithm of the original data (Altman, 1991a; Bland, 1995). In many practical situations, non-normality is accompanied by unequal variances. Using an appropriate transformation might produce data that are consistent with the requirements of both normality and homogeneity of variance.

When no appropriate transformation can be found, or when the data are measured at an ordinal or nominal level, statistical tests are selected that do not require assumptions about the distribution of values in the population. Statistical methods based on distributional assumptions are called *parametric* and those that do not depend on distributional assumptions are called *nonparametric* (Pett, 1997) or *distribution-free* (Neave and Worthington, 1988). Many nonparametric procedures are based on sums of ranks. The ranks are relative positions of the values associated with the variable being investigated or the 'numerical' order of data with respect to a variable. When the sample size is large, we can use the central limit theorem to assume that the sum of ranks closely follows a normal distribution (Section 13.2.2). In this situation, a normal distribution is a good approximation to the sampling distribution of the sum of ranks and, therefore, the nonparametric method might be performed through a *normal approximation* (Altman, 1991a; Conover, 1999). This is not to say, however, that the data are consistent with values in a random sample from a normal population. Further discussion of parametric and nonparametric methods is given in Section 13.7.

13.4.6 The test statistic and p value

In the hypothetical example outlined in Section 13.4.1, the population mean was 100 and its standard deviation was known to be 28 units. A random sample of 64 units produced a mean score of 110.5 units, corresponding to a standardized score of 3. This standardized score was calculated assuming the population mean value of 100 and using the properties of a normal sampling distribution. It is called a *test statistic* and forms the basis for statistical decision making. In general, a test statistic is some quantity that is calculated from a sample of data, using the information in the null hypothesis and the sampling distribution of the test statistic. For the above example,

$$\text{test statistic} = \frac{\text{sample mean} - \text{hypothesized population mean}}{\text{standard error of the sample mean}}$$

$$= \frac{110.5 - 100}{28 / \sqrt{64}}$$

$$= 3$$

Hence, the test statistic is a value that can be compared with the distribution that we expect to see if the null hypothesis is true. Large magnitudes are unlikely; small ones are likely.

The p value is the probability of the obtained value, or a more extreme value, of the test statistic which would occur if the null hypothesis were true, given a random sample of the specified size. The p value therefore represents a conditional probability (Section 13.1.3).

13.4.7 Significance level and making a decision

Traditionally, the decision made in relation to a statistical hypothesis test has been based on a cut-off value that divides the p values into 'low' and 'high'. Low p values are smaller than or equal to the cut-off value. These cast doubt on the null hypothesis, leading to the decision to reject it; the result is called *statistically significant*. High p values are those that are larger than the cut-off value. These do not cast doubt on the null hypothesis, leading to the decision not to reject the null hypothesis and the result is said to be 'statistically non-significant' (Figure 13.7).

The cut-off value is specified before any data are collected and is called the *significance level*. The usual levels of significance are .05 (5%), .01 (1%) and .001 (0.1%). These are arbitrary levels and have no specific importance; hence, a decision to 'reject' or 'not reject' does not necessarily provide any guidance in practical situations (Altman, 1991a; Bland, 1995). The exact p values give only slightly more information.

It is worth noting that the word 'significant' is associated with the result from a hypothesis test and not with the null hypothesis that is being tested. Hence, a null hypothesis should be worded as 'there is no difference in effectiveness of two medications, A and B', rather than 'there is no significant difference in effectiveness of two medications, A and B'.

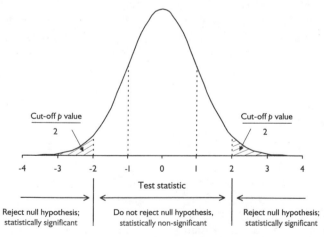

Figure 13.7 *Use of a cut-off value (significance level) to make a decision in statistical hypothesis testing based on a normal distribution.*

13.4.8 Significance level, power and sample size

Significance level and types of error

The significance level is chosen at the design stage of a study and, as seen in the previous section, is the cut-off value for statistical decision making. The null hypothesis is rejected (when the p value is smaller than or equal to the significance level) or not rejected (when the p value is larger than the significance level) based on the evidence in a random sample from the population. There are two errors possible here (Table 13.3): rejecting a true null hypothesis (called a Type I error) and not rejecting a false null hypothesis (called a Type II error). The symbols α (alpha) and β (beta) are frequently used to denote the probabilities of Type I and Type II errors, respectively. The relationship between these errors is illustrated in Figure 13.8 (see also Box 13.6).

Box 13.6   *An analogy with judicial decision making*

An analogy with judicial verdicts can be used to illustrate Type I and Type II errors. In a criminal trial, the initial presumption of innocence equates with the null hypothesis. At the end of the trial, the accused may be found guilty when he or she is really innocent; this is equivalent to rejecting the null hypothesis when it is true (Type I error). Alternatively, the accused may be acquitted when he or she is really guilty; this corresponds to retaining the null hypothesis when it is false (Type II error). The likelihood of convicting the accused can be increased by adopting a less stringent standard of proof (such as 'on the balance of probabilities', rather than 'beyond reasonable doubt'); this is equivalent to increasing alpha (e.g. from $p = .05$ to $p = .10$). Doing so increases the likelihood of finding innocent people guilty or, equivalently, of rejecting null hypotheses that are true.

Table 13.3   *Possible results in statistical decision making based on a significance level α*

Statistical decision	True situation (unknown)	
	H_0 true	H_0 false
H_0 rejected	Type I error (probability α)	Correct decision (probability $1 - \beta$)
H_0 not rejected	Correct decision (probability $1 - \alpha$)	Type II error (probability β)

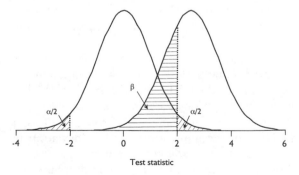

Figure 13.8   *Relationship between Type I and Type II errors.*

In reality, the true situation regarding the truth of the null hypothesis is unknown (the research would be unnecessary otherwise) and therefore we do not know when an incorrect decision has been made, or indeed a correct decision. Further, depending upon the sampling error, a second sample from the same population might result in a different decision. Thus, although steps can be taken to restrict the likelihood of either a Type I or a Type II error, we can never know whether either error has been committed in any one study.

This has implications for the wording of conclusions drawn from statistical tests. An accurate statement would be either that 'the data in this study provide evidence to doubt the null hypothesis', or that 'the data in this study provide no evidence to doubt the null hypothesis'; the latter is preferable to referring to 'accepting' the null hypothesis, although the term 'retain' might be used (Calder, 1996; Huck and Cormier, 1996); see also Box 2.2.

Power

The probability of a Type I error is controlled by the researcher; it is the significance level, commonly $\alpha = .05$. That is, the researcher decides an acceptable risk of rejecting a true null hypothesis (or finding a 'false positive' result) in a particular study. The probability of a Type II error (or finding a 'false negative' result) is controlled through the sample size. Larger sample sizes are associated with smaller sampling errors, and hence smaller Type II errors. It is more usual to consider the complement of the Type II error, which is correctly rejecting a false hypothesis or finding a significant result when an effect does indeed exist in the population. The probability of correctly rejecting a false null hypothesis is called the *power* of a test and is denoted by $(1 - \beta)$, or $100(1 - \beta)\%$. A power of 80% or 90% is normally considered acceptable in most studies.

Sample size

The sample size is chosen so that an observed effect in the sample – equal in magnitude to a population effect considered important by the researcher – can be discerned as statistically significant (at the selected significance level and with the specified power). Any other sample size might be viewed as unethical (Section 7.5.2). A smaller sample size might fail to detect a clinically meaningful effect in the population. A larger sample size is wasteful on resources, having the power to statistically discern an effect that is too small to be important in practice. Calculations for the sample size are usually based on the most important outcome variable or combination of outcome variables, and require information on the hypothesis test to be performed, an estimate of what effect size (or difference) is important and an estimate of the variability of the outcome values. These estimates might exist from previous studies or they might be obtained through a pilot study. Section 17.3.1 contains a discussion of effect size statistics, and further details of sample size calculation can be found in Section 18.6.

13.4.9 Presenting results from statistical analyses

Reporting results only as 'significant' or 'not significant' provides no indication of the importance of findings with respect to professional practice. The common practice of reporting the p value and (where applicable) the value of the test statistic for each statistical test is little better. These values provide no information about the magnitude of an effect or strength of an association, irrespective of whether or not it is significant. Summary statistics and confidence intervals, however, provide information about the magnitude of an effect, enabling a judgement to be made concerning the clinical importance of results. The summaries can be presented for each outcome variable, for change over time, for differences between groups, and for subgroups. Producing and examining summary statistics was recommended as an important element within Step 8 in the general procedure for performing hypothesis tests (Figure 13.6).

13.4.10 Interpretation and clinical implications

Hypothesis tests (also sometimes called 'significance tests') lead to 'significant' or 'non-significant' results. Confusion often occurs over the word 'significant' because, in everyday parlance, it is used to denote something of importance. A statistically significant result is not necessarily important in practice – health professionals must determine what size of effect (e.g. what magnitude of difference or what degree of association) is clinically meaningful in any specific context.

Although the term 'statistically significant' is accepted usage, 'statistically discernible' might be less misleading. The magnitude of effect that is discernible through a statistical hypothesis test is affected by the sampling error, which is a function of the population standard deviation (a measure of the variability of individual values around the mean in the population) and the sample size. Larger sample sizes enable smaller effects in a population to be statistically discernible in random samples from that population. However, larger sample sizes also have the power to detect as statistically significant some differences that might not be practically meaningful (Di Fabio, 1999). That is, small effects present in the random sample might be discerned as statistically significant. The converse situation is that small samples might lack the power to detect population effects that are practically important. The practitioner should not equate 'non-significance' with absence of an effect in the population. 'Non-significance' implies that the variability expected as a consequence of sampling error can reasonably account for the size of effect obtained in the random sample. It does not imply that no effect exists in the population; that is, 'absence of evidence is not evidence of absence' (Altman and Bland, 1995; Tarnow-Mordi and Healy, 1999).

Thus, an effect may exist in the population despite the fact that no effect has been demonstrated in the sample. It is equally the case that if an effect is demonstrated in a sample, this does not in itself indicate an effect of the same magnitude in the corresponding population parameter, as the effect in the sample might be due to sampling error. It might therefore reasonably be argued that, in such a situation, the effect is not a real one (Rothstein, 1995). However, it is important to realize that although the effect may not be 'real' for the population, it is still 'real' for the sample (assuming a valid method of measurement has been employed).

Health professionals need to be critical of the findings from statistical hypothesis tests and not base their clinical interpretation of the results solely upon the p values. They need to examine the summary statistics, including confidence intervals or effect sizes where applicable, and draw upon their professional knowledge to determine the practical importance of such statistics.

13.4.11 Influence of aberrant values

Descriptive statistics, such as frequency distributions, and graphs, such as boxplots, provide a simple visual check for aberrant values or outliers (Section 12.6). *Outliers* are cases with extreme values on one or more variables which appear to be incompatible with the rest of the data. They are important because they can have a marked influence on the results from statistical analyses. For example, one very large value in a small data set will produce a mean value that is much larger than the median.

There are several possible reasons for the presence of outliers (Tabachnick and Fidell, 1996):

- an incorrect data entry – the entry in the computer file should be checked against the data sheet, which in turn is checked against the original record or questionnaire
- forgetting to set the missing value codes within the computing package, so that missing value indicators appear as real data
- inadvertent inclusion of a case that does not satisfy the inclusion and exclusion criteria for the study – the case should be omitted
- a case has been recorded that has extreme values within the population being studied.

The last of these is a difficult situation to resolve. First, the records should be checked for any information that identifies the reason for this extreme value; for example, a problem with the measurement procedure for this case, or the occurrence of a major life event during the study that might have affected the variable for the individual concerned. If a reason of this kind exists, the case can justifiably be omitted. Similarly, a case can be omitted if, when the profile of values across all variables is considered, the case is found to be extreme on every variable.

Alternatively, if there is evidence that the distribution is skewed, a transformation might be applied to the data. Apparent outliers on one scale might be typical values on another more appropriate scale. Finally, if no plausible reason can be found for the atypical value, the analysis might be repeated both with and without the case. Similar results indicate that the outlier has had a minimal influence. Very different results indicate that the outlier has had an undue influence and an alternative analysis should be performed (perhaps using nonparametric statistical procedures that utilize ranks rather than the actual variate scores).

13.5 APPLICATION OF CONFIDENCE INTERVALS AND HYPOTHESIS TESTING

Confidence interval estimation and hypothesis testing involve drawing inferences about population characteristics from the information contained in a random sample (or samples) from that population. The medical and biomedical literature appears to suggest that beginners in research use statistical hypothesis testing as the preferred method of data analysis (Altman, 1991a; Sim and Reid, 1999). The move towards reporting confidence intervals was greatly influenced by the encouragement or requirement of several leading medical journals that authors present confidence intervals with their main findings (Altman *et al.*, 1989). Articles discussing the key concepts of statistical inference (Abrams and Scragg, 1996; Maclaren, 1998) and the use and merits of confidence intervals in the context of medical and biomedical research (Altman, 1991a; Chinn, 1991a; Sim and Reid, 1999) have provided further encouragement to researchers.

The main difference between the two approaches to statistical inference lies in the information that derives from their use. The *p* value is central to hypothesis testing and the declaration of a result as 'significant' or 'not significant'. However, it provides no information about the magnitude of any effect, difference, change or association in the population being investigated. On that basis, it is difficult to consider the clinical importance of any findings. Even non-significant results might be important in practice (Altman, 1991a; Sim and Reid, 1999). To some extent, the sample size determines what is detectable as statistically significant. Some quantification of the magnitude of effect, difference, change or association is needed to inform the practitioner about what is probably happening in the population. This can be provided in terms of a point estimate, or

more usefully, through a confidence interval. Further, the confidence limits could be used in a cost-effectiveness analysis to evaluate the likely minimum and maximum effects associated with two therapies.

Further comparisons of the properties of hypothesis testing and confidence interval estimation are given in Table 13.4.

13.6 RANDOM AND NON-RANDOM SAMPLES

The discussion hitherto on inferential statistics has assumed that the data being analysed are from a random sample from some well-defined population. This assumption is required for the strict validity of the statistical procedures. There are many investigations in which it is unrealistic or impossible to achieve random sampling, or for which no well-defined population can be specified. For example, convenience sampling is used in many student projects as a result of difficulties in accessing research participants and various resource constraints. Similarly, projects that evaluate educational interventions might be reliant on volunteers as participants, and routine patterns of practice might be observed over a specified number of consecutive patients attending a clinic. In all of these situations, the individual items of data are likely to vary in a haphazard way. The issue is whether we can argue that, although the data do not derive from a random sample, they are nonetheless subject to random, unsystematic variation that makes them compatible with data from a random sample (Armitage and Berry, 1994).

A reasoned argument can be made that data from comparative experiments, such as randomized controlled trials, are compatible with those from a random sample. The participants are not usually randomly selected from a well-defined population; rather, they are consecutive, willing persons who satisfy inclusion and exclusion criteria. However, the participants are allocated at random to various groups (a minimum of two) to receive different treatments (Section 7.2.1). Comparison of the treatment

Table 13.4 *Comparison of the properties of hypothesis testing and confidence interval estimation with respect to the effectiveness of an intervention*

Hypothesis testing	Confidence interval estimation
• Usually, tests an assumption of no effect in the population (null hypothesis, H_0) against an assumption of some effect (alternative hypothesis, H_1).	• Produces an interval that, with a specified level of confidence, contains the population mean effect. Requires no assumption about the magnitude of the effect in the population.
• Uses data from a random sample of the population.	• Uses data from a random sample of the population.
• Makes an assumption about the distribution of the sample mean effect, e.g. a normal distribution for large samples.	• Makes an assumption about the distribution of the sample mean effect, e.g. a normal distribution for large samples.
• The researcher selects the significance level (α) and the power for the statistical test.	• The researcher selects the confidence level ($1 - \alpha$) for the confidence interval (CI).
• The sample size is calculated from the significance level, the power, and the magnitude of effect that the researcher wants to be able to detect as statistically significant.	• The sample size is calculated from the confidence level and the precision with which the researcher wants to estimate the magnitude of the effect in the population.
• Provides a p value – the probability, when the population mean effect is zero, that a random sample from the population would produce a mean effect at least as extreme as that obtained from the collected sample.	• Provides an interval estimate for the magnitude of the mean effect in the population. The interval is associated with a confidence of ($1 - \alpha$) that it contains the population mean effect.
• Produces a decision based on the p value and the significance level. The decision is either to 'reject' or 'not reject' H_0, the assumption that the mean effect is zero in the population.	• A hypothesis test, with significance level, could be performed using the CI. H_0 would be rejected when the confidence interval did not contain the assumed mean effect; otherwise, H_0 would not be rejected.
• The p value provides no information about the magnitude of the effect in the population.	• Any value between the lower and upper confidence limits is a plausible value for the mean effect in the population.
• The p value does not indicate clinical importance, irrespective of its value.	• Clinical importance may be assessed by considering the confidence limits.
• Larger samples lead to smaller p values.	• Larger samples lead to narrower CIs (i.e. higher precision), for a given confidence level.
• Smaller sampling error leads to smaller p values, for a given sample size.	• Smaller sampling error leads to narrower CIs (i.e. higher precision), for a given confidence level and a given sample size.
• A larger mean effect in the population leads to smaller p values, for a given sample size.	• A larger mean effect in the population will cause the CI to shift further from the null value, for a given sample size and a given sample variance.
• Other things being equal, a smaller value of α leads to fewer false rejections of H_0, but more false retentions.	• Other things being equal, a higher value of ($1 - \alpha$) leads to a wider interval, reflecting a higher confidence of containing the population mean effect.

effects is a primary objective of such a study, and requires an assessment of the extent to which the between-group contrasts are affected by random variation. The random allocation of participants to groups ensures that the differences between groups behave like differences between random samples – irrespective of the presence of any treatment effects. Thus, although random *sampling* may be absent, the presence of random *allocation* means that infer-

ential statistical procedures are valid for the analysis of comparative experiments (Daniel, 1991; Armitage and Berry, 1994).

For other situations, we try to visualize the shape of the sampling distribution that would be produced if we could collect an infinitely large sample exhibiting the same pattern of variation as those in the available data. If this distribution is deemed compatible with that produced through random sampling, then inferential procedures are performed. This decision is based on non-statistical considerations, including the method of sampling, known features of the population being sampled, and the researcher's judgement concerning the representativeness of the sample (Maclaren, 1998). The assumption of no systematic error should be scrutinized. Assuming that the data behave like a random sample when they do not can lead to grossly misleading conclusions. In published studies, a careful examination of the participants' characteristics might provide some indication of systematic error.

13.7 PARAMETRIC AND NONPARAMETRIC STATISTICAL METHODS

The relative merits of parametric and nonparametric inferential procedures have been debated for more than 60 years. Parametric inferential procedures concern testing hypotheses about one or more population parameters and require knowledge of, or assumptions about, the distribution of values in the population. Nonparametric inferential procedures are not based on assumptions about population parameters. These 'distribution-free' inferential procedures (Neave and Worthington, 1988) make no assumptions about the distribution of the population. It is common practice to use the terms 'nonparametric and 'distribution-free' interchangeably (Box 13.7).

The choice between parametric and nonparametric procedures is not an easy one. Common characteristics of the two approaches are given in Table 13.5. Section 13.4.5 discussed determinants of test choice, such as the research objective, type of random process employed, level of measurement, validity of assumptions underlying a test, and robustness of the findings to departures from these assumptions. When all the assumptions hold, for a fixed sample size and significance level, parametric tests are considered more powerful than nonparametric tests based on ranks or a nominal level of measurement (Siegel and Castellan, 1988; May *et al.*, 1990; Hunter and May, 1993; Pett, 1997). Monte

Box 13.7 *'Nonparametric' and data*

It is fairly common, but incorrect, practice to refer to '(non)parametric data'. Since the data come from a sample and parameters are properties of a population, this is illogical usage. Furthermore, it is the assumptions made by a statistical procedure about the nature and distribution of the values in the population from which the data are selected that are parametric or nonparametric, not the data themselves. Any data based on a sample that has been drawn from a population will have population parameters associated with them, and to that extent all such data could be described as 'parametric'; the issue is whether or not a statistical procedure has to make assumptions about these parameters.

Carlo simulations have indicated that, under random sampling, the relative power of parametric and nonparametric tests is dependent upon sample size and the distribution of values from which the samples were drawn (Lehmann and D'Abrera, 1975; Blair and Higgins, 1985). nonparametric tests were shown to be the more powerful in situations involving non-normal distributions. Hunter and May (1993) argue that it is a rare situation in which all assumptions hold, with non-normality and non-random sampling, in particular, being common occurrences. Further, the researcher should remember that procedures used to test assumptions are themselves based upon assumptions that need checking.

Choosing a test is sometimes considered in terms of *relative efficiency* (also called 'power efficiency'). The relative efficiency of a test B with respect to another test A is defined as the ratio of the sample sizes needed for both tests to achieve the same power. That is,

$$\text{relative efficiency} = \left(\frac{n_A}{n_B}\right) \times 100\%$$

For example, if tests A and B require 45 and 50 cases, respectively, to achieve the same

Table 13.5 *Common characteristics of statistical tests*

Parametric tests	Nonparametric tests
Suitable for data measured on at least an interval level.	Suitable for data measured on at least a nominal level. That is, some procedures are applicable for data comprising classifications or rankings. Some require underlying continuity of the variable under study.
Require assumptions about the distribution of population values.	Require no assumptions about the distribution of population values.
Many are based on the assumption that the data comprise values from a normally distributed population.	Many are based on sums of ranks. Some require symmetrical distributions.
Based on the assumption that a random process is employed, e.g. random sampling or random allocation to groups.	Do not require the assumption of random sampling (Hunter and May, 1993), but need independence between cases.
Use a sample size determined to statistically discern an important difference at a given significance level with specified power, i.e. Type I error and power are controlled.	Use a sample size determined to statistically discern an important difference at a given significance level with specified power, i.e. Type I error and power are controlled.
Most are based on equal sample sizes.	Most cope with unequal sample sizes.
Can be used on small samples ($n < 30$) only when the assumptions are known to hold.	Can be used with small samples ($n < 30$).
For large samples, the central limit theorem can be invoked to assume that means, totals, proportions follow a normal distribution.	For large samples, the central limit theorem can be invoked to assume that the normal distribution is a good approximation to the sampling distribution of ranks.
Data values might be unrelated (not matched or unpaired) or related (matched or paired).	Data values might be unrelated (not matched or unpaired) or related (matched or paired).
Many require data to be values from populations having equal variances.	Can cope with unequal variances across groups.
Results are affected by gross outliers.	Results are insensitive to gross outliers.

power, at a specified significance level, test B is said to have a relative efficiency of 90% (45/50 × 100). In other words, to achieve the same power with both tests (at a specified significance level and when all assumptions are met) we would need to select ten cases for use in test B for every nine cases required for test A. The relative efficiency of specific parametric and nonparametric tests will be discussed in Chapters 14 and 18.

13.8 CONCLUSION

This chapter has discussed the role and use of inferential statistics. Basic principles of probability, the normal distribution and sampling distributions were introduced to explain the precepts upon which inferential procedures and methods are based. An understanding of them is fundamental to a real understanding of hypothesis tests and confidence interval estimation. This understanding enables the researcher to appraise published statistical analyses, to select appropriate statistical analyses for use in his or her own research, and to report results in an appropriate and informative manner without confusing or misleading the reader.

There is ongoing debate about when parametric and nonparametric tests should be used and about the reporting of p values. What is not subject to debate is the need for the researcher to pursue descriptive analyses on the data before rushing into performing hypothesis tests, and to report summary statistics as well as p values.

The next chapter will consider some hypothesis tests and interval estimates that are frequently used by health care researchers.

14 ANALYSING DATA FROM DESCRIPTIVE AND EXPLANATORY STUDIES: PROCEDURES

SUMMARY

This chapter explores the following topics:

- a selection of statistical methods for the analysis of associations between two variables, or between two sets of data on a single variable:
  - Pearson's chi-square test of independence
  - Pearson's product moment correlation coefficient
  - Spearman's rank order correlation coefficient
- a selection of statistical methods for the analysis of differences between two sets of data on a single variable:
  - the related *t* test and the Wilcoxon signed-ranks test
  - the unrelated *t* test and the Wilcoxon rank sum test
- estimation of differences between two sets of data on a single variable

The previous chapter has explored some of the general principles that underlie statistical inference. In this chapter, we describe some of the specific procedures that can be used to test for associations or differences between two variables, or two sets of data on a single variable. These sections will enable a researcher to identify an appropriate analysis for his or her own data and to judge the appropriateness of the tests used and the findings reported in many published articles. More advanced procedures – e.g. those that deal with more than two sets of data – are considered in Chapter 18.

There is a lot of debate both within and between different professions and disciplines about the use of statistical tests and what they are able to demonstrate. We will discuss their

strengths and weaknesses so that the reader may make an informed choice about what test to use. Each procedure is presented under a standard series of subheadings to assist this process:

- research question
- data
- assumptions
- checking the assumptions
- statistical hypotheses
- rationale for test
- results and their interpretation
- further analyses or statistics (where applicable)
- other comments
- alternative procedures.

In many cases, examples of analyses will be taken from the Rheumatoid Arthritis Study and the Low Back Pain Study. These analyses are for illustrative purposes, and they will not in all cases necessarily represent the optimum way in which either of these studies as a whole would be analysed.

14.1 TESTING ASSOCIATION: TWO VARIABLES, OR TWO SETS OF DATA ON A SINGLE VARIABLE

Many descriptive and explanatory studies are concerned with associations between variables – the tendency for values on one variable to be related to values on a second variable. Sample data are used to investigate the existence of, and to assess the strength of, such associations. The researcher's interest often lies in generalizing from an observed association in a sample to the population from which the sample was drawn. For example, can an observed association between side of stroke with respect to lateral dominance and success or failure of a rehabilitation programme be generalized to all patients

Table 14.1 *Methods for testing associations between two variables or two sets of data on a single variable. The kappa coefficient is considered in Chapter 18*

Level of measurement		Statistical method
First variable	**Second variable**	
Nominal	Nominal	*Unrelated measures:* Fisher's exact test (2 × 2); chi-square test (r × c) and phi or Cramér's V
		Related or repeated measures: McNemar's test (2 × 2); kappa coefficient
Nominal	Ordinal	Mantel-Haenszel test for trends
Ordinal	Ordinal	Spearman's rho; Kendall's tau; Kendall's W
Ordinal	Interval or ratio	Spearman's rho; Kendall's tau; Kendall's W
Interval or ratio	Interval or ratio	*Both normal:* Pearson's r
		Normal or non-normal: Spearman's rho; Kendall's tau

who have experienced a stroke? Generalization is achieved through statistical methods such those indicated in Table 14.1.

14.1.1 Pearson's chi-square test of independence

In surveys, it is usual to record many attributes against each participant. In the Rheumatoid Arthritis Study, for example, the requested information included profession of therapist, profile of workload, source of patient referrals, approaches to assessment and treatment, and perceived responsiveness of patients to therapy. A researcher is often interested in how many participants fall into the subgroups defined by jointly considering two of the measured attributes; for example, whether occupational therapists and physiotherapists differ in their use of general and specific rehabilitation programmes for patients with rheumatoid arthritis.

That is, we wish to test an assumption about the independence of two attributes in a specified accessible population when the response options against the attributes are recorded at a nominal level of measurement in a representative sample. This is achieved through a chi-square (χ^2) test of association (also called a 'chi-square independence-of-attributes test'), which is a commonly used nonparametric test. Counts are set up according to the joint levels of the two attributes and are presented in tables referred to variously as *cross-tabulations*, *contingency tables*, *cross-*

classifications, or *frequency tables*. The question at issue is whether the attributes are independent or interact in some way. If the attributes are independent, for any case in the sample, its value on one attribute will not influence, and will not be influenced by, its value on the other attribute (see Section 13.1.3). Independent factors can be studied separately, whereas dependent factors work together and need to be studied together. An observed association indicates dependency between two attributes, but it neither indicates nor implies that a causal relationship exists between them. Other factors (which might not be measured in the study) could influence both attributes. To consider causation, the data need to be collected through an experimental or quasi-experimental design (see also Box 14.2).

Research question

This is a suitable test when investigating the association (or lack of association) between two attributes. The pattern of any association is not specified or formulated. For example, in the Rheumatoid Arthritis Study: do occupational therapists (OTs) and physiotherapists (PTs) differ in their use of general and specific programmes for patients with rheumatoid arthritis (RA)?

Data

The cases comprise a representative sample of

Table 14.2 *Cross-tabulation of observed number of therapists using each approach for patients. Figures in parentheses are percentages*

Approach	Profession OT	Profession PT	Approach total
No specific programme	15 (37.5)	23 (29.9)	38 (32.5)
Yes, in general for rheumatology	15 (37.5)	27 (35.1)	42 (35.9)
Yes, specifically for RA patients	10 (25.0)	27 (35.1)	37 (31.6)
Profession total	40 (100)	77 (100)	117 (100)

OT = occupational therapist; PT = physiotherapist.

the population of interest (e.g. all PTs and OTs who treat people with RA). The data comprise counts of the cases with respect to the two attributes of interest (e.g. profession and therapeutic approach to individuals with RA). They are presented in a cross-tabulation (often referred to as an $r \times c$ table, having r rows and c columns). Table 14.2 shows the 3×2 cross-tabulation of profession and approach. A percentage stacked bar chart (Figure 14.1) provides a visual comparison of the patterns of cases with respect to each attribute (similar patterns indicate no difference in approach to patients with RA).

Assumptions

The following assumptions are required to perform a chi-square test of association:

- The entry for each cross-classification or subcategory is a count (and not, for example, a percentage, a rank, or a mean value).
- Each attribute is measured on a nominal scale with at least two response options.
- The attributes define mutually exclusive and collectively exhaustive categories so that every case can be assigned to one, and only one, cross-classification (i.e. to one cell in the table).
- The attributes are recorded on independent participants or cases.
- No participant is counted more than once, i.e. no participant contributes to the count in more than one cell.

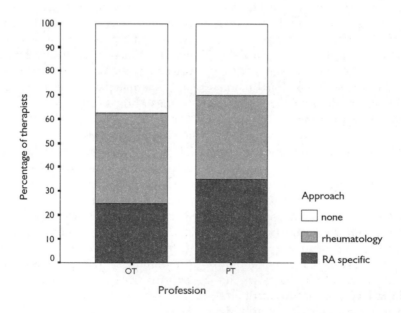

Figure 14.1 *Association between profession and approach. OT = occupational therapy; PT = physiotherapy.*

- The sample size is sufficiently large (see 'Checking the assumptions' below).

In terms of the present example, these assumptions might be written as:

- The data comprise counts in respect of profession and approach, both measured at a nominal level.
- Every respondent is either an OT or a PT, but not both.
- The approaches constitute mutually exclusive categories.
- A particular therapist uses only one of the specified approaches.
- The approach adopted by one therapist is not influenced by that used by any other therapist in the sample.
- The sample size ($n = 117$) is sufficient for the proposed analysis.

Checking the assumptions

Appraisal of the sampling method, the actual context in which the sampling was performed, the measurement tool and the achieved levels of measurement will enable most assumptions to be checked – which is the situation for the present example. Common situations in which a chi-square test is invalid include: using attributes that correspond to multiple-response questions, checklists with multiple endorsements or ipsative scales, and responses from the same participants at more than one point in time; in each case, the data will not be independent (see Section 15.1.5 for a definition of an *ipsative scale*). Incorrect use of the chi-square test for data that are not independent will normally inflate the Type I error rate (Ottenbacher, 1995).

Deciding whether the sample size is sufficient is based on a rule of thumb attributed to Cochran (1952). He recommended the use of chi-square tests:

- for a 2 × 2 table when no cells have expected counts less than 5
- for an $r \times c$ table (either r or c or both being greater than 2) when no more than 20% of the cells have expected counts of

less than 5, and no cell has an expected count of less than 1.

Cochran's rule is said to be conservative, but is the only unambiguous rule that appears in the literature (Siegel and Castellan, 1988; Bland, 1995; Pett, 1997; Conover, 1999). Furthermore, a chi-square test performed under less conservative requirements would have very little statistical power (Delucchi, 1993). The words 'expected counts' should be noted – these are the counts that we expect to see in each cell if the null hypothesis is true and the other assumptions hold. They are not the 'observed counts' in the cross-tabulation from the sample. Most statistical computing packages report the number and percentage of cells that do not satisfy Cochran's rule. In some instances, it might be possible to satisfy this rule by combining categories of an attribute and, thereby, reducing the number of cells. This is acceptable as long as the new categories so created have a meaningful interpretation with regard to the study objectives (Jordan *et al.*, 1998).

Statistical hypotheses

The null hypothesis states that no association exists between the two attributes and the alternative hypothesis that an association does exist. For example,

Null hypothesis: the approach adopted is independent of the therapist's profession.
Alternative hypothesis: the approach adopted is dependent upon the therapist's profession.

Equivalently, the null hypothesis might be phrased in terms of independence between attributes, or, for a 2 × c table, in terms of no difference in the proportion of cases that fall into the two 'row' categories when considered across the 'column' categories. Thus, we might state the null hypothesis as: there is no difference between the proportions of OTs and PTs using each type of approach for their patients with RA. The alternative hypothesis would then state that a difference exists across the proportions.

Rationale for test
Assuming

- independence between the two attributes (profession and approach in our example), and
- that the number of cases in every category (for each attribute separately) is a fixed quantity (e.g. 40 OTs, 77 PTs),

the probability of a randomly selected case possessing a particular combination of categories is given by using the relative frequency approach to probability (Section 13.1.2). For example, the probability of a randomly selected therapist being an OT who follows no specific programme for the management of patients with RA is given by (40/117 × 38/117). The expected count in a cell is simply this probability times the total sample size ($n = 117$). If the assumption of independence between the two attributes is true, then the expected count in each cell should differ from the observed count through the influence of sampling error alone. This is judged through the use of the chi-square statistic, a standardized measure of the difference between the observed and expected cell counts, which under all the assumptions listed follows a chi-square distribution.

Results and their interpretation
Statistical computing packages will produce tables of the observed and expected counts,

percentage values, Pearson's chi-square test statistic (χ^2), the p value and many other pieces of information such as standardized residuals (i.e. standardized differences between the observed and expected cell counts). The observed and expected numbers of therapists in the example from the Rheumatoid Arthritis Study are shown in Table 14.3. The χ^2 test statistic is 1.36, with a p value of .507.

The statistical decision is based on the p value. When the null hypothesis is retained (p value > chosen significance level), there is no evidence of any association between the two attributes and, in general, no further analysis is performed. In this example, using a significance level of .05, there is no reason to reject the null hypothesis (since .507 > .05). That is, on the basis of this sample, there is no evidence of an association between therapist's profession and the use of specific approaches for patients with rheumatoid arthritis.

Had the null hypothesis been rejected (p value ≤ chosen significance level), there would be evidence of an association between the attributes, and further analyses would be performed to determine the strength of the association and to identify the cells that contribute most towards the significance. A causal relationship between the attributes would not be indicated, however, unless one had been designated as an intervention variable and the other as an outcome variable within an experimental design.

Table 14.3 *Observed and expected numbers of therapists. Figures in parentheses are percentages*

Approach	Observed number OT	Observed number PT	Expected number OT	Expected number PT	Approach total
No specific programme	15	23	13.0 (32.5)	25.0 (32.5)	38 (32.5)
Yes, in general for rheumatology	15	27	14.4 (35.9)	27.6 (35.9)	42 (35.9)
Yes, specifically for RA patients	10	27	12.6 (31.6)	24.4 (31.6)	37 (31.6)
Profession total	40	77	40 (100)	77 (100)	117 (100)

OT = occupational therapist; PT = physiotherapist.

Further analyses or statistics

Neither the p value nor the value of the test statistic, χ^2, indicates the strength of any association. Other things remaining the same, a larger sample size will lead to a smaller p value and a larger χ^2. That is, a large sample provides the capability of statistically detecting a weak association. There are several coefficients that measure the strength of the association between two attributes recorded at a nominal level and most statistical packages include a choice within the options of the chi-square test. Values of these coefficients lie between 0 (no association) and 1 (a perfect association when both attributes possess the same number of categories, otherwise an 'asymmetrical' perfect association (Siegel and Castellan, 1988)). For a 2×2 cross-tabulation, the phi coefficient (ϕ) is usually calculated; for a $r \times c$ cross-tabulation, Cramér's V coefficient is calculated. Cramér's V enables the researcher to compare the strengths of associations based on different sample sizes and across tables with differing numbers of rows and columns (Norušis, 1997).

The cells that contribute most towards a significant result can be identified by examining *standardized residuals*. The standardized residual for a cell is defined here as the difference between the observed and expected counts, divided by the square root of the expected count for that cell. Negative residuals indicate that fewer occurrences were observed than expected, whereas positive residuals indicate that more occurrences were observed than expected. The largest standardized residuals (ignoring their signs) identify the cells on which the interpretation of the association should be focused. Further information about significant associations can be found through partitioning the cross-tabulation into a series of independent 2×2 tables. This is explained in Siegel and Castellan (1988) and Pett (1997).

Other comments

1. It is sometimes suggested that *Yates's continuity correction* should be used for the chi-square test in 2×2 contingency tables for small samples, so as to gain a better approximation of the discrete observed frequencies to the continuous distribution of the χ^2 test statistic (Portney and Watkins, 1993; Munro, 1997). The difference between the normal Pearson χ^2 statistic and that obtained with Yates's correction is minimal with large samples. With small samples, it decreases the value of χ^2, and hence raises the obtained p value, making the test more conservative. However, the use of the correction may make the test *too* conservative, and a number of authorities argue against its use (e.g. Neave and Worthington, 1988; Howell, 1997; Norušis, 1997).

2. More specialized applications of the chi-square test are described in Box 14.1.

Alternative procedures

1. On some occasions, the chi-square test is inappropriate. A 2×2 cross-tabulation containing one or more cells with an expected frequency of less than 5 will fail to meet one of the stipulations of Cochran's rules (i.e. that no more than 20% of cells have an expected frequency of less than 5). In such a situation, a 2×2 cross-tabulation can be analysed using *Fisher's exact test* (Siegel and Castellan, 1988). With a sample of less than 20, a 2×2 cross-tabulation will automatically fail to meet Cochran's requirement, so Fisher's exact test should always be used for a 2×2 cross-tabulation of this size.

2. There are many instances in health care research when data are collected from the same participants at two points in time in order to answer a research question. Van Sant (1993, p. 237) gives the following example: are physical therapists just as likely to change their work setting from hospital to non-hospital settings as they are to change from non-hospital to hospital settings? Such a study would involve repeated measures on a dichotomous variable; the same therapists are surveyed on two occasions to determine any change in their work setting. The data are

Box 14.1 *Specialized applications of the chi-square test*

1. When random samples of a fixed size are drawn from each of a number of different populations, and the cases in each sample are categorized according to the nominal levels of a given attribute, the chi-square test can be used to test the hypothesis that the probability of a random case being in a particular category is the same for all populations. Details are given in Conover (1999).

2. The above test can be modified to examine whether three or more independent samples have been drawn from populations with equal median values (Siegel and Castellan, 1988). In this instance the attribute is measured on at least an ordinal level.

3. When one attribute is measured at a nominal level and the other at an ordinal level, the *Mantel–Haenszel test* for trends is preferred over the chi-square test of independence (Pett, 1997). The latter does not account for any ordering across categories and therefore can lose potentially important information. The Mantel–Haenszel trend test should not be confused with the Mantel–Haenszel method for combining 2 × 2 tables (Mantel, 1963; Bland, 1995).

4. A *chi-square goodness-of-fit test* can be used to determine whether the proportion of cases in each of a set of nominal categories departs from an equal distribution of proportions (e.g. 20% in each of five categories). It can also be used to test for departure from a specific hypothesized distribution of proportions (e.g. 10%, 15%, 25%, 10%, 40%). Goodness-of-fit tests are defined in Section 13.4.2.

not therefore independent. The data can be summarized as counts in a 2 × 2 table, with rows representing pre-intervention categories and columns post-intervention categories. *McNemar's test* is a form of the chi-square statistic that can be used to test the hypothesis of no change (or no difference) before and after an intervention (Siegel and Castellan, 1988).

14.1.2 Correlation

Researchers often wish to study the association between two variables when data are collected on at least an ordinal level of measurement and values are recorded on both variables for every participant or case in the sample. Interest might centre on how paired measurements relate to each other; as values increase from low to high on one variable is there a corresponding move on the other variable from low to high values, or from high to low values, or no discernible pattern? For example, in the Rheumatoid Arthritis Study, is the amount of their working week that therapists spend on the care of patients with rheumatoid arthritis related to their rating of these patients' responsiveness to treatment? In the Low Back Pain Study, is a patient's reported measure of pain affect related to the measure of pain intensity?

Correlation is also an appropriate means of assessing the concurrent validity of a scale in relation to another scale whose validity has already been established (the criterion measure), where the scales in question have differing numbers of scale points (Box 9.2).

The term 'correlation' is used to describe an association between variables measured on at least an ordinal scale (and should not, therefore, be used with data at a nominal level). The direction and strength of the correlation is quantified in a *correlation coefficient*. The general characteristics and properties of correlation coefficients are discussed in this section, and some commonly used correlation coefficients are considered in subsequent sections.

Scatter diagrams

A useful starting point in an investigation of the correlation between two variables is to draw a scatter diagram (or 'scatterplot'). This is a plot of the pairs of measurements on a simple graph. Values of one variable are plotted on the vertical axis (often referred to as the 'Y axis') and those of the second variable on the horizontal axis (often referred to as the 'X axis'). Each cross on the plot is the intersection of an X, Y pair of values and represents a case.

Given sufficient cases and a sufficient number of scale points on an ordinal scale, scatter diagrams visually display the direction and strength of association between two variables. The direction can be positive (the value of Y increases as the value of X increases, e.g. Figure 14.2, plots a, d and f) or negative (the value of Y decreases as the value of X increases, e.g. Figure 14.2, plots b and c). The strength of association is indicated by the amount of scatter of the crosses (i.e. cases) around a perfect pattern. Thus, plots a, b and f in Figure 14.2 indicate perfect associations, whereas plots c, d and e indicate progressively less perfect or weaker associations. In fact, plot e would indicate no association between the two variables, since there is a complete lack of pattern to the crosses.

General characteristics of correlation coefficients

A correlation coefficient is a quantitative measure of the association between two variables such that:

- it is a standardized index, and hence does not lie on a particular scale (i.e. it is dimensionless)
- its sign indicates the direction of the association
- its magnitude indicates the strength or degree of association
- its value falls between -1 and $+1$
- a value of $+1$ indicates a perfect positive association, with the value of Y increasing as the value of X increases, and the value of Y decreasing as the value of X decreases (e.g. plot a in Figure 14.2 and, depending upon the choice of correlation coefficient, plot f)
- a value of -1 indicates a perfect negative association, with the value of Y decreasing as the value of X increases, and vice versa (e.g. plot b in Figure 14.2)
- a value of 0 indicates no correlation (plot e in Figure 14.2); this needs careful interpretation:

- it does not necessarily indicate no association
- it might indicate that an inappropriate correlation coefficient has been used
- a scatter diagram will provide a visual display of the pattern of association between X and Y.

Use of correlation coefficients

Correlation coefficients are widely reported in the literature and are frequently misused. It is important, therefore, to use and interpret them critically. Some of the issues to consider are those presented in Table 14.4.

Interpretation of correlation coefficients

Correlation coefficients need to be interpreted with care. In particular, the magnitude of the coefficient needs to be assessed carefully. According to Pett (1997), magnitudes between

- .00 and .25 indicate weak or no association
- .26 and .50 indicate a low degree of association
- .51 and .75 indicate a moderate to strong degree of association
- .76 and 1.00 indicate a very strong degree of association.

In assessing magnitude, the sign of the correlation coefficient is ignored. Hence, $-.75$ and $.75$ have the same magnitude. It is also important to remember that the values of correlation coefficients are not proportions (Gravetter and Wallnau, 1988); therefore, differences between values and ratios of values are not easily interpreted. We cannot say, for example, that a correlation coefficient of .6 represents an association that is twice as strong as an association having a correlation coefficient of .3. Note that, because the coefficient cannot lie above 1 or below -1, no zero is placed before the decimal point (see Box 13.2).

A statistical hypothesis test is often performed to determine whether the degree of association present in the sample data could have occurred by chance. The null hypothesis states that the

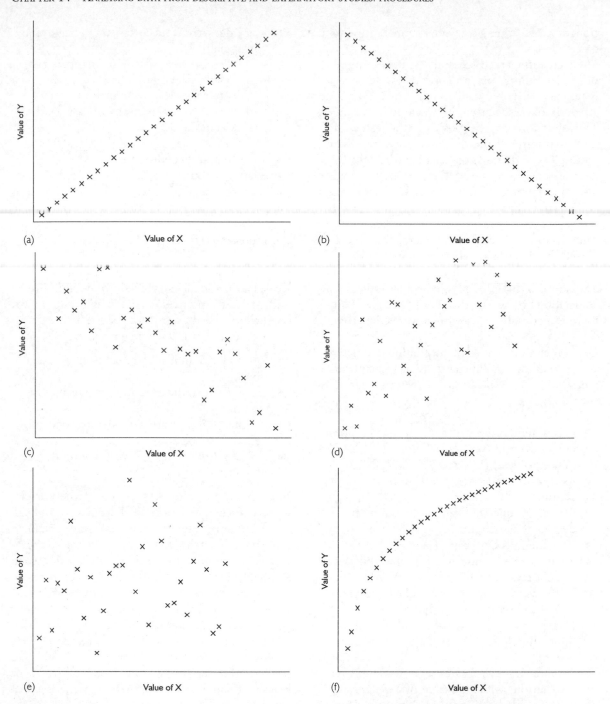

Figure 14.2 *Examples of scatter diagrams. (a) Perfect association: rank-order agreement; positive linear association. (b) Perfect association: rank-order disagreement; negative linear association. (c) Strong association: rank-order disagreement; negative linear association. (d) Weak association: rank-order agreement; positive linear association. (e) No association: no rank-order agreement; no linear association. (f) Perfect association: rank-order agreement; but a non-linear association.*

Table 14.4 *Potentially troublesome issues associated with the use and interpretation of correlation coefficients*

Issue	Comments
Appropriateness	There are several correlation indices; each one quantifies the degree of association between two variables. The choice of an appropriate index depends upon the levels of measurement of X and Y, the distribution followed by the measurement errors, and the type of association to be described (Nunnally and Bernstein, 1994).
Assessing agreement of measurement tools	Correlation coefficients measure the degree of association and not how closely the actual values of the two variables agree (Altman, 1991a); that is, they do not investigate differences across the paired values of X and Y. They are, therefore, inappropriate for the comparison of two tools that purportedly measure the same quantity (Box 9.2, Section 18.3.1).
Sample selection	Deliberately restricting the range of X or Y values in the sample might seriously affect the size of the correlation coefficient. If the objective is to generalize from the sample data to a population, then random samples should be selected that cover the range of interest for the X and Y values.
Extrapolation	It is potentially misleading to assume that associations identified within a specific region of X and Y are valid outside that region. For example, there is a strong correlation between height and weight for 6-9-year-olds, but a weak association for 20-23-year-olds.
Subsets of data	The strength of association identified over the whole sampled X-Y region is, in general, higher than that measured within a subset of the region; e.g. the correlation between height and weight for 6-9-year-olds compared with a subset of 6-7-year-olds.
Subgroups of data	If data from two or more subgroups are combined, the resulting correlation coefficient may differ considerably from those of the individual subgroups. Depending on how the distribution of the two variables in the subgroups differs from that of the combined group, the correlation coefficient in the latter may be either larger or smaller than those of the subgroups, and may even change direction, such that negative correlations in the subgroups become positive in the combined group, or vice versa (Myers and Well, 1995).
Extreme cases	Deliberately omitting or including extreme cases on each variable from the sample might seriously affect the size of the correlation coefficient.
Component variables	It is misleading to calculate a correlation coefficient when one variable represents a constituent of the other variable. A high correlation is almost inevitable; e.g. correlating the time spent by patients in the waiting area with the total time that they spend in a clinic.

population correlation coefficient is zero and the alternative hypothesis states that the population correlation coefficient is not zero; i.e. an association exists. Based on certain theoretical propositions, it may sometimes be justified to propose a positive (population correlation coefficient >0) or a negative (population correlation coefficient <0) association in the alternative hypothesis. Thus, it might be argued that if any association exists between pain intensity and pain affect, this will be a positive one. However, we would urge caution in using such directional hypotheses (Box 13.5). Statistical computing packages produce the value of the sample correlation coefficient and a p value for making a decision about its statistical significance. If there is no violation of the assumptions underlying such a test, the null hypothesis is rejected when the p value is less than or equal to the chosen significance level, and retained otherwise (Section 13.4.7).

The effect of sample size should be borne in mind. Large sample sizes enable weak associations to be detected as statistically significant (Section 13.4.8). Put another way, smaller correlation coefficients are statistically significant when derived from larger sample sizes.

Regardless of the strength of the observed association in the sample data, causation is not implied (Nolan, 1994). There are numerous examples of spurious correlations that illustrate this. For example, it has been demonstrated that there is a positive correlation between the number of toys sold and the amount of alcohol sold, between the number of television licences issued and the number of mental breakdowns, and between the number of telephones and infant mortality. A strong correlation between two variables X and Y might be due to one of four explanations: (1) chance occurrence; (2) X influences Y; (3) Y influences X; (4) both X and Y are influenced by one or more other variables (Box 14.2). The last explanation often accounts for the misleading strength of correlation coefficients between two variables whose values have been recorded repeatedly over time. It also accounts for one of the spurious correlations cited earlier:

If you compare country statistics, you find a negative correlation of about -.9 between the number of telephones per capita and the infant mortality rate. However much fun it is to speculate that the reason is because mums with phones can call their husbands or the taxis and get to the hospital faster, most people would recognize that the underlying cause of both is degree of development.

(Norman and Streiner, 1994, p. 105)

Above all, there is the basic issue of practical importance. A statistically significant correlation coefficient does not imply that a practically important association has been identified (Section 13.4.10).

14.1.3 Pearson's product moment correlation coefficient

Pearson's product moment correlation coefficient is the most frequently reported correlation coefficient. It was developed by Karl Pearson to measure the degree of *linear* association between two continuous variables (Section 12.2.6) that are measured on at least an interval scale. The symbol ρ (rho) is used to denote the population parameter (the degree of linear association in the population of interest) and r the sample statistic (an estimate of ρ calculated from a random sample drawn from the population). A perfect positive linear association

Box 14.2 *Recursive relationships*

Attempts are sometimes made to infer causation from correlation on the basis of a recursive model; that is, a theoretical proposition to the effect that the direction of causation can only be one way. For example, if height (X) and educational attainment (Y) are shown to be correlated, it might be argued that height causes educational achievement because there is no way that achievement could determine one's height. However, although Y cannot be determined by X, it is still possible that Y can be determined by a third factor Z (such as genetic make-up) which also influences X. So, even in the presence of a recursive model, causation still cannot be conclusively inferred from correlation.

implies that the values of Y increase in exact proportion to the values of X; sample data are represented on a scatter diagram by crosses that fall exactly on a straight line with a positive slope (plot a in Figure 14.2), and $r = 1.00$. A perfect negative linear association implies that the values of Y decrease in exact proportion to the values of X; a scatter diagram would exhibit a straight line with a negative slope (plot b in Figure 14.2), and $r = -1.00$. A perfect *nonlinear* association implies that there is some functional relationship between the values of Y and X, but one that is not exactly proportional; a scatter diagram would exhibit a curve (for example, plot f in Figure 14.2). Pearson's product moment correlation coefficient is an inappropriate measure of association for nonlinear relationships. If calculated, the value of r could be very misleading, with some curves giving $r = 0$. For the curve in plot f in Figure 14.2, $r = .93$.

In reality, less than perfect associations are observed between variables. This is a consequence of measurement error, sampling error, the influence of random effects, and the effects of other variables on the values of Y and X. A scatter diagram would exhibit crosses scattered around a straight line (plots c and d in Figures 14.2).

Research question

The research question proposes a specific pattern (i.e. linear) for the association between two variables. For example, in the Low Back Pain Study: are patients' reported measures of pain affect linearly related to reported measures of pain intensity?

Data

The data comprise pairs of measures on X and Y from a random sample of cases, and are visually depicted in a scatter diagram. Figure 14.3 shows the data on pain affect and pain intensity for each patient in the Low Back Pain Study.

Assumptions

The following assumptions are required to use Pearson's r:

- It is appropriate to consider the linear association between two variables, X and Y.
- The pairs of values on X and Y are measured on at least an interval scale.
- The pairs of values on X and Y are independent, i.e. only one pair of values is recorded from each case in the study.

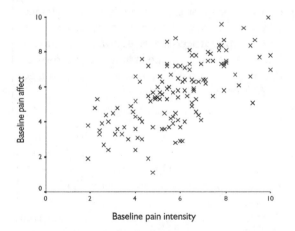

Figure 14.3   *Association between pain affect and pain intensity, 1 week before attendance on a low back pain management programme. Each cross represents the scores on a visual analogue scale (in cm) for both pain affect (vertical axis) and pain intensity (horizontal axis), for an individual participant.*

If generalization to the sampled population is desired, further assumptions are required in order to perform a valid hypothesis test:

- The cases in the study represent a random sample from some specified population.
- The spread of errors about the straight line is approximately the same at all values of X and of Y (i.e. homoscedasticity).
- The errors affecting each variable (X and Y) must be normally distributed (Nunnally and Bernstein, 1994).

Checking the assumptions

Examining the sampling method, the context in which the sampling was performed and the measurement tools utilized will enable most of the assumptions to be checked. Normality can be demonstrated through any of the methods referred to in Box 14.3. For the current example from the Low Back Pain Study,

- the scatter diagram appears to indicate a linear association between pain affect and intensity 1 week before attendance on a low back pain management programme
- Dr Buckley assumed that scores from a visual analogue scale satisfy the requirements of at least an interval level of measurement (Price and Harkins, 1992)
- only one pair of values for pain affect and pain intensity is considered per patient
- the patients might be considered to be a random sample of those likely to attend such programmes
- normal probability plots provide no indication of non-normality in pain affect or pain intensity scores.

Statistical hypotheses

The null hypothesis states that no linear association exists between the two variables in the population ($\rho = 0$). The alternative hypothesis states that a linear association exists in the population ($\rho \neq 0$). In some situations, theoretical or experiential considerations might support a test against a prior selected value for the correlation coefficient in preference to zero.

Box 14.3 *Testing for normality and homogeneity*

Normality
Normality might be demonstrated through a normal probability plot (Pett, 1997), summarized through measures of skewness and kurtosis (Altman, 1991a; Pett, 1997), or tested using Kolmogorov–Smirnov, Shapiro–Wilks or Lilliefors tests (Pett, 1997; Conover, 1999). The normal probability plot provides a visual assessment of the normality of a distribution by plotting each datapoint against its expected value if the distribution were in fact normal.

Homogeneity
The homogeneity of two population variances can be tested using the F distribution, and that of several populations using the Levene test or Bartlett's test (Armitage and Berry, 1994). However, these tests are not robust to non-normality (Winer et al., 1991). A rule of thumb commonly employed is that homogeneity is not doubted if variances differ by less than a factor of two (Pett, 1997).

Rationale for test
Pearson's r measures the degree of proportional consistency in the paired values of X and Y (see also Box 14.4).

Results and their interpretation
In the Low Back Pain example, the 130 data pairs on pain affect and pain intensity (1 week before attendance on a course) gave $r = .67$, with a p value $<.0005$ (see Box 14.5). At a significance level of .05, this represents a statistically significant result. On the basis of these data, there is evidence of a moderate linear association between pain affect and pain intensity for RA patients.

General points about the results of correlation coefficients and their interpretation were considered in Section 14.1.2. There, it was pointed out that we cannot interpret the relative magnitude of two correlation coefficients, since the coefficient does not lie on a

Box 14.4 *Pearson's product moment correlation and deviation*

Pearson's r is based on the concept of *covariance*, that is, how the X and Y values vary with respect to each other, or covary. For a strong positive linear association, high values of X occur with high values of Y, and low values of X occur with low values of Y; that is, there is a strong covariance. In Section 12.4.3, the standard deviation was introduced as a measure of the variability of individual values around their mean. Similarly, in the Pearson correlation statistic the measure of covariance is formulated in terms of deviations around mean values – more specifically, the product of the deviation around the mean for the X values and the corresponding deviation around the mean for the Y values; i.e. the product of moments. The units and the size of the covariance depend upon the units and standard deviations of X and Y. For example, the covariance between height and weight would be numerically larger if weight were measured in grams rather than kilograms, as would the standard deviation of weight. A standardized index of covariance (i.e. a correlation coefficient) is formulated by dividing the covariance by the product of the standard deviations of X and Y. This procedure is equivalent to taking the mean product of the standardized scores of X and Y (Section 13.2.1 discusses standardized scores).

ratio scale. If, however, the correlation coefficient is squared, this gives the *coefficient of determination* (r^2). This statistic expresses the proportion of variation on one variable which is accounted for by a linear association with the other variable. For example, for a correlation between pain intensity and pain affect of .67, r^2 is .45; hence 45% of the variation in pain intensity is accountable for by variation in pain affect (and vice versa). If the coefficient of determination is subtracted from one (i.e. $1 - .45 = .55$), this gives the *coefficient of aliena-*

Box 14.5 *Interpreting p values in computer output*

Statistical computing packages round figures before printing them. A *p* value of .000 on a computer output – such as was produced for this Pearson's correlation coefficient – implies a value of less than .0005 (a chance of less than 5 in 10,000), not zero (which is an impossibility; see Section 13.1.3). Note that any value of the fourth decimal place that was greater than 5 would have been rounded up to .001. Hence, a *p* value reported by a computer package as .000 should be reported as $p < .0005$, not as $p < .001$.

tion – the proportion of unexplained variation (i.e. the variation in one variable unaccounted for by variation in the other variable). Unlike the correlation coefficient, the coefficient of determination lies on a ratio scale, and it is therefore appropriate to say that an r^2 of .90 is twice as large as an r^2 of .45. The coefficient of determination plays an important part in the context of linear regression (see 'Other comments' in Section 18.4.3).

Other comments

1. Pearson's r is very sensitive to the existence of extreme data values. A scatter diagram will alert the researcher to this situation.
2. Confidence intervals can be computed for the population parameter (Altman, 1991a), and are more informative than the p value (Section 13.5).
3. A measure of non-linear association between two variables is given by *eta*, which takes values between 0 and 1. Large differences between the magnitudes of *eta* and r might arise through serious violation of the assumptions of linearity, normality of errors, or homoscedasticity; or through *ceiling effects* (Nunnally and Bernstein, 1994). A ceiling effect occurs when several participants respond at the highest score on a particular scale but, given a wider scale, would have responded against a higher score.

14.1.4 Spearman's rho (Spearman's rank-order correlation coefficient)

Spearman's rank-order correlation coefficient quantifies the degree of association between two variables that are measured on at least an ordinal level. Thus, it can be used when two variables are measured on an ordinal scale, or as an alternative to Pearson's product moment correlation coefficient when some of its assumptions are seriously violated.

Spearman's rho assesses the degree of *monotonicity* between two variables; that is, the degree of consistency in the rank ordering of cases with respect to X and Y. The symbol ρ_S denotes the population parameter and r_S the sample statistic. A perfect rank-order agreement ($r_S = 1$) implies that the values of Y increase as the values of X increase (plots a and f in Figure 14.2). Complete rank-order disagreement ($r_S = -1$) implies that the values of Y decrease as the values of X increase (plot b in Figure 14.2). As might be expected, less than perfect associations are nearly always observed in practice.

Research question

The research question considers the association between two variables. To take the example considered in the previous section, had the distribution of pain affect and/or pain intensity been non-normal, the assumptions of Pearson's r would not have been satisfied. The correlation between these variables could have been performed with Spearman's rho.

To take another example from the Low Back Pain Study, the following research question was posed: what is the association between pain affect scores, measured at baseline, and participants' self-rated symptomatic change at 3 months?

Data

The data comprise paired measures recorded for every case in the study. The rank orders of the data are used to compute r_S. A scatter diagram usefully depicts the association between the two variables as long as the number of points on an ordinal scale exceeds about seven.

Assumptions

The following assumptions are required to use Spearman's rho:

- The pairs of values on X and Y are measured to at least an ordinal level.
- The data comprise independent pairs of values.

Checking the assumptions

The assumptions are easily checked from the sampling procedure and the reported data. For the Low Back Pain example, pain affect is measured on a visual analogue scale, which is at least an ordinal level of measurement. Self-rated symptomatic change is measured on a five-point scale (see Table 7.1), which constitutes an ordinal level of measurement. The data are independent, since only one pair of values is considered per patient.

Statistical hypotheses

The null hypothesis states that no association exists between X and Y in the population (or that X and Y are mutually independent). The alternative hypothesis states either that there is a tendency for larger values of Y to be associated with larger values of X, or that there is a tendency for smaller values of Y to be associated with larger values of X. Incidentally, the null hypothesis has not been written as '$\rho_S = 0$', since, when the distribution of errors is non-normal, a zero correlation does not necessarily imply that the variables are independent, but independence implies a zero correlation (Siegel and Castellan, 1988).

Rationale for test

The sample statistic, r_S, is equivalent to Pearson's r with the rank orders replacing the data values.

Results and their interpretation

The general points discussed in Section 14.1.2 are relevant here.

Other comments

1. Sometimes, two or more cases have the same value on the same variable; that is, the scores are tied. If the proportion of ties is small, their effect on r_S will be negligible. However, when the proportion of ties is moderate, a correction factor should be incorporated into the computation (Siegel and Castellan, 1988). Researchers who use a statistical computing package to perform the computations should check that this adjustment is made. A large number of ties invalidates the use of r_S.
2. When the number of cases is greater than 20, a normal approximation can be used to compute the p value in a statistical hypothesis test; otherwise, an exact test should be used (Siegel and Castellan, 1988).
3. Spearman's rho has a relative efficiency of 91% compared with Pearson's r (Siegel and Castellan, 1988) when the assumptions for Pearson's r are satisfied.

Alternative procedures

1. Kendall's rank-order correlation coefficient, also called *Kendall's tau* (τ), is an alternative to Spearman's rho; it too requires the data to be measured on at least an ordinal scale. Kendall's tau is used to assess the degree of association between two variables (X and Y), or to determine the degree of correspondence (or concordance) between rankings assigned to the same cases by two raters (X and Y). For each pair of cases, their ordering on X and Y is defined as *concordant* (ordered the same way), *discordant* (ordered in opposite directions), or *tied* (equal for either X or Y). Kendall's tau is defined as 'the proportion of concordant pairs minus the proportion of discordant pairs' (Bland, 1995, p. 218). This definition is used to interpret the strength of the association. In general, the value of r_S is larger than the value of Kendall's tau (Norman and Streiner, 1994); for example, values of .67 and .48, respectively, were obtained for the association between pain affect and pain intensity in the Low Back Pain Study. The power of the two tests is

comparable, however (Sprent, 1993; Conover, 1999). There are three versions of Kendall's tau (named *a*, *b* and *c*). Kendall's tau-*b* takes account of tied ranks, and copes rather better with a large number of ties (such as may occur when there is a limited number of scale points and the sample size is large) than does Spearman's rho (Bland, 1995). Neave and Worthington (1988) recommend Spearman's rho over Kendall's tau when the sample size is less than about 20. Kendall's tau, like Spearman's rho, may be used in tests of significance. Further details may be found in Siegel and Castellan (1988), Pett (1997) or Conover (1999).

2. Spearman's rho and Kendall's tau deal with two variables or two sets of rankings. *Kendall's coefficient of concordance* (W) assesses the degree of overall correspondence between rankings assigned to the same cases by more than two raters. It may be used in statistical significance tests. A significant result can be interpreted in terms of the degree of consensus in the ordering of cases across raters. Hence, Kendall's W assesses the degree of agreement in ranks, and is a nonparametric analogue to the intraclass correlation coefficient (Section 18.3.2) when conducting reliability studies (Norman and Streiner, 1994). However, it provides no information about actual agreement in scores (when data are collected at an interval or ratio level of measurement), or about the correctness of the ordering if a true order exists.

3. The *Olmstead-Tukey C test* can be used in place of either the Spearman or the Kendall correlation coefficient, and is easy to compute by hand (Neave and Worthington, 1988). Its power approaches that of the Spearman and Kendall tests.

4. In some studies, several raters might categorize the cases according to some nominal measure rather than assigning ranks to them. The intention might be to assess agreement across the raters' assignments of cases to the categories; that is, the research question is 'Do raters agree with each other about the category membership of each case?' The data comprise the number of raters who assign a specific case to a particular category, considered over all cases and all categories. These numbers can be presented in a table whose rows are defined by the cases and columns defined by the categories. Spearman's rho and Kendall's tau are inappropriate statistics in this situation. The *kappa* statistic (Section 18.3.5) assesses the agreement of case assignment to categories, corrected for chance agreement (Dunn, 1989; Haas, 1991a).

14.2 TESTING DIFFERENCES: TWO SETS OF DATA ON A SINGLE VARIABLE

All explanatory studies and some descriptive studies address research questions that involve comparisons across sets of data corresponding to groups of cases or points in time. For example, in the Low Back Pain Study, what impact does participation in a group-based approach have on pain affect compared with participation in an individual-based approach? Is the impact of low back pain on health status reduced following participation in a group-based cognitive-behavioural programme for the management of low back pain?

Such research questions are usually posed in relation to a population from which the available data have been randomly sampled. Confidence intervals and hypothesis tests enable inferences to be made about this population. The process for computing a confidence interval or performing a hypothesis test is selected according to:

- the level of measurement for values of the variable
- the achieved sample size for each set of data
- the nature of cases with respect to the two sets of data:
  - two measurements made on every case (repeated measures), usually at two points in time

- matched pairs of cases across the two sets of data
- independent cases in the two sets of data
• the assumptions, if any, that can be made about the distribution of sampling error.

The sign test, Wilcoxon signed-ranks test, Wilcoxon rank sum test (Mann–Whitney U), related t test and unrelated t test are statistical methods commonly employed for testing differences between two sets of data on one variable (Table 14.5). Most of these procedures provide information on *average* differences (i.e. in terms of means or medians). It should be remembered, however, that a small or moderate average difference may conceal large differences for individual cases (see Section 7.4). This underlines the importance of displaying data graphically before undertaking further descriptive or inferential analyses.

14.2.1 Tests for matched cases or repeated measures

Repeated measures and matched designs are often employed to assess the effectiveness of an intervention. Their aim is to eliminate the effects of extraneous variables in a study by using each case (participant) as his or her own control, or by using cases that are matched with respect to important attributes. The data analysis involves making comparisons across the repeated measures or matched pairs of values.

The related t test (or paired t test) is a para-metric test used for such comparisons. It is also appropriate for comparing matched pairs of values that have been collected cross-sectionally in a survey. The Wilcoxon signed-ranks test is the nonparametric equivalent of the related t test. It is particularly useful when the sample size is small ($n < 30$) and the distribution of differences in values for related cases is markedly non-normal (but, fairly symmetrical). In this situation, neither t nor z is an appropriate test statistic.

Research hypothesis

Typically, a research hypothesis in an explanatory study such as a randomized controlled trial states that a particular intervention has a beneficial effect on some condition. The effect is quantified through change in the value of a chosen outcome variable. For example, in the Low Back Pain Study, the research hypothesis might postulate that participation in a group-based cognitive-behavioural programme for the management of low back pain reduces its impact on a person's health status.

Data

The data comprise pairs of values that are either repeated measures on the same cases, or measures on matched cases. The statistical test analyses the differences in the paired values. In the low back pain example, the Aberdeen Back Pain Scale (ABPS) score was recorded for each participant one week before attendance and one week after attendance on a group-based

Table 14.5 *Statistical methods for testing differences between two sets of data on one variable*

| Nature of cases | Level of measurement | | |
	Nominal	Ordinal	Interval or ratio
Matched cases, or repeated measures on the same cases	Sign test	Sign test	*Normal distribution*: related t test *Any distribution*: Wilcoxon signed-ranks; z test for large samples
Independent cases		Wilcoxon rank sum (Mann-Whitney U)	*Normal distribution*: unrelated t test *Any distribution*: Wilcoxon rank sum; z test for large samples

programme. These data are summarized (for those patients who responded both before and after attendance) in Table 14.6 and depicted in a boxplot in Figure 14.4.

The assumptions, statistical hypotheses, results and their interpretation differ for the related *t* test and Wilcoxon signed-ranks test and are presented in separate sections (14.2.2 and 14.2.3, respectively).

14.2.2 Related *t* test

An introduction to the related *t* test, an example research hypothesis and associated data were given in Section 14.2.1.

Table 14.6 *Aberdeen Back Pain Scale scores, 1 week before and after attendance at a group-based low back pain management programme*

Statistic	Pre-attendance	Post-attendance
n	56	56
Mean (standard deviation)	41.51 (1.93)	38.76 (2.31)
Median (minimum, maximum)	41.30 (37.30, 45.70)	38.45 (34.20, 44.30)

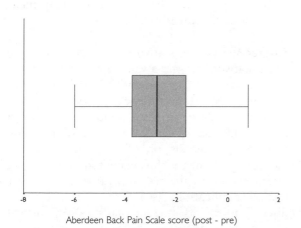

Aberdeen Back Pain Scale score (post - pre)

Figure 14.4 *Differences in Aberdeen Back Pain Scale scores after a group-based management programme (scores 1 week post-programme minus baseline scores); n = 56.*

Assumptions

The assumptions for the related *t* test are:

- The data constitute values from a random sample of cases, each with two measurements (which might represent two points in time); or the data constitute values from a sample of matched pairs of cases with random allocation into two groups.
- The differences in values for related cases constitute a random sample from a normally distributed population with unknown mean and unknown standard deviation.
- The underlying random variable of interest is continuous.
- The data are measured on an interval or ratio scale.

Checking the assumptions

The assumptions are checked by reference to the sampling method, details of the employed measurement tool, and the use of any recognized method for checking normality (Box 14.3). In the Low Back Pain Study example currently being considered,

- patients attending the group-based programme were randomly assigned to that approach
- Aberdeen Back Pain Scale scores are recorded for the same patients at two points in time
- a normal probability plot of the differences in Aberdeen Back Pain Scale scores (i.e. scores 1 week post-attendance minus scores 1 week pre-attendance) cast no doubt on the assumption of normality of differences in the population and indicated no extreme values
- a person's health status is essentially a continuous variable
- Dr Buckley accepts the assumption that Aberdeen Back Pain Scale scores satisfy the requirements of at least an interval level of measurement

Statistical hypotheses

The null hypothesis states that the intervention has no effect on the condition: the mean effect in the population is zero and there is no difference (or change) in the population mean values of the chosen outcome variable. For example, participation in a group-based cognitive-behavioural programme for the management of low back pain does not change the impact that low back pain has on a person's health – or population mean Aberdeen Back Pain Scale scores are the same before and after participation on the given programme.

The alternative hypothesis states that the intervention has some effect on the condition, as indicated by difference or change in the chosen outcome variable; the mean effect in the population is not zero. For example, participation in the given programme changes the impact of low back pain on a person's health status – or there is a difference in the population mean Aberdeen Back Pain Scale scores before and after participation. Note that although the *research* hypothesis was directional, in terms of the *statistical* hypotheses we have stated a non-directional alternative hypothesis (see Section 13.4.4).

Rationale for test

Under the null hypothesis of no difference and the specified assumptions, the standardized mean difference in the paired values (i.e. the mean difference divided by the standard error of the paired differences) follows a normal distribution (Section 13.2.1).

In reality, the population standard deviation is unknown and is replaced by s, the sample standard deviation (Section 12.4.3). The resultant standardized score is called a *t statistic* and follows a statistical distribution called 'Student's t'. This distribution has a similar shape to the standard normal distribution but has longer tails to take account of the variation of s from sample to sample. The t distribution is really a family of curves; each curve reflects the different amount of independent information (called *degrees of freedom*) that is used to estimate the standard error of the sample mean

difference. Degrees of freedom are linked to the sample size.

Results and their interpretation

It is usual to report the sample size, the mean and standard deviation of outcome values for each group or time point, the mean and standard deviation of the difference in paired values, the t statistic, and the p value.

The p value is used to make a statistical decision about the null hypothesis. When the p value is greater than the chosen significance level, the null hypothesis is not rejected; there is no evidence to doubt a zero mean effect in the population. When the p value is less than or equal to the significance level, the null hypothesis is rejected; there is evidence to doubt a zero mean effect in the population.

From the information in Table 14.7, and using a significance level of .05, the null hypothesis is rejected ($.0005 < .05$); that is, there is evidence to doubt the assumption of no effect of the programme on Aberdeen Back Pain Scale scores. The mean Aberdeen Back Pain Scale score decreased by 2.75 units (from 41.51 to 38.76 units) following attendance. Therefore, based on this study there is evidence that the mean impact of low back pain on a person's health status is lower following participation in a group-based low back pain management programme (however, see Section 7.2.8).

Further analyses or statistics

The t statistic and the p value are affected by the sample size and the variability of values on the outcome measure and, hence, provide no direct information about the magnitude of any effect in the population (Section 13.4.9). Calculating confidence intervals or effect sizes is recommended to indicate this magnitude and to aid interpretation of the results with regard to their clinical implications (see Section 17.3.1 for a discussion of effect size statistics). Statistical computing packages produce confidence intervals, but most do not compute effect sizes.

For the current example, the 95% confidence interval for the mean difference in Aberdeen

Table 14.7 *Change in Aberdeen Back Pain Scale (ABPS) scores following participation on a group-based low back pain management programme (n = 56)*

Variable	1 week pre-attendance mean (s.d.)	1 week post-attendance mean (s.d.)	Difference (post – pre) mean (s.d.)	*t* statistic	*p* value
ABPS score	41.51 (1.93)	38.76 (2.31)	−2.75 (1.64)	−12.57	< .0005

s.d. = standard deviation.

Back Pain Scale scores following participation on a group-based programme is −3.18 to −2.31 units (post minus pre scores). This might be interpreted as: 'based on this study of 56 patients, participation in a group-based cognitive-behavioural low back pain management programme lessens the mean impact of low back pain on a person's health status by between 2.31 and 3.18 units (95% confidence interval)'. The clinical importance of this finding might be discussed in relation to these values rather than the mean difference of 2.75 units only. The interval could have been computed on pre-attendance minus post-attendance scores, in which case the 95% confidence interval would have been 2.31 to 3.18 units, but the interpretation would be unchanged. Similarly, the *t* statistic would have been 12.57 rather than −12.57, but this too would not affect the associated *p* value. It is important to note that the confidence interval that is relevant here is that for the mean of the paired differences, not the confidence intervals for the means of the two sets of scores.

It should also be noted that although the estimated mean change is that expected for an individual patient, it will not be achieved for every patient. Some patients might not perceive a change or might report a worsening of the impact of low back pain on their health. Assuming that all other factors remain the same as during the study period, the mean change will be achieved on average in the long term when many patients have been assessed.

Other comments

There is debate about the robustness of the related *t* test to departures from the assumption of normally distributed paired differences. Bland (1995) asserts that the test is robust to all but large departures.

Alternative procedures

1. For large sample sizes, the standardized mean difference follows a standard normal distribution and a *z* test can be used to test the null hypothesis, with the sample standard deviation of differences replacing the population parameter. The distribution of paired differences is unimportant in this situation. 'Large' is defined as *n* > 30 according to Daniel (1991) and *n* > 50 according to Bland (1995).
2. When the sample size is small and the assumptions or the related *t* test are not met, then a Wilcoxon signed-ranks test (Section 14.2.3) is recommended.

14.2.3 Wilcoxon signed-ranks test

An introduction to this test, research hypotheses, and data were covered in Section 14.2.1; the Wilcoxon signed-ranks test will be applied to the same research hypothesis as the related *t* test, but under a somewhat different set of assumptions.

Assumptions

The assumptions for the Wilcoxon signed-ranks test are:

- The data constitute values from a sample of independent cases, each with two measurements (which might represent two points in time); or the data constitute values from a sample of matched pairs of cases with random allocation into two groups.

- The underlying population of differences between the values of paired cases is approximately symmetrical (in which case the mean and median differences are equal).
- The data are measured on at least an interval scale, so that differences are meaningful (see Box 14.6).
- The sample size is not too large (to prevent too many differences of the same value).

Box 14.6 *Measurement assumptions of the Wilcoxon signed-ranks test*

It is sometimes claimed that the Wilcoxon signed-ranks test is appropriate for ordinal data (Greene and D'Oliveira, 1982; Hurlburt, 1994; McCall, 1996; Hicks, 1999). In contrast, Blalock (1972), Daniel (1990), Bland (1995), Cliff (1996) and Wright (1997) stipulate an interval level of measurement for this test. The latter is the more accurate view, since any test that is based on difference scores will assume that numerically equal differences have the same mathematical meaning. It is true to say that, for the purposes of the test, the difference scores will be ordinal (Haber and Runyon, 1977), but for this to be the case the data on which they are calculated must be at an interval or ratio level. Therefore, unless the raw data in question are at least interval (or a sound argument can be mounted that the data can be treated as such), a test such as the sign test should be used, rather than the Wilcoxon signed-ranks test. Incidentally, this illustrates the fact that not all nonparametric tests for variate data can be used with ordinal data.

Checking the assumptions

The assumptions are checked by reference to the sampling method, details of the employed measurement tool, and a histogram or box plot. In the Low Back Pain Study example presented in Section 14.2.1,

- patients have been randomly assigned to the group-based programme
- each patient was requested to complete an Aberdeen Back Pain Scale score at two points in time
- a boxplot of the differences in Aberdeen Back Pain Scale scores (1 week post-attendance minus 1 week pre-attendance) cast no doubt on the assumption of symmetry of differences in the population, and indicated no extreme differences
- Dr Buckley accepts the assumption that Aberdeen Back Pain Scale scores satisfy the requirements of at least an interval level of measurement

Statistical hypotheses

The null hypothesis states that there is no difference (or change) in the population median values of the chosen outcome variable; the alternative hypothesis states that there is such a difference (or change).

In the Low Back Pain Study example, the null hypothesis is that participation in a group-based cognitive-behavioural programme for the management of low back pain does not change the impact that low back pain has on a person's health. More explicitly, this is worded as: there is no difference in the population median Aberdeen Back Pain Scale scores before and after participation on the programme. The alternative hypothesis would be that there is a difference in the population median Aberdeen Back Pain Scale scores before and after participation.

Rationale for test

Differences between the paired values are assigned ranks without regard to sign – the smallest difference (ignoring signs) having a rank of 1, the next smallest a rank of 2, and so forth. Some of the differences will be positive and others negative. Under the assumption that the null hypothesis is true, we expect a balance of smaller and larger ranks across the positive and negative differences; that is, the sum of ranks assigned to positive differences is expected to be equal to the sum of ranks assigned to negative differences. If the two sums of ranks are very different (or equivalently, if the smaller of the sums of ranks is very small) then the null hypothesis is rejected.

Results and their interpretation

The sample size, median, minimum and maximum outcome values for each point in time or each group are usually reported, as are the median, minimum and maximum difference in paired values, and the p value. Sometimes, the smaller sum of ranks (often denoted by T) or the z value (see Note 1 under 'Alternative procedures' below) is also reported.

As usual, the p value is used to make a statistical decision about the null hypothesis. A decision not to reject is made when a p value is greater than the chosen significance level and leads to the conclusion that there is no evidence to doubt the assumption of equal population median values.

The results for the low back pain example are shown in Table 14.8. With a significance level of .05, a p value less than .0005 indicates rejection of the null hypothesis; that is, there is evidence to doubt the assumption of no effect of the programme on Aberdeen Back Pain Scale scores. The median Aberdeen Back Pain Scale score decreased by 2.8 units following attendance; therefore, based on this study there is evidence that the median impact that low back pain has on a person's health status is lower following participation on a group-based cognitive-behavioural management programme (however, see Section 7.2.8).

Further analyses or statistics

Whether the null hypothesis is rejected or not, the Wilcoxon signed-ranks test provides no indication of the size of any median difference. This might be conveyed through a confidence interval for the population median difference; the calculation of confidence intervals for median values is described in Gibbons (1985), Neave and Worthington (1988) and Conover (1999).

Sometimes, it is informative to consider the proportion of individual differences in paired values that are positive or negative. A confidence interval might be presented for the population proportion of cases for whom an 'improvement' is likely (Daniel, 1991; Note 4 in 'Other comments' below) based on the reported outcomes in the sample. Clearly, the direction of change denoting an 'improvement' depends upon the outcome variable; for example, an increase in mobility but a decrease in anxiety scores would signify improvement. The researcher might equally be interested in estimating the proportion of cases for whom a 'deterioration' is likely.

Other comments

1. The Wilcoxon signed-ranks test, sometimes called a 'test of symmetry' (Conover, 1999), is based on differences in values for paired cases and is therefore suitable for outcome variables measured on at least an interval scale. It is, however, also appropriate for situations in which both the direction and rank order (ignoring the direction) of differences in values for paired cases are known although the values themselves are unknown.

Table 14.8 *Comparison of Aberdeen Back Pain Scale (ABPS) scores following participation on a group-based low back pain management programme (n = 56)*

Variable	1 week pre-attendance median (min, max)	1 week post-attendance median (min, max)	Difference (post – pre) median (min, max)	T (-ve ranks)	p value
ABPS score	41.3 (37.3, 45.7)	38.5 (34.2, 44.3)	–2.8 (–6.0, 0.8)	12	<.0005

2. When there are tied ranks (equal differences across the values of paired cases), it is necessary to adjust the computations to take account of the reduced variability in values of the test statistic (Conover, 1999). Most statistical computing packages report adjusted test statistics.

3. Many packages (and hand calculations) completely ignore zero differences across the values of paired cases. However, when there are several zero differences, this would appear to support the decision not to reject the null hypothesis. In such a situation, the results from the Wilcoxon signed-ranks hypothesis test might be grossly misleading (Bland, 1995). As always, one should always look carefully at the data before performing any hypothesis test (Section 12.1).

4. The Wilcoxon signed-ranks test does not indicate in what proportion of cases the differences are positive, zero or negative. For large samples ($n > 30$) and a proportion between .05 and .95, calculation of the confidence interval for the proportion of positive values is based on a normal distribution; otherwise a binomial distribution might be used (Gardner and Altman, 1989b; Daniel, 1991).

5. When the assumptions are met for a related t test, the relative efficiency of Wilcoxon's signed-ranks test is about 95%, and will be at least 86% for any symmetrical distribution (Gibbons, 1985; Conover, 1999). When the assumptions are not met, Wilcoxon's test is more powerful, and often vastly so, than a related t test (Siegel and Castellan, 1988; Pett, 1997).

Alternative procedures

1. For sample sizes larger than 15, the sum of ranks is approximately normally distributed and a z test is used as an approximation to the Wilcoxon signed-ranks test (Siegel and Castellan, 1988). Most statistical computing packages indicate when this approximation has been reported.

2. When the data are recorded on an ordinal level of measurement, the *sign test* can be used to test the null hypothesis that the populations from which the two set of related cases have been drawn have the same median value (Pett, 1997; Conover, 1999). This is the oldest nonparametric test. It assumes that each pair of values is from an independent case. The test analyses the signs (plus or minus) of the differences between pairs of scores and, therefore, is also suitable for situations in which the data comprise rank orders, or direction of preference between two options. The sign test ignores zero differences between scores and might, therefore, produce misleading results if many zeros occur. When the distributional assumptions of the related t test or of the Wilcoxon signed-ranks test are satisfied, the relative efficiency of the sign test is about 64% and 66%, respectively. With a markedly skewed distribution, however, the power of the sign test will be considerably greater; 200% relative to the related t test and 133% relative to the Wilcoxon signed-ranks (Gibbons, 1985; Conover, 1999).

3. An alternative procedure for dealing with data recorded at an ordinal level is to utilize the *Friedman test* (Section 18.1.8). Although this test is commonly used for more than two sets of data on a single variable, and is essentially an extension of the sign test (Conover, 1999), it can be used for just two sets of data. Its power in this situation is similar to that of the sign test.

14.2.4 Tests for independent cases

Unrelated designs are employed to assess differences in response variables or outcome measures across groups comprising independent cases (see Section 13.1.3). Such groups might be generated in two ways:

1. Two groups might be created by random assignment of cases to two arms of a randomized controlled trial. This random allocation of cases effectively produces two random samples from the same population and,

initially, any between-group differences in characteristics can be assumed to be due to sampling error (Section 7.2.1). Other factors remaining the same, comparisons across the groups following intervention can be ascribed to the effect of the intervention, and the groups can be considered to represent random samples from two populations.

2. Alternatively, the two groups might arise from the selection of random samples from two populations, or by some other sampling method that produces independent groups. The researcher is interested in comparing characteristics across the two populations.

In both cases, there might be different numbers of cases per group.

The unrelated t test is a parametric test used for comparing mean response or outcome values across two independent groups, thereby testing an assumption about the difference between the mean values of two populations. The Wilcoxon rank sum test (Mann-Whitney U test) is the non-parametric equivalent of the unrelated t test. It is useful when the sample sizes are small (i.e. both groups have fewer than 20 cases) and the assumptions for use of the t test are not met (Section 14.2.6). It tests an assumption about the difference between median values in two populations.

Research hypothesis
A typical research hypothesis refers to a directional comparison across populations; for example, pain intensity is lower following participation in an individual-based approach to low back pain management than following a group-based approach.

14.2.5 Unrelated t test
The unrelated t test is appropriate for the situations described in Section 14.2.4; further details for use of the test are given below.

Data
The data comprise values associated with independent cases in two groups. For example, pain intensity was recorded for each participant 1 week after completion of a low back pain management programme for patients randomly assigned to a group-based and an individual-based approach. These data are summarized in Table 14.9 and in a boxplot in Figure 14.5.

Assumptions
The assumptions for the unrelated t test are:

- The observed data constitute values from two random samples from two normally distributed populations with unknown means and unknown standard deviations (hence, unknown variances).
- The underlying random variable of interest is continuous.
- The data are measured on an interval or ratio scale.

One of two further assumptions is required (see under 'Rationale for test' below):

- The unknown population variances are equal (homogeneity of variance, or homoscedasticity).
- The unknown population variances are unequal (heterogeneity of variance, or heteroscedasticity).

Checking the assumptions
The assumptions are checked by reference to the sampling method, details of the measurement tool, and any recognized methods for checking normality, outliers, and homogeneity of variance (Box 14.3). In the example on pain intensity,

- the patients were randomly assigned to a group-based or individual-based approach;

Table 14.9 Pain intensity scores 1 week after completion of low back pain management programme

| Statistic | Approach | |
	Individual	Group
n	53	56
Mean (standard deviation)	5.29 (1.93)	5.15 (2.01)
Minimum	0.90	1.30
Maximum	9.80	9.90

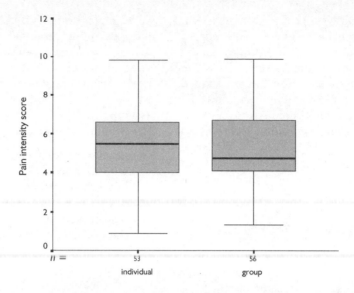

Figure 14.5   *Pain intensity, on a visual analogue scale (in cm), one week after completing a low back pain management programme, for individual and group approaches.*

hence, effectively, there are two random samples post intervention (see Section 13.6)

- Dr Buckley assumes that pain intensity scores measured on a visual analogue scale are on at least an interval level of measurement
- normal probability plots for each group cast no doubt on the assumption of normally distributed populations and indicated no extreme values
- Levene's test for equality of population variances indicated no reason to doubt the assumption of equal population variances ($F = 0.05$, p value = .82).

Statistical hypotheses

The null hypothesis states equality of the two population mean values; that is, no difference in the mean values of the two populations from which cases in the groups are sampled. A non-directional alternative hypothesis states that there is a difference between mean values in the two populations. The null hypothesis might be: there is no difference in mean pain intensity

scores for patients following completion of an individual-based or a group-based approach to the management of low back pain. The alternative hypothesis might be that there is some difference in mean pain intensity scores across the two approaches. Note that although the *research* hypothesis was directional, in terms of the *statistical* hypotheses we have stated a non-directional alternative hypothesis (see Section 13.4.4).

Rationale for test

The difference between the two group means is influenced by the actual difference between the population means that it estimates and by sampling error. If the population means are equal, the difference between the group means reflects solely sampling error. The null hypothesis can be tested, therefore, by calculating the probability of getting a difference of the obtained magnitude or larger when random samples of the chosen size are drawn from populations having equal means. When the samples are drawn from normally distributed populations, the standardized mean difference

Table 14.10 *Comparison of pain intensity scores following individual-based and group-based approaches to low back pain management*

| | Approach | | | | |
Variable	Individual-based ($n = 53$) mean (s.d.)	Group-based ($n = 56$) mean (s.d.)	Difference (individual – group) mean (s.d.)	t statistic	p value
Pain intensity	5.29 (1.93)	5.15 (2.01)	0.14 (3.92)	0.37	.72

s.d. = standard deviation.

(difference in sample mean values divided by the standard error of the difference between the means) follows a normal distribution and the probability is easy to calculate (Section 13.2.1). In reality, the variances of the two populations are unknown and the standard error of differences is estimated from the sample variances. This estimation differs according to whether the two populations have equal or unequal variances and affects the distribution of the resultant standardized score. Under the assumption of homogeneity, the standard error is estimated by combining information across both samples and the resultant standardized mean difference follows a t distribution. When the variances are unequal, the standard error is estimated by using the separate variances in the two groups and the resultant test statistic approximately follows a t distribution (Portney and Watkins, 1993; Daniel, 1991).

Results and their interpretation

The sample size, mean and standard deviation of the variable of interest are usually reported for each group, together with the mean, standard deviation, t statistic and p value for the between-group differences. Statistical computing packages provide options for performing the test under the assumption of either homogeneity or heterogeneity of population variances.

The p value is used to make a statistical decision about the null hypothesis, with a decision to reject being made for p values less than or equal to the chosen significance level.

From the results in Table 14.10, using a significance level of .05, the null hypothesis is not rejected (.72 > .05); that is, there is no evidence to doubt the assumption of zero difference in the effect of individual-based and group-based approaches on mean pain intensity scores.

Further analyses or statistics

The sample sizes and variances influence the t statistic and p value. An estimate of the difference in population mean values is given by a confidence interval. Most statistical computing packages produce confidence intervals under the assumptions of homogeneity and heterogeneity. In the pain intensity example, the 95% confidence interval was (–0.612 to 0.889); i.e. the mean pain intensity score for patients following an individual-based approach was estimated to be between 0.6 units lower and 0.9 units higher than for patients following a group-based approach (95% confidence interval; sample sizes: $n_1 = 53$, $n_2 = 56$).

Other comments

1. There is debate about the robustness of the unrelated t test to departures from the assumption of normality of the two populations. The related t test tends to be more robust than the unrelated t test, since it assumes the normality of the difference scores, not that of the raw scores in the two sets of data; the distribution of difference scores will usually be closer to normality than the raw scores on which they are based (Bland, 1995). Robustness of the unrelated t test to departures from normality is greater when sample sizes of the two groups are

equal and fairly large (Sawilowsky and Blair, 1992).

2. In most situations, the unrelated t test is more robust to departures from normality than to departures from homogeneity of variance. As in the case of normality, robustness to departures from homogeneity of variance is greater when sample sizes of the two groups are equal and fairly large (Myers and Well, 1995).

3. The unrelated t test is sensitive to the presence of extremely large or small values in one or both groups (Conover, 1999).

Alternative procedures

1. When the sample sizes are large (both samples comprising more than 30 cases), the central limit theorem (Section 13.2.2) can be invoked to assume that the sample means follow normal distributions. In this situation, a z test can be used, with population standard deviations being estimated by the sample standard deviations (Daniel, 1991).

2. When one or both sample sizes are small and the assumptions of the unrelated t test are not met, a Wilcoxon rank sum test (Section 14.2.6) is recommended.

3. The unrelated t test is a special case of the more general methods called 'analysis of variance', which are discussed in Section 18.1.

4. In the pain intensity example, the post-intervention mean scores were analysed, but pre-intervention mean scores were also measured. It was assumed that the random assignment of patients to the two approaches produced balanced groups with respect to pre-intervention scores on pain intensity. Alternative analyses might have been followed, for example: (1) a repeated measures analysis of variance with one within-subjects factor and one between-subjects factor (Section 18.1.6); (2) an unrelated t test on change scores (post-intervention minus pre-intervention); (3) an unrelated t test to compare pre-intervention mean pain intensity scores and patient char-

acteristics such as age and duration of illness. Altman says that this last procedure merely forms a check on the random allocation of cases to groups and does not recommend it (Altman, 1991a). However, an analysis that ignores major differences (pre-intervention) between groups might produce misleading results. Analysis of covariance (ANCOVA; Section 18.5) is often used to adjust analyses for such baseline differences.

14.2.6 Wilcoxon rank sum test

The Wilcoxon rank sum test is appropriate for the situations described in Section 14.2.4. This test is essentially the same as the Mann–Whitney test (Neave and Worthington, 1988).

Data

The data comprise values associated with non-matched cases in two groups. Researchers who dispute the claim that visual analogue scales produce data on an interval level of measurement might use the Wilcoxon rank sum test to compare differences in pain intensity scores following completion of individual-based and group-based approaches to the management of low back pain.

Assumptions

The assumptions for use of the Wilcoxon rank sum test are:

- The data constitute values of cases in two samples (or groups) independently drawn from their respective populations; or the data constitute values of cases independently drawn from one population and then randomly assigned to two groups.
- The underlying population of differences is approximately symmetrical.
- The data are measured on at least an ordinal scale.

Checking the assumptions

The assumptions are checked by reference to the sampling method, details of the employed measurement tool and a boxplot for each group. In the current example,

- the patients are randomly assigned to the two approaches
- the assumption that the underlying population of differences is approximately symmetrical is difficult to check, but the boxplots (Figure 14.5) do not exhibit markedly skewed distributions and, therefore, this assumption appears reasonable
- pain intensity was measured on a visual analogue scale, i.e. on at least an ordinal level of measurement.

Statistical hypotheses

The null hypothesis states that the two population have equal median values, and the alternative hypothesis states that they are different. Hence, in the pain intensity example, the null hypothesis is that there is no difference in population median pain intensity scores for patients following either an individual-based or a group-based approach to management of low back pain. The alternative hypothesis is that there is a difference between the population median pain intensity scores for patients following either an individual-based or a group-based approach.

Rationale for test

Interest is centred on the comparison of median scores across groups. Data from the two samples are jointly ordered from smallest to largest and the values are assigned ranks without regard to group membership – the smallest value is assigned a rank of 1, the next smallest a rank of 2, and so forth. If the population median values are equal, we expect each sample to contain a mix of low, medium and high ranks. If the population median values are very different, we expect one sample to contain low and medium ranks, whereas the other sample would contain medium and high ranks. Hence, if the sum of ranks for the values in one of the groups is too small (or too large), the null hypothesis of no difference in population median values is rejected.

Results and their interpretation

For each group, the sample size, median, minimum and maximum values are reported for the variable of interest. The p value and test statistic (U, W or z) are also reported. The W statistic is associated with the Wilcoxon rank sum test and represents the sum of ranks for the smaller sample. The U statistic is associated with the Mann–Whitney test, and represents the number of times that a value in one sample is smaller than values in the other sample, taken over all values in the first sample. If U is divided by the product of the two sample sizes, the resultant number estimates the probability that an additional value randomly selected from the first population will be smaller than an additional value randomly selected from the second population (Altman, 1991a). Finally, z refers to the standardized z score, which is reported when the sample sizes are large (see Note 1 under 'Alternative procedures' below).

As usual, the p value is used to make a statistical decision, with values smaller than or equal to the chosen significance level leading to rejection of the null hypothesis and a conclusion that there is evidence to doubt the assumption of equal median values in the two populations.

From the results shown in Table 14.11, at a significance level of .05, a p value of .71 indicates that the null hypothesis is not rejected. That is, there is no evidence to doubt the assumption of no difference between the median pain intensity scores for patients following an individual-based or a group-based approach to low back pain management. Based on this study, there is no evidence that one approach is more effective than the other with respect to pain intensity scores. The conclusion requires careful wording, since change over time has not been explicitly considered in this analysis.

Further analyses or statistics

Whether the null hypothesis is rejected or not, the Wilcoxon rank sum test provides no indication of the size of any median difference. A confidence interval can be calculated for the difference in median values; Sprent (1993) provides details.

Table 14.11 *Comparison of pain intensity scores following individual-based and group-based approaches to low back pain management*

Variable	Approach		Median difference (Individual-Group)	W statistic	p value
	Individual-based (*n* = 53) median (min, max)	**Group-based** (*n* = 56) median (min, max)			
Pain intensity	5.50 (0.90, 9.80)	4.75 (1.30, 9.90)	0.75	2977	.71

Other comments

1. The Wilcoxon rank sum test might be used for comparison of change scores across groups (Pett, 1997); for example, a comparison of the change in pain intensity scores (post-intervention minus pre-intervention scores) across individual-based and group-based approaches. This analysis is appropriate when the data are measured on at least an interval level (otherwise, differences denoting change over time are meaningless), but not all the assumptions for the unrelated *t* test are met.

2. The test is fairly insensitive to a few tied ranks (more than one case having the same value). However, the power of the test diminishes as the number of ties increases, and a modified statistic is recommended when there are many ties. Details are given in Siegel and Castellan (1988), Daniel, (1991) and Conover (1999).

3. In theory, the test is appropriate for ordinal scales containing two or more response categories. However, the number of tied ranks is likely to increase as the number of scale points decreases, with a resultant loss of power. Chi-square, Fisher's exact and Mantel-Haenszel tests might more appropriately be considered when the number of response categories is small (two or three). Of these, only the Mantel–Haenszel test would preserve the ranked nature of the data.

4. When the assumptions are met for the unrelated *t* test, the relative efficiency of the Wilcoxon rank sum test is about 95%, and is always at least 86% if the distributions are symmetrical (Gibbons, 1985; Conover, 1999). When the assumptions are not met, Wilcoxon's is the more powerful test (Siegel and Castellan, 1988).

5. The test is also appropriate for data that comprise rank order across two groups for some variable of interest.

Alternative procedures

1. When the sample sizes are both large, the sum of ranks is approximately normally distributed and a *z* test is used as an approximation to the Wilcoxon rank sum test. 'Large' is given as greater than 20 according to Daniel (1991) and 10 according to Siegel and Castellan (1988). Most statistical computing packages indicate when this approximation has been reported.

2. The *Kolmogorov–Smirnov test* is a nonparametric procedure that tests for differences between unrelated samples in terms of both the median values and the distribution (i.e. dispersion and skewness) of the two samples. The Kolmogorov–Smirnov test can also be used as a goodness-of-fit test (Section 13.4.2, Box 14.3). Neave and Worthington (1988), Siegel and Castellan (1988), and Pett (1997) provide details.

14.3 ESTIMATING DIFFERENCES: TWO SETS OF DATA ON A SINGLE VARIABLE

Many research questions involve comparisons across sets of data corresponding to groups of cases or points in time, for example, those posed at the beginning of Section 14.2. These research questions might be investigated through the use of confidence intervals, which will provide an interval estimate for the magnitude of the population effect of an intervention, the population mean difference in some characteristic across two groups, or the difference in proportions satisfying some condition in two populations.

The construction of commonly used confidence intervals follows a simple rule: the lower and upper limits are given by, respectively, subtracting from and adding to the sample statistic a multiple of its standard error (Section 13.3). The standard error reflects sampling error (Section 8.5), but does not account for non-sampling errors. The 'multiple' reflects the chosen confidence that the interval contains the population parameter that is being estimated and is a standardized score from the appropriate sampling distribution (Sections 13.2.2 and 13.3). A possible interpretation is that the parameter value is estimated to be greater than or equal to the lower limit and smaller than or equal to the upper limit, with the specified confidence. That is, any value in the interval is a plausible value for the population parameter. This interpretation reveals a link with hypothesis testing (assuming a non-directional alternative hypothesis). If the parameter value stated by the null hypothesis falls within the interval, then the null hypothesis is retained. By the same token, if the parameter value of the null hypothesis is excluded from the interval, the null hypothesis is rejected. This also indicates that the use of a confidence interval is subject to the same assumptions as the equivalent hypothesis test (Section 14.2).

However, confidence intervals convey more information than hypothesis testing (Section 13.5). Most statistical computing packages have options to calculate confidence intervals using standard distributions such as t, normal, chi-square and Fisher's F, but few compute confidence intervals associated with the distribution of ranks (for example, for median values). Details and examples of hand calculations are given in Gardner and Altman (1989a) and Conover (1999).

14.4 CONCLUSION

This chapter has considered some hypothesis tests that are frequently used by health care professionals. It has presented the rationale for each test and the assumptions that support drawing generalizations from the results. Presentation of results has also been covered, since the dissemination of findings to other researchers is an important element in any research.

Although statistical hypothesis testing has received most attention, the use of confidence intervals is strongly recommended when investigating change over two points in time or differences between two groups. Confidence intervals estimate the magnitude of effects, enabling practitioners to distinguish between clinically important findings and statistically significant findings.

Many studies will involve more than two sets of data. Chapter 18 will consider more advanced statistical analyses that are suitable for these situations.

PART FIVE

MORE SPECIALIZED ISSUES

15 Issues in questionnaire design and attitude measurement

SUMMARY

This chapter explores the following topics:

- methods commonly used for the measurement of attitudes, beliefs and reported behaviour
- testing attitude scales for reliability
- sources of bias in attitude measurement
- issues of question wording and construction
- the presentation and layout of questionnaires

Questionnaires are a common means of measuring attitudes and beliefs in health care research. The methodological demands of questionnaires are crucial if valid and reliable data are to be gained, but are sometimes underestimated by health care researchers (Layte and Jenkinson, 1997). Perhaps this is because, in contrast to students of the social and behavioural sciences, most student health professionals receive little education in *psychometrics*. Psychometrics is the theory underlying the measurement of psychological variables such as attitudes, beliefs and aspects of intelligence (Rust and Golombok, 1999).

This chapter will address some of the principal issues to be considered when designing questionnaires and similar instruments, and will build upon the topics addressed in Chapter 6.

15.1 SCALES AND RESPONSE FORMATS

There are a number of ways in which facts, attitudes, beliefs or self-reported behaviour can be measured. All scales and other response formats will consist of one or more *items*. The items that find their way into a questionnaire will have been selected from an initial *pool* of such items, which will either have been composed by the researcher or have been gleaned from existing instruments.

These items very often take the form of questions, but may be phrased as an instruction (e.g. asking respondents to tick a certain option, or to enter certain information in a space provided). Questionnaire items may be either *closed ended* or *open ended*. A closed-ended item requires the respondent to select one or more of a series of predetermined response categories. In contrast, an open-ended item does not provide predetermined response options, but allows the respondent to respond in his or her own words (see Section 15.1.6 for more details).

Items that seek to quantify a particular entity or variable are known as *scales*. Sometimes a scale may consist of a single item (a uni-item scale), or may be composed of a number of items (a multi-item scale). A questionnaire should not therefore be described as a multi-item instrument unless it consists of one or more multi-item scales, as defined in this way.

This section will consider some of the more straightforward response formats. More complex formats – especially multi-item scales – will be reserved for the following section.

15.1.1 Numerical rating scales

A numerical rating scale, with anchors at each end, is often used as a means of measuring attitudes and beliefs (Figure 15.1). It is considered that such a scale should normally consist of at least seven scale points (Finn, 1972). However, the optimum number may vary from context to context. As a general principle, Streiner and Norman (1995) argue that if the number of scale points is less than the individual's ability to discriminate, information will be lost. An odd number of scale points provides a neutral midpoint. It is important that respondents understand the rela-

Please indicate how helpful you have found the information leaflet provided by the midwife
(please circle the appropriate number between 1 and 7 on the scale below):

'Not at all helpful'   1   2   3   4   5   6   7   'Very helpful'

Figure 15.1 *Numerical rating scale.*

tionship of the scale points to the two anchors, and if a number of such items are to be used together it is useful to provide an explanation, and possibly an example, at the beginning of this section of the questionnaire.

The use of negative numbers in a scale (e.g. using −5 to +5 rather than 0 to 10 for an 11-point scale) will tend to change the way in which the scale is perceived. Using negative numbers for the lower half of a scale may make it appear more 'negative' than if positive numbers were used throughout the scale (Schwartz *et al.*, 1991).

15.1.2 Visual analogue scales

Whereas a numerical rating scale is discrete, with a predetermined number of scale points, a visual analogue scale (VAS) is continuous, with an almost infinite number of possible points. Conventionally, the VAS consists of a 10 cm line, anchored at each end, on which the respondent puts a mark corresponding to his or her attitude or belief (Figure 15.2). A VAS was used to measure pain intensity and pain affect in the Low Back Pain Study (Table 7.1).

A score is generated by measuring from the left-hand end of the line to the mark made by the respondent; this measurement is usually rounded up to the nearest millimetre (McQuay and Moore, 1999). Sometimes, researchers round the score to the nearest centimetre, but this seems to offer no advantages over a ten-point numerical scale, which is likely to be easier to use. The relationship of the anchors to the line is crucial, and

the VAS is cognitively quite demanding for some individuals (Waterfield and Sim, 1996). Although some researchers use labels for intermediate points on the scale, as well as for the anchors at each end, this is probably ill advised. A VAS that only has anchors at each end is likely to encourage greater use of the extremes of the scale, and will thus discriminate between respondents more effectively. Moreover, responses that lie between the extremes of the scale are likely to be focused on the intermediate labels (Streiner and Norman, 1995); this effectively reduces a continuous scale to a discrete scale.

Given that the scale is continuous, data yielded by a VAS are generally considered to be at an interval level of measurement (McGuire, 1984; Price *et al.*, 1983; Price and Harkins, 1992), though there is some debate on this issue (B. May, 1991; Sim and Waterfield, 1997). The decision that a researcher takes on this question should be based upon a consideration of the likely isomorphism between the scale and the construct it is measuring, and a judgement as to the appropriate role of assumptions of isomorphism in determining statistical operations (Box 15.1).

When using a VAS or a numerical rating scale to measure serial change – e.g. when asking how much pain relief has been experienced since the last assessment – it is important to remember that each measurement is based on the amount of pain present, and also on the amount of pain relief reported, on the previous occasion. It is not anchored to a fixed quantity, as in the example

Please indicate the *average* severity of your pain over the last 7 days by placing a vertical mark on the line below:

'No pain' |————————————————————| 'Worst pain imaginable'

Figure 15.2 *Visual analogue scale for pain intensity. (Not to scale; actual length of line would be 10 cm.)*

Box 15.1 *The question of isomorphism*

When a scale is being used to measure an underlying attitude or other psychological construct, the question arises as to whether the structure of the scale matches that of the construct; i.e. whether the scale and the construct are *isomorphic*. This has a particular bearing on the measurement properties that are ascribed to the scale. If a scale is isomorphic with respect to the construct it is measuring, this means that small changes on the scale should represent proportionately small changes in terms of quantities of the underlying construct (and correspondingly for large changes). Thus, a movement of two points on a ten point scale should represent a corresponding magnitude of change in the construct, wherever on the scale this two-point change occurs. If, however, a two-point change might represent a small change in the underlying construct when it occurs near the middle of the scale but a noticeably larger change when it occurs at one or other end of the scale, this suggests that the scale and the construct are not isomorphic. The visual analogue scale exemplifies this issue. Streiner and Norman (1995) argue that, although measurements on the scale can be made with a high degree of discrimination (e.g. to the nearest millimetre on a 10 cm scale), it does not necessarily follow that these responses represent the underlying construct with the same degree of resolution. When it comes to determining the measurement properties of a scale, some researchers take a strict view of isomorphism, and argue that data from a scale can be treated as interval only if the assumption of isomorphism can be justified. Others take a more liberal view, and claim that as long as the data derived from the scale appear to possess the property of interval data, they can be treated as such statistically, almost irrespective of the precise structural relationship between the scale and the underlying construct (Nunnally and Bernstein, 1994). This controversy is not easily resolved (Knapp, 1990). However, researchers should be aware of the issues at stake in this debate when considering their own use and subsequent analysis of psychological and attitudinal measures.

in Figure 15.2. Moreover, as further pain relief is achieved, the scope for further relief is restricted correspondingly. Consequently, the meaning of a given distance on the scale will change from measurement to measurement.

15.1.3 Adjectival and adverbial rating scales

Some scales are made up of a series of adjectives or adverbs, arranged hierarchically. Examples of such scales from the questionnaire used in the Rheumatoid Arthritis Study are shown in Figure 15.3.

Note that although a numerical score corresponds to each response category, responses should be elicited from respondents in terms of the adjectives or adverbs provided. It is clearly important that the hierarchy of the words is not open to debate. This may be the case in the example in Figure 15.4, since some respondents might disagree about the relative strength of 'somewhat' and 'moderately', regardless of any dictionary definitions.

Although this sort of adverbial scale is quite similar to a Likert scale (see Section 15.2.1), the latter term should be reserved for scales in which the responses are framed in terms of either agreement/disagreement or approval/disapproval.

It is important to realize that the meaning of an adjectival or adverbial response is not fixed, but is determined by the other categories in the scale (Fowler, 1995). Compare, for example, the scales in Figure 15.5. It will be noted that the meaning of a word like 'good' depends on its relationship to the alternative adjectives provided, and becomes progressively weaker from scale A to scale C. It would, therefore, be hazardous to compare responses to a question using scale A with those to a question using scale C.

A final point of caution is that respondents

Generally speaking, how responsive do you find rheumatoid arthritis patients are to therapy?

Extremely responsive 5	Very responsive 4	Moderately responsive 3	Quite unresponsive 2	Extremely unresponsive 1
☐	☐	☐	☐	☐

Please indicate the frequency with which patients with rheumatoid arthritis are referred to you from each of the following sources:

	Very often 5	Often 4	Sometimes 3	Seldom 2	Never or almost never 1
Rheumatologist	☐	☐	☐	☐	☐
Orthopaedic surgeon	☐	☐	☐	☐	☐
Other therapist	☐	☐	☐	☐	☐
[.........]	☐	☐	☐	☐	☐

Figure 15.3 *Examples of adjectival and adverbial rating scales. The small-font numbers are for coding (see Section 15.5.3).*

How much does your back pain bother you in relation to each of the following?

	Not at all 5	Somewhat 4	Moderately 3	Very much 2	Extremely 1
Self-care (e.g. washing and dressing)	☐	☐	☐	☐	☐
Mobility outside the home	☐	☐	☐	☐	☐
Normal leisure activities	☐	☐	☐	☐	☐
[.........]	☐	☐	☐	☐	☐

Figure 15.4 *Adverbial rating scale with questionable descriptors.*

A

Good	Fair	Poor
☐	☐	☐

B

Very good	Good	Fair	Poor
☐	☐	☐	☐

C

Excellent	Very good	Good	Fair	Poor
☐	☐	☐	☐	☐

Figure 15.5 *The effect of scale length and structure on the meaning of an adjectival descriptor.*

may use a particular abstract description of frequency, such as 'very often', to refer to different rates of occurrence (Bradburn and Sudman, 1980). Individuals will have different views of the appropriate frequency with which something should occur – taking vigorous exercise four times a week may be 'very often' to some people, but only 'quite often' to other more energetically disposed individuals. The topic concerned is another source of variation: Foddy (1993) points out that a frequency of 'once a day' may be considered 'very often' when talking about a haircut but not 'very often' when talking about brushing one's teeth. Asking for a precise frequency (e.g. 'twice a week') can avoid such ambiguity in cases where the actual rate of occurrence of an action or event is desired. However, it does not capture the respondent's subjective notion of frequency. The researcher's interest may be more in *perception* of frequency than in actual rate of occurrence.

15.1.4 Checklists

In a checklist, the respondent is provided with a list of possible answers, and is required to endorse one or more of these, as in the example in Figure 15.6, which is taken from the questionnaire used in the Rheumatoid Arthritis Study.

Two important aspects of questionnaire design are illustrated here. First, it is necessary to make it explicit whether respondents are to endorse one answer only, or as many answers as apply. Note, however, that if a respondent fails to check a box in the example in Fig 15.6, this

may indicate that the item is not applicable, or it may be that the respondent was unsure, or perhaps overlooked the item. Hence, an alternative, favoured by Sudman and Bradburn (1982), is to require a 'yes' or 'no' response to each item (and a 'don't know' category if appropriate). Second, a residual ('other' or 'not applicable') category should be included if it is foreseeable that some respondents will wish to reply in terms of a category not provided for in the list, or if the question as a whole will not be applicable to some respondents. Hence, therapists who use an instrument other than those listed have a response option available to them, as do those who are not involved in measuring pain intensity. Krosnick (1999) suggests, however, that, despite the presence of a residual category, respondents tend to confine their answers to the listed options, even if none of these is wholly appropriate. A checklist should therefore be as comprehensive as possible in relation to anticipated response categories.

15.1.5 Ranking procedures

Sometimes, respondents may be given a list of items and asked to rank them in order of preference, importance, familiarity, frequency of use, and so forth (Figure 15.7). Some people find this fairly demanding, and the number of items should be kept to a minimum, or else respondents should be asked to rank only a few items (e.g. the top three items). Moreover, a ranking procedure may force respondents to express a hierarchy of preference in respect of some items

By what means do you assess the *intensity* of the rheumatoid arthritis patient's pain (please tick all that apply)?

Numerical rating scale (e.g. 1–10)	☐ 1
Verbal rating scale (e.g. 'severe, moderate...')	☐ 2
Visual analogue scale	☐ 3
McGill Pain Questionnaire (long or short form)	☐ 4
Other (please state below)	☐ 5
None of the above because I do not routinely assess pain intensity	☐ 6

Figure 15.6 Checklist.

From the following list, please choose the *three* factors that you find *most* stressful at work and rank them in order from 1 to 3 (with 1 indicating the most stress factor). Please do not use any rank more than once.

	Rank	
Handling issues I have not previously dealt with	☐	A
Dealing with dissatisfied or irate members of the public	☐	B
Deadlines by which work has to be completed	☐	C
Being unable to control my own time	☐	D
Conflict with colleagues	☐	E
Shortage of equipment, facilities and other work resources	☐	F
Working within inflexible procedures	☐	G

Figure 15.7   *A ranking item. The small-font letters are for coding (Section 15.5.3).*

that they may not really hold (Converse and Presser, 1994); people tend to find it particularly hard to rank items in the middle of their order of preferences (Sudman and Bradburn, 1982). The difficulties of ranking are heightened if a questionnaire is administered over the telephone, when the respondent does not have a visible list of items to which to refer (Dillman, 1978). Respondents should be specifically instructed not to give tied rankings (Henerson *et al.*, 1987), since these are very hard to analyse.

The data resulting from ranking form an *ipsative* scale, in which a particular scale point can be used only once by a single respondent (in a ranking procedure, each rank can be assigned to only one item). Statistically, scores on ipsative scales are not independent; i.e. the choice of a certain rank for one item determines the ranks that remain available for other items. This may have implications for the type of statistical analysis that can be performed on such data.

15.1.6 Open-ended items

Hitherto, we have considered closed-ended items, i.e. those in which there is a range of responses specified in advance by the researcher and listed for the respondent to choose from. An alternative approach is to leave open the nature and form of the response to an item – for the respondent to respond in his or her own words. The data gained in this way will often be qualitative, and must be coded by the researcher. As this will demand case-by-case judgements, the

inter-rater reliability of open-ended items is likely to be poorer than that of closed-ended items. Open-ended items are also more time consuming for the researcher to analyse, and for the respondent to complete in the first place. Against this, it should be pointed out that a large number of closed-ended items may be tedious to complete, and respondents appreciate the opportunity to respond to at least some questions in their own words (Fowler, 1993). When asking respondents to recall types of behaviour (e.g. 'In the last seven days, which of the following foods have you eaten?'), or their familiarity with certain items (e.g. 'Which of the following drugs have you prescribed?'), there may be important differences in the data yielded by open-ended responses as compared with checklists. In particular, data collected by the two methods should not be brought together in a comparative analysis (Belson and Duncan, 1962). When constructing open-ended questions, careful judgement must be made as to how much space to provide for the response, bearing in mind that this may communicate to the respondent an appropriate or acceptable length of response.

There is evidence that, in respect of potentially threatening or sensitive topics, open-ended questions may elicit higher levels of reported behaviour than closed-ended questions (Bradburn and Sudman, 1980). The respective roles of open-ended and closed-ended questions in collecting different forms of information are summarized in Table 15.1.

15.2 SPECIALIZED MEANS OF MEASURING ATTITUDES

One of the purposes of a questionnaire is frequently to measure respondents' attitudes or beliefs on one or more topics, and some questionnaires take the form of specialized attitude inventories. It is important, therefore, to consider some of the methods available for measuring attitudes. Four main techniques – Likert scales, Guttman scales, Thurstone scales and the semantic differential scale – will be examined in this section.

Table 15.1   *Respective roles of open-ended and closed-ended questions*

Purpose	Closed-ended questions	Open-ended questions
Identifying issues that are of personal interest or relevance to individual respondents		✓
Determining whether a respondent has opinions/knowledge on the issue	✓	
Eliciting general attitudes on the issue in question		✓
Eliciting specific views on particular aspects of the issue	✓	
Determining respondents' reasons for their attitudes	✓	✓
Determining the strength with which an attitude is held	✓	
Determining responses on a very wide variety of items, or on a list of items which cannot be fully specified in advance		✓
Determining responses on a limited number of items which can be specified in advance	✓	
Obtaining exact numerical quantities (e.g. income, age)		✓
Obtaining quantities in bands (e.g. 0–10, 11–20, etc.), where respondents may be unable or reluctant to give exact numerical quantities	✓	

15.2.1 Likert scales

The Likert scale is a very common means of attitude measurement and will therefore be considered in some detail. The scale provides a measurement of attitude by asking the respondent to indicate his or her agreement or disagreement (or in some cases, approval or disapproval) with one or more statements. The Likert scale can therefore be used as either a uni-item or a multi-item scale (Moser and Kalton, 1971). When used as a multi-item scale, it may be used either to provide a single indicator for each of a number of attitude dimensions (i.e. one Likert item per dimension), or to provide multiple indicators of a single attitude dimension (i.e. several items for one dimension), or to provide multiple indicators of each of a number of dimensions (i.e. several items for each of several dimensions). When a multi-item scale is used, responses on individual items are summed (usually with subtotals if the scale is measuring separate dimensions). In such a case a Likert scale is known as a *summative* scale. Likert himself advocated that scores be treated in this way (Likert, 1932). When a number of items are used to tap a concept, higher reliability will be obtained than if a single item were used, though

there comes a point where the gain in reliability tails off with increasing number of items (Smith, 1975). The items in Figure 15.8, which are taken from the questionnaire used in the Rheumatoid Arthritis Study, form uni-item Likert scales, since each item is the sole indicator of a separate attitude.

The statement, or stem, can be worded either positively or negatively (hence, the second item in Figure 15.8 could be worded 'These patients are generally ill-informed on their condition'). A mixture of positive and negative items helps to counteract the effects of *acquiescence bias* (i.e. the tendency to agree with a statement) and a *response set* (i.e. the tendency to respond in a similar way to successive items, irrespective of their content). The midpoint category (where present) may appear variously as 'neither', 'undecided' or 'no opinion'. Responses can be scored numerically, such that 'strongly agree' scores 5 and 'strongly disagree' scores 1, as in the present example. The resulting data are strictly on an ordinal level of measurement, since the difference between, say, 'strongly agree' and 'agree' is not necessarily of the same magnitude as that between 'agree' and 'neither'. Although the five-point scale (or four-point, if there is no midpoint) is most common, a seven-point scale

	Strongly agree 5	Agree 4	Neither 3	Disagree 2	Strongly disagree 1
Restoring function is more important than treating pain	☐	☐	☐	☐	☐
These patients are generally well informed on their condition	☐	☐	☐	☐	☐
The therapist should attend to patients' psychological needs as much as to their physical needs	☐	☐	☐	☐	☐

Figure 15.8 *Likert items.*

(or six-point, if there is no midpoint) can be utilized, as in Figure 15.9.

The process by which a multi-item Likert scale is constructed and administered is normally as follows:

1. A pool of items is obtained, preferably of equal strength and of both positive and negative content. Nunnally (1967) suggests that the item pool should consist of around 40 such items and Reckase (1990) takes the view that approximately twice as many items are required as are intended to be in the final scale. Scales that will be tapping a number of dimensions will clearly require proportionately more items that those addressing a single dimension.
2. The items are examined for clarity and ambiguity; some are likely to be discarded as a result.
3. A selection of items are put together to form the scale, with approximately equal numbers of positive and negative items. At this stage, the homogeneity of the scale should normally be tested through a preliminary study (see Section 15.3).
4. The items are administered to the sample for the main study, and the resulting scores are computed and, if appropriate, summated.

For a multi-item Likert scale measuring a specific attitude dimension, assuming the scale is scored 1–5 on each item, the minimum score possible is equal to the number of items, and the maximum possible is the number of items multiplied by five. There are, however, certain caveats that should be borne in mind here. First, summation of scores is strictly only appropriate for interval data, and it is important to consider whether the data from a particular Likert scale, which are in strict terms ordinal, can be treated as though they are interval (Reckase, 1990; see Box 15.1). Second, summation also assumes that responses are equally weighted, since the same score on different items contributes equally to the total score. However, although Likert items are in theory supposed to be of equal strength (Kerlinger, 1986), in practice some items are likely to be stronger indicators, or more central to the topic concerned, than others, and thus it is strictly inappropriate that they should count equally in the summated score. Foddy (1993) points out that 'strongly agree' in relation to a weak item may actually have the same meaning as 'agree' in relation to a stronger item, but the score for the items will differ. If items are weighted in proportion to their strength or importance (e.g. scores on some items might be multiplied by 1.5, and others by 2.0, and so forth), this may par-

	Completely agree 7	Mostly agree 6	Slightly agree 5	Undecided 4	Slightly disagree 3	Mostly disagree 2	Completely disagree 1
	☐	☐	☐	☐	☐	☐	☐

Figure 15.9 *Response categories for a seven-point Likert item.*

Table 15.2 *Hypothetical scores on a Likert scale for two respondents*

Item	Respondent One's score	Respondent Two's score
1	4	3
2	2	4
3	5	4
4	3	3
5	5	4
6	1	2
Total	20	20

tially counteract this difficulty. Determining the appropriate weights is, however, a difficult issue.

Third, because there are many different ways of achieving a specific score on a scale consisting of a number of Likert items, such a score can represent various profiles of response. For example, Table 15.2 shows hypothetical scores on six items for two respondents; the total score is the same in both cases, but their attitude profiles, as expressed by the individual item scores, differ. However, if the scale is homogeneous, it is the total score that is of primary interest, so that small differences for individual items are not necessarily problematic.

Fourth, care must be taken to reverse-score negative items so that they contribute appropriately to the summated score (Loewenthal, 1996). Hence, if 'strongly agree' on a positive item is to be scored 5, 'strongly agree' on a negative item should be scored 1 in order to attain equivalence of meaning. Similarly, 'agree' would be scored 4 for a positive item, and 2 for a negative item.

The above points should be carefully considered when using Likert items summatively. In this way, a scale will be produced that provides the information required while observing basic psychometric principles.

There are also important issues to consider in the wording, construction and ordering of individual Likert items. When these items are constructed, the stem must not represent a neutral or middling attitude; otherwise it is not possible to interpret disagreement. If respondents disagree with the statement 'My health is

fair', you cannot tell in which direction they are disagreeing (Fowler, 1993): is their health better, or worse, than fair? Items should not, however, be too extreme, or respondents will all tend to polarize to the 'strongly disagree' end of the scale, with the result that their responses cannot be differentiated (Nunnally, 1967). Similarly, items that are too mild and uncontroversial will tend to polarize respondents to the 'strongly agree' end of the scale.

A similar problem may occur if items on which respondents have strong feelings follow items that are of less concern to them. Respondents who have answered 'strongly agree' to these earlier items and then come to items with which they are in greater agreement have no means of indicating this stronger agreement (Foddy, 1993). This is an example of a *context effect* (see Section 15.5.2).

As with numerical rating scales, a decision must be made on whether to have an odd or even number of scale points; an even number excludes the midpoint 'undecided' option. Some feel you should force the respondent to commit himself or herself to either agree or disagree, others feel that if there is likely to be a genuine neutrality of opinion on the topic concerned, you should cater for it. The choice here is not straightforward. On the one hand, having a midpoint may discourage the person from thinking the response through, and the meaning to be attached to such a response is not in fact self-evident; does it represent an intermediate attitude between 'agree' and 'disagree', or does it represent an unknown or indeterminate attitude? On the other hand, not having a midpoint excludes information on the degree of ignorance or indifference that exists on the issue (Sudman and Bradburn, 1982). It may also lead to a high level of item non-response (Tull and Albaum, 1973). Also, if respondents do not have a neutral category available to them, they may guess (producing random error), and are more likely to fall into a response set (producing systematic error). Whether or not a neutral category is included will affect the *number* of responses falling into the other categories, but not necessarily the *ratio* of the responses in these categories (Converse and Presser, 1994). Which approach is adopted is really a matter of judgement, in relation to the topic concerned and the likely responses of the sample. Pre-testing the scale both with and without the midpoint may provide useful information (Fink, 1995b).

The structure of the Likert scale is established and well validated; the researcher merely provides the content. There is therefore no need to use a panel of experts to construct the scale (though it will usually need pre-testing or piloting, and experts may of course be enlisted when creating the individual items in the scale). It is easy to create subscales of Likert items, and thereby cover different dimensions of a topic.

15.2.2 Guttman scales

The Guttman scale is less common than the Likert scale, and is a *cumulative* rather than a summative scale. In a Guttman scale, a number of dichotomous items of different strength are constructed on a single dimension and in a hierarchy, such that endorsement of a particular item automatically implies endorsement of all weaker items (Guttman, 1944). An example of such a scale is shown in Figure 15.10.

The process by which a Guttman scale is constructed and administered is roughly as follows:

1. A pool of items of varying strengths is obtained. The items are administered to a panel of judges, representative of the study sample, who are asked to agree or disagree with them.

2. A *scalogram analysis* is carried out on the responses from the previous stage. This determines the order of the items in terms of most to least agreement: the item with which almost everybody agrees will tend to be a very 'weak' item; the one with which the least people agree will tend to be a very 'strong' one.

3. Reproducibility is checked by making sure that, for each judge, agreement with a 'strong' item is accompanied by agreement with all the 'weaker' items (here, 'reproducibility' refers to the ability to predict a respondent's responses to individual items from knowing his or her overall score). The scale is usually considered acceptable if this occurs with at least 90% of the subjects – this known as the *coefficient of reproducibility* (Babbie, 1989).

4. The final scale should include a representative selection of items of different degrees of popularity (i.e. with different frequencies of endorsement). The popularity of an item is an index of its intensity (the most popular are the weakest), and a spread of items across the range of intensity of opinion is therefore required.

5. The respondent is asked to tick 'yes' or 'no' to each item, and the score for that individual is simply the number of items endorsed.

On a given scale there is (with a degree of confidence equivalent to the scale's coefficient of

	Yes	No	
	1	0	
I can walk around my home if I have help	☐	☐	A
I can walk around my home without help	☐	☐	B
I can walk one block without help	☐	☐	C
I can walk several blocks without help	☐	☐	D
I can walk at normal pace with no restriction	☐	☐	E
I can walk at a fast pace with no restriction	☐	☐	F

Figure 15.10 *Guttman scale.*

reproducibility) only one way to get a given score: thus one can predict a respondent's specific responses from his or her total score with this level of confidence. In contrast to the Likert scale, any given score therefore has only one meaning. The Guttman scale lies at an ordinal level of measurement (van der Ven, 1980; Streiner and Norman, 1995). A recent discussion of the use of a Guttman scale to measure degrees of functional capacity can be found in De Souza (1999).

15.2.3 Thurstone scales

Thurstone scales (Thurstone and Chave, 1929) are similar to Guttman scales in that respondents give a dichotomous 'agree'/'disagree' or 'yes'/'no' response to each item. However, the Thurstone scale differs from both the Likert and the Guttman scales in providing an interval (or quasi-interval) scale. It is known as a *differential* scale, in that respondents 'differentiate' themselves by agreeing with only those items that correspond approximately to their own attitude and disagreeing with those that are more extreme in either direction (Moser and Kalton, 1971). Thurstone items differ, therefore, from Likert items, which are designed so that a respondent who disagrees with an item does so in one direction only (Procter, 1993a).

The process by which a Thurstone scale is constructed and administered is roughly as follows:

1. A pool of items (usually at least 100) of varying strengths is obtained. These items each require a dichotomous 'agree'/'disagree' response. However, although they are of varying strengths, Thurstone items are not designed to be cumulative in the way that Guttman items are.
2. The items are presented in random order to the panel of judges, each of whom is asked to sort them into 11 piles in order of perceived strength (not in terms of their own personal opinion or belief), scoring the piles from 11 (most favourable) to 1 (least favourable).
3. The score value of each items is taken to be

its median pile position, and the items are resorted into piles according to this score (such that all items with a median pile position of 1 are placed in the first pile, and so forth). Items whose dispersion of scores is too great are eliminated.
4. A scale is compiled with items evenly spread across the range of median scores (usually two items from each of the 11 piles), but presented in random order.
5. Respondents are instructed to endorse all items with which they agree, and the respondent's score is the median of all the scores on the individual items endorsed. Each respondent should endorse only a small number of items, since only a small number will lie at his or her own strength of opinion on the issue.

The process by which items are accorded a score value is designed to secure equal intervals between adjacent scale points. Hence the Thurstone scale is considered to lie at an interval level of measurement (Kerlinger, 1986), though whether this is strictly true is debated (Moser and Kalton, 1971). As with the Likert scale, a given score can be derived from the endorsement of a variety of items and does not represent a unique pattern of responses to individual items. However, because a respondent is expected to endorse a small number of items of similar strength, this gives a rough indication of the pattern of scores. Thurstone scales are generally considered to be rather less reliable than Likert scales; i.e. a greater number of scale items are usually required in a Thurstone scale to obtain the same level of reliability (Seiler and Hough, 1970).

Comparative features of Likert, Guttman and Likert scales are shown in Table 15.3. For small or medium-sized studies, the Likert scale is probably the simplest and most efficient method.

15.2.4 Semantic differential scale

The semantic differential scale was originally developed by Osgood and his colleagues (Osgood *et al.*, 1957), and is a means of measuring attitudes by asking respondents to

Table 15.3   *Principal points of comparison between Likert, Guttman and Thurstone scales*

	Likert	Scale Guttman	Thurstone
Level of measurement	Ordinal	Ordinal	Interval
Ease of construction	Easy	Laborious	Very laborious
Panel of judges	Not required	Required	Required
Reliability	Needs to be tested separately	Tested in the process of scale construction	Tested in the process of scale construction
Dimensionality	Readily adapted for multidimensional measurement by means of subscales	Designed for measuring a unidimensional construct	Designed for measuring a unidimensional construct
Meaning of scores	Score does not indicate the pattern of responses to individual items	Score indicates the pattern of responses to individual items	Score indicates the pattern of responses to individual items to a limited extent
Analysis	Individual items can be analysed as well as the scale as a whole	Scale is analysed as a whole	Scale is analysed as a whole
Frequency of use	Common	Rare	Rare

place themselves on a continuum between two polar opposites (Figure 15.11). Both the direction and the intensity of the respondent's attitude are tapped (Heise, 1970). As its name suggests, and in common with the Thurstone scale, the semantic differential scale is a form of differential scale: respondents differentiate themselves by choosing one end of the scale rather than the other.

Items tend to fall into one of three broad categories: evaluation (e.g. clean/dirty, warm/cold); potency (e.g. firm/soft, strong/weak); activity

(e.g. fast/slow, active/passive). The semantic differential scale therefore lends itself to multidimensional scaling, and scores can be derived for the scale as a whole or for subscales of evaluation, potency and activity.

Care must be taken that the scale does not interact with the concepts it is designed to rate (Nunnally, 1967). It may be, for example, that adjectives change their evaluative meaning when applied to different objects: on an 'active'/'passive' scale, 'active' might be positive when applied to a student but negative when applied

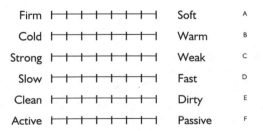

A person who smokes marijuana is:

Firm	├─┼─┼─┼─┼─┼─┼─┤ Soft	A
Cold	├─┼─┼─┼─┼─┼─┼─┤ Warm	B
Strong	├─┼─┼─┼─┼─┼─┼─┤ Weak	C
Slow	├─┼─┼─┼─┼─┼─┼─┤ Fast	D
Clean	├─┼─┼─┼─┼─┼─┼─┤ Dirty	E
Active	├─┼─┼─┼─┼─┼─┼─┤ Passive	F

Figure 15.11   *Items from a semantic differential scale.*

It is important not to confuse issues that relate to the *content* of a questionnaire with those that relate to its *form* – which is not to say, of course, that there is not a very important relationship between form and content. The researcher is well advised to determine the necessary content of the questionnaire, in terms of the specific items of information that it should yield, *before* starting to word specific questions. Otherwise, it is very easy to lose sight of what one wants to find out, in the complex process of constructing and wording individual questionnaire items. Worse still, the form chosen for an item may even alter the nature of the information gained from that originally intended.

Pre testing and piloting (Section 6.1) are particularly important here. More in-depth testing procedures can also be utilized. Foddy (1996) discusses the value of these procedures. Elsewhere, he summarizes much of the more general empirical work that has been done in relation to question construction (Foddy, 1993).

15.4.1 Constructing questionnaire items

A number of fundamental rules should be followed in order to ensure that questionnaire items are valid and reliable (Smith, 1975; Converse and Presser, 1994; Fowler, 1995):

- The terminology used should be non-technical as far as possible (unless, of course, the potential respondents are expert in the area concerned) and should generally consist of concrete rather than abstract words.
- An item should carry the same meaning for all respondents – ambiguity in *items* should be eliminated as far as possible.
- The meaning of a response should be clear to the researcher – ambiguity in *responses* should be eliminated as far as possible.
- Answers to a given question should be given in the same terms – a question that produces a mixture of factual and attitudinal data will be very hard to analyse.

- Respondents should be clear whether a particular question requires an answer from them and, if so, should understand exactly how to respond.
- Respondents should be competent to respond to each item – items that use obscure or specialist terminology, or that demand knowledge or experience unlikely to be shared by all respondents, should be avoided.

Space does not permit a detailed consideration of all aspects of question wording and construction. Instead, a number of examples are provided in Figure 15.12.

15.4.2 Bias in attitude measurement

Because they are very personal phenomena that are closely associated with an individual's social and psychological identity, attitudes are very prone to various forms of bias:

Fear, misunderstanding, the desire to place oneself in a more favourable light, social taboos, dislike for the research worker and other motives may all play a part in distorting the results and may lead to outright refusal.

(Oppenheim, 1992, p. 210)

Such systematic error undermines measurement validity, and must therefore be minimized in order to gain a valid measurement of respondents' attitudes (but see Box 15.2). There are two main sources of bias in attitude measurement. First, owing to certain cognitive or other psychological mechanisms, respondents may respond in a particular pattern that is unrelated to their true attitudes. An example would be the response set (Table 15.5). Second, most methods for measuring attitudes or recording behaviour convey to the respondent certain expectations as to what they should believe or how they should behave. A number of examples of such cues – which are known as *demand characteristics* (Orne, 1962) – are included in Table 15.5.

Questionnaire item	Comment
How often do you observe correct manual handling procedures? Always ☐ Usually ☐ Sometimes ☐ Seldom ☐ Never ☐	The word 'observe' is ambiguous: it could mean 'witness' or 'practise in accordance with'. The meaning of 'correct' is also debatable unless the criterion of 'correctness' is provided. Also, absolute categories such as 'never' and 'always' rarely apply in a strict sense, and should usually be replaced by 'never or hardly ever' and 'always or nearly always'.
Soft drugs such as marijuana should not be decriminalized Strongly Agree ☐ Agree ☐ Undecided ☐ Disagree ☐ Strongly Disagree ☐	The double negative in the stem is likely to confuse some respondents, especially when they try to work out what it means to disagree with a proposition containing two negatives! Note, however, that apparently equivalent words or phrases can have different meanings or connotations (Rugg, 1941; Converse and Presser, 1994). A phrase such as 'the Government should permit...' may elicit less agreement than 'the Government should not forbid...', as the latter phrase appeals to respondents' sense of personal liberty. Similarly, to ask if somebody 'likes' a particular practice is not the same as asking if they 'approve of' that practice
Have you suffered from headaches or nausea in the last seven days? Yes ☐ No ☐	An example of a double-barreled question. Two questions are asked in one and the respondent cannot respond meaningfully if his or her answers to the two questions differ. A 'one-and-a-half barreled' question is one in which, although the content of the question stem is restricted to a single issue, one or more of the responses provided introduce an additional issue (Sudman and Bradburn, 1982).
What is the average number of new patients you see per week? Under 10 ☐ 10 - 20 ☐ 20 - 30 ☐ 30 - 40 ☐	The categories in a question such as this should be mutually exclusive and collectively exhaustive. As it is the categories overlap. A similar problem occurs with categories that subsume previous ones; for example 'less than 1 week; less than 1 month; less than 2 months; less than 6 months etc'. An additional problem with this item is that the possibility that some respondents might see more than 40 patients per week is not catered for.

Figure 15.12 *Examples of flawed questionnaire items.*

When did you start to experiment with illegal drugs?

Some open questions may not make it clear what sort of response is required. Possible responses to this question might be 'in 1989', 'five years ago', 'in my first year at college', 'when I was 19', 'shortly after my girlfriend started', 'when I got disillusioned with my career', etc. Some such responses specify dates, others indicate life-stages, and others convey motives. The wording of the question should give a better indication as to which of these is required (e.g. 'in what year did you...', 'how old were you when...', 'what prompted you to...'). Note also that this is a presumptive question (see Table 15.5), and would be inappropriate unless it has already been established that the respondent has taken illegal drugs.

How helpful would you find it to be able to contact the occupational therapist directly?

Very helpful	helpful	unhelpful	Very unhelpful
☐	☐	☐	☐

The range of response categories is inappropriate. Although an ability to contact one's therapist may not be helpful, it is unlikely ever to be unhelpful. The categories should probably range from 'Very helpful' to 'Not at all helpful'. The words in the middle of the stem do not read very easily. An improvement might be 'If you were able to contact your occupational therapist directly, how helpful would this be?'

How many painkiller tablets have you needed recently?

Many more than usual ☐
More than usual ☐
Same number as usual ☐
Fewer than usual ☐
Many fewer than usual ☐

The word 'recently' may mean different things to different people. A standardized period should be specified, e.g. 'in the last four weeks'. This period of time should be of a length appropriate to the topic of the question, bearing in mind that long periods introduce the problem of poor recall.

Please indicate the average time after diagnosis that these patients are referred to you:

Minimum time after diagnosis _____
Maximum time after diagnosis _____

In this item, the responses required are at variance with the instruction given to the respondent. The stem asks for an average, but the available categories are in terms of minimum and maximum. The researcher probably used the word 'average' in the hope of gaining some sense of usual practice. It would have been better to say: 'Please state the minimum and maximum periods after diagnosis that these patients are normally referred to you'. If respondents are asked to write an answer, rather than circle an alternative or tick a box, 'state' is probably a better instruction than 'indicate'. Also, no indication is given of the units in which the answer should be given – days, weeks or months?

Figure 15.12 Continued.

Do you ever feel jealous of your colleagues' success?					As it stands, this question is liable to suffer from a social desirability bias – most people would not readily admit to feelings of jealousy, even in an anonymous questionnaire. In cases such as this it may be advisable to rephrase this item as an indirect question, in such a way as this 'All of us have somewhat negative emotions towards others from time to time. Do you ever feel jealous of your colleagues' success?' In this way, the respondent is, as it were, given permission to express what might otherwise seem to be unacceptable feelings. Although the question may now appear to be a leading one, any such effect probably only counterbalances the effect of the social desirability bias. A further drawback with this item is that the most socially acceptable response option appears first. This may encourage respondents to opt immediately for this response, and it is probably better to put the least acceptable option first (Sudman and Bradburn, 1982; Fink, 1995a).
Never or almost never ☐	Seldom ☐	Sometimes ☐	Usually ☐	Always or almost always ☐	
Are you satisfied with the service provided by the physical therapy department?					This question only has two response categories and in most cases will not adequately differentiate respondents (Streiner and Norman, 1995). In place of the dichotomous 'yes/no' alternatives, a range of ordinal categories (e.g. from 'very satisfied' to 'very dissatisfied') should be provided. This will not only provide a more revealing distribution of responses, but will open up more possibilities in terms of statistical analysis. Assuming this is the only question on this topic, one should also consider whether it is sufficient to have an overall rating of the service. Often, it is important to know respondents' views on different aspects of the service. If, however, a global rating is indeed what is required, it is advisable to indicate this with a phrase such as 'in general', 'all things considered' or 'overall', otherwise respondents who feel differently about various aspects of the service may be unsure how to respond (Czaja and Blair, 1996).
Yes ☐ No ☐					

Figure 15.12 Continued.

Box 15.2 *Bias in attitude measurement*

When we speak of 'bias' and seeking to measure the 'true attitude' of a respondent, it is important to remember that we are making certain epistemological assumptions. We are assuming, for example, that beneath what people say or do there is a stable underlying attitude that transcends any particular context, and that adopting the correct measurement techniques will allow us to measure this attitude objectively. We further assume that we can make some sort of distinction between what people *say* they think, feel and believe, and what they *really* think, feel and believe. Hence Staples (1991) argues that the answers to items in a questionnaire may be 'incorrect', owing to ignorance, unwillingness to disclose, or actual lying. These assumptions are central to the survey approach to research and the practice of psychometrics, but would be contested by researchers working within a phenomenological framework. From the latter perspective, the idea that a respondent could express his or her beliefs or attitudes 'incorrectly' would be seen as fundamentally misconceived (see Sections 2.3.3 and 9.4).

Careful attention to the wording, construction and sequencing of attitude items may counteract many of these biases. For example, questions can be worded so as not to suggest one direction of response (e.g. 'Are you in favour of, or do you oppose, mandatory HIV testing for emergency room staff?'). The use of neutral vocabulary will help to eliminate loaded questions. Similarly, a mixture of positively and negatively worded Likert items may prevent a response set.

Table 15.5 *Some sources of bias in attitude measurement*

Category of bias	Description
Social desirability bias	Respondents may choose the response that they feel is correct or social desirable, and thus expected of them.
Conformity ('me too') bias	Respondents may choose the response that they feel is in keeping with the majority view.
Denial ('not me') bias	Respondents may fail to endorse an opinion or report a behaviour because it is considered threatening, embarrassing or taboo (e.g. they may fail to endorse apparently discriminatory attitudes or fail to report deviant behaviour).
Leading questions	Questions that imply a certain answer (e.g. 'Would you not agree that . . .').
Acquiescence ('yea-saying') bias	Respondents may tend to agree with a statement, largely irrespective of its content.
Loaded terminology	Words or phrases whose connotations tend to elicit either favourable or unfavourable responses, regardless of their context (e.g. 'natural', 'interference', 'exploitation', 'respectful', 'excessive', 'bureaucracy', 'the problem of . . .', 'come to terms with . . .').
Response set	Respondents may fall into a pattern of response, largely irrespective of the content of individual items.
Halo effect	Respondents may rate items according to their overall attitude to the issue or topic, rather than in terms of particular aspects of the issue or topic.
Presumptive ('spouse-beating') questions	A question that presumes a particular fact, attitude or belief and thereby obliges the respondent to give a particular commitment, regardless of his or her response. The classic example, and the source of the alternative description, is 'Have you stopped beating your spouse?' – however respondents answer the question, the implication is that they have previously beaten their spouse.
Central tendency bias	Respondents may tend to avoid the extremes of a scale.
Severity bias	Certain respondents may take a strong stance on an issue.
Leniency bias	Certain respondents may avoid taking a strong stance on an issue.

Moreover, using items in this way will also serve to detect a bias when it occurs. One would expect responses to positively and negatively worded items on a given topic to be the mirror image of each other (e.g. a person who agrees with the positive item should disagree with the negative item). If all such items receive the same response, this suggests that the respondent's underlying attitude is not being tapped consistently.

A more specific strategy often employed to counteract biases in attitude measurement is the use of indirect methods of attitude measurement, known as *projective techniques*. In a projective test, a respondent is usually presented with some form of stimulus, and the nature of his or her response is taken to represent an underlying attitude (Oppenheim, 1992). Because this attitude was not elicited directly, many of the usual demand characteristics are likely to be avoided. Examples of projective techniques are:

- word association techniques: the respondent is asked to say the first thing that comes to mind
- sentence completion techniques: the respondent is asked to complete a sentence in his or her own words
- cartoons: the respondent is given a cartoon and is asked to suggest what the characters in the cartoon might be saying
- pictures or vignettes: the respondent is asked to explain what is happening in a picture, or is read a story and asked to explain an aspect of it (e.g. to supply the reason why a character in the story took a certain action).

These specialized procedures may offer distinct advantages over more conventional methods of measuring attitudes. Vignettes, for example, allow the expression of attitudes or beliefs to be placed in a context in a way that traditional attitude scales fail to (Finch, 1987). Since the situation portrayed in a vignette is often hypothetical, the details in the vignette can be finely manipulated so as to tap complex or sensitive attitudes (Gould, 1996), or to elicit

differences in response across subgroups of respondents (Wilson and While, 1998). However, some of these projective techniques require a considerable degree of skill to utilize and interpret – in particular, word association techniques and sentence completion techniques – and the assistance of a psychologist experienced in their use is advisable.

15.5 QUESTIONNAIRE LAYOUT AND PRESENTATION

When conducting a study based on a questionnaire, it is vital to address the following tasks:

- to maximize the potential response rate
- to minimize bias between responders and non-responders
- to ensure that questions are clear and unambiguous
- to ensure that responses to these questions are also clear and unambiguous
- to ensure that the questionnaire, and any subsections within it, are filled in correctly and completely.

Judicious use of layout and presentation can help to secure each of these goals.

15.5.1 Presentation and delivery of a questionnaire

Most of the issues to be addressed in terms of presentation are purely practical ones, and are generally a matter of common sense or courtesy. However, apparently trivial considerations can have a major impact on the quality of the data gathered through questionnaires.

For postal questionnaires, the accompanying letter should be courteous, and should explain clearly to potential respondents the purpose of the study, the basis on which they have been selected for participation, and what is being asked of them. Assurances of anonymity or confidentiality should be given where appropriate, and it is helpful to provide an estimate as to how long the questionnaire will take to complete. Researchers sometimes promise to provide respondents with the results of the study. Unfortunately, this promise is often broken, with the result that some respondents may feel disappointed and disillusioned. Consequently, Sieber (1992) questions the wisdom of giving such assurances. It is advisable to indicate the date by which questionnaires should be returned; this should be far enough ahead to give a reasonable amount of time for the questionnaire to be completed, but not so far ahead that potential respondents merely put it to one side. Chesson (1993) recommends 7 to 10 days. Unless the return date is an absolute deadline, a phrase such as 'please return by . . .' is preferable to one such as 'the last date for receipt is . . .', as in the latter case those respondents who have just missed the due date may feel that it is pointless in returning the questionnaire and discard it. A statement to the effect that reminders will be sent may increase the first-time response rate (Green, 1996).

If it is possible to address the envelope and the letter to each potential respondent by name, this may increase the response rate. Indications that the respondent's name was obtained from a standard alphabetical list – e.g. an obviously pre-printed label on which the surname appears before the forename – should be avoided (Dillman, 1978). A postage stamp on the envelope is preferable to automated stamping (franking) of envelopes (Oppenheim, 1992; Mangione, 1998). Dillman (1978) recommends using stamps at the first class postage rate. Certified or registered mailing may also assist response rates (Rimm et al., 1990). Signing each letter by hand and providing a reply-paid or, preferably, stamped self-addressed envelope for the return of the questionnaire are also important in this regard.

The questionnaire itself should be clearly legible and attractively laid out. It is often advisable to use coloured paper, for a number of reasons. First, coloured paper may increase response rates (though there seems to be no empirical evidence for this as yet). Certain colours are perceived as warmer and more congenial than others, and white paper is often associated in the respondent's mind with routine

or tedious items of paperwork. Second, a coloured questionnaire is also easier to locate (Chesson, 1993), and may serve as a visible reminder that it needs to be completed. Third, different colours can be used to distinguish responses from different groups in the study sample, or different forms of questionnaire (Woodward, 1988). Dark colours should be avoided, however, since they reduce the contrast between the paper and the print, and some colours may be difficult for people who are colour blind to read (Bourque and Fielder, 1995). Chesson (1993) suggests that black print on yellow paper is particularly easy to read.

A suitable, easy-to-read typeface should be used, and this should not be too small. Although it is desirable to limit the number of pages occupied by a questionnaire – for reasons of economy and so as not to create the impression of a lengthy questionnaire – questions that appear very densely on the page in a small font size are rather daunting and are more prone to completion or analysis errors (Sudman and Bradburn, 1982). No question should straddle two pages, but should always begin and end on the same page. A lengthy, multipart question should not be followed by a short question at the end of the page – the short question is likely to be overlooked (Sudman and Bradburn, 1982). If a key or specific instructions are given for a particular type of item and similar items occur on the next page, the instructions should be repeated. For example, if Likert categories are named above columns of boxes, these should be repeated on each subsequent page of such items.

A decision should be made as to whether or not to print the questionnaire on both sides of the paper. Using one side of the paper minimizes the chance that a page will be missed by the respondent and may make analysis of the completed questionnaires somewhat easier. However, it adds to the bulk, and thereby the perceived length, of the questionnaire (Mangione, 1998). If double-sided printing is chosen, steps should be taken to ensure that the respondent does not omit sections of the questionnaire. It is, for example, preferable to avoid stapling the questionnaire in the top left-hand corner, since pages are especially likely be passed over when turning the sheets. Instead, two or more staples should be inserted on the left-hand side of the page, or the questionnaire should be printed on double-sized paper and made into a booklet (Sudman and Bradburn, 1982; Woodward, 1988). An instruction such as 'please turn over' should appear at the bottom of each page, whatever method of presentation is chosen. It is important that the return address appears on the questionnaire, in case some respondents mislay both the self-addressed envelope and the accompanying letter (Thomas *et al.*, 1997).

If a questionnaire is anonymous, this can create difficulties in following up non-responders. Moreover, it makes it difficult to gauge the characteristics of responders and non-responders; it is usually important to know whether these differ systematically. One strategy is simply to remail the questionnaire to the whole sample, but this is expensive and bothersome to those who have already responded. Some may even respond a second time unintentionally. Moreover, this approach does not solve the problem of identifying the characteristics of those who still fail to respond. Other strategies that have been used to deal with follow-up of anonymous questionnaires are as follows:

- Respondents can be asked to mail a separate reply-paid postcard with their name on at the same time as returning the completed anonymous questionnaire (Sieber, 1992).
- A code number can be written on the return envelope, but not on the questionnaire. The accompanying letter can explain that this will be used only to verify that the individual has responded, and that the respondent can remove the number if desired. Note that even if a number is not assigned to a questionnaire when it is sent, returned questionnaires must be numbered on receipt, so that any anomalies or suspected errors that arise during data analysis can be traced back to the questionnaires concerned.

- Questionnaires can be returned to a third party, uninvolved in the analysis of the data, who can provide the researcher with a list of those who have responded, but no indication as to the origin of individual questionnaires.

Each of these strategies not only facilitates follow-up, but also identifies non-responders. However, only the first of these strategies maintains total anonymity.

The question of an appropriate length for a questionnaire is a common one, but one to which there is no exact answer. Essentially, a questionnaire should be as short as it can possibly be made, while still gaining the necessary information (Lund and Gram, 1998). Questions of the 'it might be interesting to know ...' variety are therefore generally to be avoided. Needless to say, the more interesting and personally relevant the topic of the questionnaire is to the respondent, the longer he or she will be prepared to take over its completion. Sudman and Bradburn (1982) suggest that questionnaires of 12–16 pages will secure good cooperation from well-educated respondents for whom the topic is a salient one, but that questionnaires on relatively low-salience topics mailed to the general population should be restricted to 2–4 pages. Fife-Schaw (1995b) suggests that only very motivated respondents will spend longer than 45 minutes on a questionnaire.

Mangione (1998) gives the following guidelines on the adequacy of response rates for mailed questionnaires: 70–80% 'very good'; 60–70% 'acceptable'; 50–60% 'barely acceptable'; below 50% 'unacceptable'. Similarly, Babbie (1990) suggests that 70% or higher is 'very good', 60% or higher is 'good' and a minimum response rate of 50% is 'adequate'. Moser and Kalton (1971, p. 268) advise that results from a study with a response rate below 30% (from postal questionnaires) is likely to be 'of little, if any, value'. However, these must not be taken as hard-and-fast criteria. What constitutes a good response rate for a mailed questionnaire will depend upon the nature of the topic and the sample. A higher response rate should be expected from individuals who have a stake in the issues addressed by the questionnaire than from those to whom the issues are of minimal interest or concern. When reminders are sent, they are likely to yield half the preceding response rate. Thus, if 60% respond to the initial mailing, approximately 30% of the non-responders will respond to the first reminder, and 15% of the remaining non-responders will reply to the next reminder, and so forth. Roberts *et al.* (1993) recommend that the first reminder should take the form of a simple postcard, which they found to be as effective as another copy of the complete questionnaire. Mangione (1998) recommends that another copy of the questionnaire should be included with the second reminder, and every alternate reminder thereafter.

It should be remembered, however, that a high response rate does not on its own secure representativeness (Krosnick, 1999). Even a small proportion of non-responders who differ systematically from the responders may introduce bias. It is useful, therefore, to examine the characteristics of the non-responders where this is possible (see the discussion of anonymity

above), and compare these with those of the responders (Sheikh and Mattingly, 1981; Barriball and While, 1999). Those who fail to respond to the primary questionnaire may respond to a shortened version, or just one or two questions designed to establish their similarity or dissimilarity to the responders; excessive badgering should be avoided, however.

15.5.2 Arrangement and sequencing of items

It is important not only to examine the internal structure of each item that makes up a questionnaire or an attitude scale, but also to consider how such items are put together to form a complete instrument.

Figure 15.13 contains part of the questionnaire used in the Rheumatoid Arthritis Study, and illustrates some aspects of questionnaire structure. It is immediately apparent that certain key words have been italicized for emphasis in these two questions. This is a helpful means of drawing the respondents' attention; however, like raising one's voice in an argument, its effect diminishes with too frequent use. Question 5 is what is known as a *filter question* – depending on whether they answer 'yes' or 'no', respon-

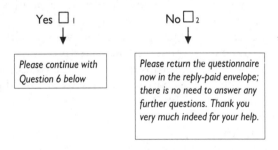

5. In the *past 12 months*, have you seen patients/clients with a confirmed diagnosis of rheumatoid arthritis (tick one)?

        Yes ☐₁   No ☐₂

        ↓   ↓

    | *Please continue with Question 6 below* | *Please return the questionnaire now in the reply-paid envelope; there is no need to answer any further questions. Thank you very much indeed for your help.* |

6. Approximately how many *new* patients fitting this definition did you see in a typical month *over the past 12 months* (tick one)?

1–5 a month ☐₁ 6–10 a month ☐₂ 11–15 a month ☐₃ more than 15 a month ☐₄

Figure 15.13 *Structuring and arranging questionnaire items*

dents are either 'filtered' to Question 6, or asked to return the questionnaire. It is very important that this is clear to respondents; otherwise some will attempt to respond to subsequent questions that are inapplicable to their clinical practice. To highlight this, arrows run from the tick boxes in Question 5 to the relevant instructions, which are set in italics to emphasize them further. The instructions must follow, not precede, the answer and should be expressed positively; i.e. the respondent should be told which question to answer, rather than which questions not to answer (Sudman and Bradburn, 1982).

A further technique for emphasis has been employed within Question 5. In order to ensure that respondents base their calculations on the previous 12 months, this figure has been placed at the beginning of the sentence, where it has more prominence than if it were buried in the middle of the sentence. Note also that 'the past twelve months' has been specified, not 'the past year'; the latter is ambiguous and could mean either 'a period of 12 months' or 'since 1 January'. The latter interpretation could be particularly problematic if a questionnaire were used over a period that bridged two calendar years (Woodward, 1988). Compared with Question 5, the format of Question 6 is poor, however. The response categories are printed close together on a single line, with the result that a respondent could easily tick the wrong box (especially in the two middle categories). If there are more than two categories, it is generally better to place each one on a new line.

The ordering of questions is an important issue. There is a widespread view that the first items in a questionnaire should be non-threatening and easy to answer (Moser and Kalton, 1971; Kidder and Judd, 1986). The respondent is made to feel confident in dealing with the questionnaire and, having answered the first few items fairly rapidly, feels that good progress is being made towards completing the questionnaire. Such advice leads some researchers to begin their questionnaire with demographic and other factual questions. However, a number of writers (Dillman, 1978; Babbie, 1989; Bourque and Fielder, 1995; Thomas et al., 1997) disagree with this practice, and point out that beginning a questionnaire with mundane items may dispel the respondent's interest and enthusiasm. Newell (1993) feels that the first few questions should be closed-ended, which are easy to answer; more demanding open-ended questions can be asked subsequently, when the respondent has become committed to answering the questionnaire. Thus, as a general rule, the first items should be easy to respond to, but should stimulate the respondent's interest.

Generally speaking, questions of a similar sort should appear together; this applies to both the content and the form of items. Respondents are likely to be put off if the response format for consecutive items is constantly changing. Equally, they may be puzzled if questions return to a topic that they perceive to have been dealt with earlier in the questionnaire. When moving from one topic to another, it may be helpful to include a *transition statement* between the two groups of items (Woodward, 1988). A transition statement is a brief comment that signals to the respondent the way in which the questionnaire is about to change direction (e.g. 'We would now like to ask you some questions about your experience of staff development in your present post').

When asking a number of attitude questions on a particular issue, *funnelling* is often advised. This is where, following a fairly broad question, questions become progressively more specific (Kerlinger, 1986). Filter questions are often used as part of the process of funnelling (Oppenheim, 1992). By this means, the respondent is encouraged to focus in on the issue concerned. The reverse process, *inverse funnelling*, can also be used if a respondent is not expected to be knowledgeable, or have clearly articulated opinions, on a subject (Frey and Oishi, 1995). Here, detailed questions precede the more general ones, so as to focus the respondent's attention on the issue. It might, for example, be easier to explore a somewhat complex topic having already encouraged the respondent, through specific questioning, to identify his or her own experience of the topic concerned.

It is important to consider *context effects*, whereby the answers to certain questions may pre-empt or bias the answers to questions that appear later in the questionnaire (Schumann and Presser, 1981). One example has been provided in Section 15.2.1. As another example, if a question were to ask of nurse educators 'Do you feel that changes should be made to the nursing curriculum in your college?', a respondent who answered in the negative would find it hard to endorse later items that were proposing specific modifications to the way in which student nurses should be educated. Having given a certain answer to a fairly categorical question on the topic, respondents would feel obliged, for reasons of consistency, to respond similarly to subsequent questions of a similar nature, even though further reflection might cause them to take a slightly different stance on the issue. Similarly, questions testing knowledge should not be preceded by items that supply some of the relevant information (Moser and Kalton, 1971); in a self-completed questionnaire, it is preferable that such information is not available anywhere in the questionnaire.

15.5.3 Precoding the questionnaire

It will probably have been noticed that in most of the examples provided in this chapter, the boxes for closed-ended items have been assigned numbers or letters in a small font. These represent the coding to be applied to the responses, and are included on the questionnaire when it is printed. Such a questionnaire is described as *precoded*. During data analysis, the researcher can immediately read off the appropriate code to be input for each item. Take Figure 15.10, for example. Assuming that this was item 7 in the questionnaire, if an individual ticked 'yes' to the statement 'I can walk around my home if I have help', this would be input on the spreadsheet as '1' in the column headed '7A'; a 'no' response to the statement 'I can walk

around my home without help' would be input as '0' in column '7B'; and so forth. This will lead to far fewer coding errors than if the analyst has to refer to a separate coding sheet. These numbers must, of course, be unobtrusive so as not to confuse the respondent. They should be in a smaller font than the text used for the item, and can also be printed in grey, rather than black. Rather than place the codes immediately next to the boxes, some researchers create a coding column on the right-hand side of the page, and specifically instruct respondents to ignore it.

If, for some reason, precoding is not possible, an alternative is to produce a copy of the questionnaire on clear acetates. Codes can then be written on the acetates next to the response options, and each page of the questionnaire can then be coded by laying the appropriate acetate on top of it.

If the equipment and resources are available, a questionnaire can be generated through specialist computer software that allows the response on the completed questionnaire to be input by an optical reader. The questionnaire is electronically precoded by the software, and the ticks in each box are automatically transferred to entries on a spreadsheet. This has huge time-saving potential, but it is important to check that the particular software to be used does not impose undue constraints on the nature and form of the information that can be gathered.

15.6 CONCLUSION

Questionnaires and attitude inventories play an important role in health care research, but are notoriously difficult to design and administer in a way that will yield valid and reliable data. Only some of the factors that need to be borne in mind when using such instruments have been addressed in this chapter, and more comprehensive texts, such as those by Moser and Kalton (1971) and Oppenheim (1992), should be consulted for more detailed discussions.

16 SINGLE INSTANCE RESEARCH

SUMMARY

This chapter explores the following topics:

- the nature and varieties of single instance research
- the design of single system quasi-experimental studies
- methods of analysing data from single system studies
- ethical issues arising from the use of single system studies
- descriptive case studies

Most of the designs considered hitherto have involved collecting data from groups of subjects or participants. In the case of the Low Back Pain Study and the Rheumatoid Arthritis Study, data were collected from a fairly large number of people, whereas fewer participants were involved in the Student Attitudes Study. Nonetheless, in each case there was a deliberate attempt to gather information from a group, or groups, of individuals (even though the extent to which this information would be aggregated was seen to vary between these studies).

On some occasions, a rather different approach is used. Data may be collected from a single individual; i.e. the research uses a sample of one. The reason for this is not that only one individual is available for study, but that the objectives of the research relate specifically to this level of analysis.

16.1 THE NATURE OF SINGLE INSTANCE RESEARCH

Research in which a sample of one is used is sometimes referred to as *single instance research*, and it may be either quasi-experimental or non-experimental in nature. Conversely, studies in which data are collected from a number of participants are sometimes referred to as *group studies*, especially in the context of experimentation (Sim, 1995b).

A single instance study that adopts a quasi-experimental design is usually known as a *single system study*, whereas a non-experimental single instance study is generally referred to simply as a *case study* (Box 16.1). In a single-system study, quantitative data are collected. In a case study, either quantitative or qualitative data (or both) may be collected, depending largely upon whether the study is descriptive or exploratory in purpose (Table 16.1). In clinical practice, a common example of a case study is the *clinical case report*, which documents the treatment management of an individual client (Rothstein, 1993b; De Souza, 1997). Whether such reports should be classified as research may depend on whether they are generated in a

Box 16.1 *Nomenclature*

Various other terms are sometimes used to describe the single system study; e.g. 'single subject study' (Robertson and Lee, 1994; Parry, 1995), 'single case study' (Riddoch and Lennon, 1991; Worthington, 1995), '*n* of 1 (or *n* = 1) trial' (Dukes, 1965; McQuay, 1991). The term 'single subject study' suggests that the unit of analysis is necessarily a person, whereas this is not always so. Sometimes, the focus of the study may be a family, a hospital ward or an institution; it is the unit of analysis, not the number of people from whom data are collected, that is 'single'. The term 'single case study' is also unsatisfactory, since it invites confusion with the descriptive case study. We therefore follow Bloom and Fischer (1982), Ottenbacher (1986a) and Domholdt (1993) in using the term 'single system study'.

Table 16.1 *Main features of case studies and single system studies*

Type of study	Unit of analysis	Research question	Data collected	Design
Case study	Single	Exploratory	Qualitative	Non-experimental
		Descriptive	Quantitative or qualitative	Non-experimental
Single system study	Single	Explanatory	Quantitative	Quasi-experimental

rigorous and systematic way, and the extent to which the practitioner seeks to draw data-based conclusions from them.

The principal characteristic of single instance research is that inferences are drawn from the analysis of a single unit, rather than from the analysis of a group of such units. A researcher may, of course, conduct a series of single system studies or case studies, but each of these will be analysed separately, such that they remain single instance studies (see Box 16.4).

16.2 THE SINGLE SYSTEM STUDY

Single system research designs first gained a firm foothold in psychological research (Barlow and Hersen, 1984). More recently, however, they have drawn the attention of researchers in health-related fields such as nursing (Sterling and McNally, 1992; Behi and Nolan, 1996c, 1997; Newell, 1998), occupational therapy (Madsen and Conte, 1980; Ottenbacher and York, 1984) and physiotherapy (Gonnella, 1989; Riolo-Quinn, 1990; Riddoch and Lennon, 1991). As was suggested in Section 7.4, single system studies can circumvent some of the shortcomings of the randomized controlled trial.

A single system study can be defined as a quasi-experimental design utilizing a sample of one and involving the sequential introduction and withdrawal (or modification) of an intervention variable to determine its effect on one or more outcome variables, through repeated measurement (Sim, 1995b). The outcome variable chosen may be a variate score on an outcome measure, such as pain intensity on a

visual analogue scale. Alternatively, it might be the frequency or duration of countable or measurable behaviours (Portney and Watkins, 1993; Perrin, 1998); for example, the incidence of aggressive gesturing, or the time spent by a client in verbal interaction.

Normally, the participant first enters a baseline (A) phase, in which serial measurements are taken but no intervention is applied (Figure 16.1). Once a sufficient number of baseline measurements have been obtained, the participant enters an intervention (B) phase and measurement is continued. Subsequent A and B phases may follow alternately. The logic of the study is therefore similar to that of the crossover design, in that the participant is exposed to each level of the intervention variable (Section 7.3.2). A particular study is

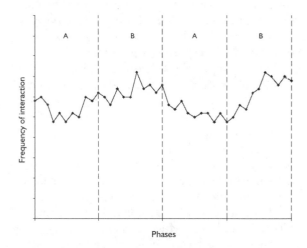

Figure 16.1 *An ABAB single system study, illustrating the effect of a behavioural intervention designed to increase the level of interaction by a withdrawn child.*

described in such a way as to indicate the number and sequence of the phases (e.g. ABA study, ABAB study, etc.). The phases in the study may on occasions follow a different order (e.g. BABA), and more than one intervention may be tested in a single study (e.g. ABAC). Alternatively, in a multiple baseline study (Box 16.2), an intervention may be applied to more than one behaviour or aspect of performance, so that a corresponding number of outcomes are measured (e.g. $AB^1B^2B^3$).

Inferences about treatment effectiveness are drawn from changes in the graph line which occur at the transition between phases. Figure 16.1 illustrates a hypothetical study in which a behavioural intervention designed to increase interaction is tested on a child showing marked symptoms of withdrawal and lack of sociability. The outcome variable is the number of episodes of interaction with the staff and/or other children in the school. On the basis of a quick visual inspection, it appears that interaction increased following the introduction of the intervention (i.e. following the transition from the first A phase to the first B phase). When the intervention is withdrawn (i.e. when the child has passed into the next A phase), there appears to be a *reversal effect*; interaction returns towards the levels observed in the initial baseline phase. However, when a further intervention phase is introduced, there is once more improvement in the child's level of interaction.

This example shows how the single system study can resist some of the threats to internal validity that are often encountered in experimental or quasi-experimental research (see Table 7.2). For example, an alternative explanation for the apparent improvement that occurred between the first A phase and the first B phase is that the child's behaviour changed spontaneously (i.e. maturation). However, the fact that the level of interaction demonstrated a reversal effect in the following A phase counters this explanation. Alternatively, it might be argued that the initial improvement following the first A–B transition was due to some other event – e.g. the relocation of the children to a room in

Box 16.2 *Variations on the basic design*

In the *multiple baseline study*, the researcher chooses aspects of performance that can be targeted independently (i.e. such that an intervention can be directed at one without thereby influencing the others). The behaviours are targeted for intervention singly in successive phases of the study, and the untreated behaviours in any one phase act as control variables for the one that is being subjected to treatment (Kratochwill, 1978). This study has only an initial baseline phase; all subsequent phases are intervention phases. In the *changing criterion study*, the level of attainment in performance that is specified in the outcome variable is raised progressively as the client improves, and the scores recorded during the preceding phase serve as the baseline for assessment of the new level of performance (Kratochwill, 1978). For example, the outcome variable might focus on higher levels of functional performance in successive phases (Perrin, 1998). The changing criterion design can be used to assess interventions with irreversible effects (Morley, 1996). Unlike most single system designs, the changing criterion study employs the same intervention across phases, but adjusts the outcome measure. If, due to certain practical constraints, an AB design is the only one possible, its susceptibility to maturation can be reduced by the use of a *control variable*. This is an outcome variable, monitored alongside the primary outcome variable, that is likely to reflect any process of spontaneous recovery but not likely to respond to the intervention being tested (Wilson, 1995). Kazdin (1982), Barlow and Hersen (1984) and Ottenbacher (1986a) provide further details on these and other variations. Backman et al. (1997) review their use in rehabilitation research.

another part of the building – that had a positive effect on the child's behaviour (i.e. a history effect). The reversal effect in the second A phase would be compatible with a history effect (just as the intervention would now probably no longer exert an effect, so the influence of the change of room might also no longer be operative). However, the fact that a further improvement occurred during the second B phase makes it unlikely that a history effect was present; it is highly improbable that such an effect would coincide with the second B phase as well as with the first.

There are, however, other threats to internal validity to which the single system study is less resistant. Owing to the serial measurement that needs to be conducted, the design is particularly prone to testing and practice effects (Bithell, 1994). For example, if a client's pain intensity is measured twice daily, this in itself may elicit a change in the outcome variable, and thus act as a confounding variable. Furthermore, the external validity of the study may be affected; frequent assessment of outcome may not constitute a realistic context in which to evaluate an intervention.

Drawing inferences from the single system study depends upon the ability to detect changes in the graph line between phases. There are circumstances in which this may be difficult to achieve, and in which the usefulness of the single system study is therefore limited. The first such situation is where the clinical feature that is chosen as the outcome variable is extremely labile. It is important to establish a fairly stable baseline against which to measure change in the B phase, and this is difficult if the graph line exhibits diurnal or more frequent variations within the baseline phase (Figure 16.2). A similar problem may occur if a condition exhibits fluctuations in severity over a longer period of time, e.g. from week to week, as may occur in some neurological conditions or pain syndromes. Although the graph line may be relatively smooth within a particular phase, these natural variations in symptomatology may coincide with the phasing of the study.

A third problem occurs when the intervention, or the condition to which it is applied, is such that a sustained or irreversible change is likely to be brought about in the first B phase. This

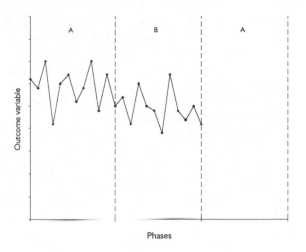

FIGURE 16.2 *A highly variable graph line, which makes it hard to discern changes in trend across phases.*

removes the possibility of a reversal effect in the following A phase (Evans, 1994), so that no additional information can be gained from the data in this phase. For example, in some cases of limitation of joint movement, any range gained by an intervention is likely to be retained after treatment has finished. Similarly, if an intervention is used to train a client in a skill or a functional activity, the change induced in the client's ability will not usually fall off once training has finished. As a general rule, all interventions should be continued for long enough to demonstrate an effect, but not so long as to make any change induced a permanent one.

The single system study can counter many of the common threats to internal validity, especially in its more sophisticated modifications (Box 16.2). However, the external validity of the single system study has also been a topic of debate, especially when compared with the group study (Riddoch and Lennon, 1991, 1994; Johannessen, 1991; Lewis, 1991; Bithell, 1994). The outcome of a single system study may indeed be a poor predictor of the way in which a category of patients will respond to a particular intervention. However, there are at least four qualifications to be made with respect to this apparent shortcoming (Sim, 1995b). First, although the findings of a group study may give a good indication of aggregate response to an intervention, they may be equally deficient when trying to predict the response of an individual client (Section 7.4). The single system study may be more informative here. Second, the single system study does not claim to generate estimates of aggregate response in the first place. It aims primarily to answer the separate question of individual response (Riddoch and Lennon, 1991; Sim, 1995b). Third, single system studies may contribute to our understanding of the theo-

retical mechanisms underlying clinical interventions, and may thereby possess some degree of theoretical, if not statistical, generalizability (Section 8.2). Finally, by means of replication (Evans, 1994), or through meta-analysis (Busk and Serlin, 1992; Faith *et al.*, 1996; see Section 17.2), some evidence of aggregate effect may be obtained from multiple single system studies. These issues have been considered in greater detail elsewhere (Sim, 1995b).

The principal design features of the single system study are shown in Figure 16.3.

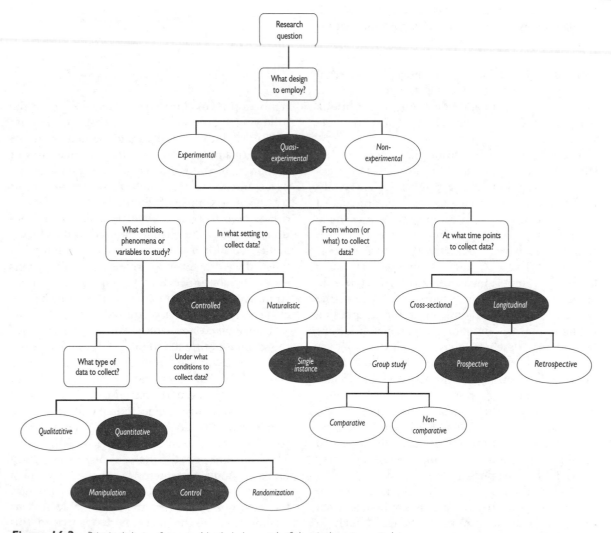

Figure 16.3   *Principal design features (shaded elements) of the single system study.*

16.2.1 Data analysis

The appropriate form of analysis for data from single system studies is still a matter of debate. The detailed pros and cons of the specific techniques available will not be examined here; these can be found in Ottenbacher (1986a), Kazdin (1982), Barlow and Hersen (1984), and Kratochwill and Levin (1992). A brief account will be given, however, of the overall approaches to data analysis and of some of the implications that these have for the measurement process.

Data from single system studies can be subjected to either visual or statistical analysis. In both cases, the objective is to distinguish systematic alterations in the graph line (deterministic changes) from those that might occur through random variability of the datapoints (random or stochastic changes).

Visual analysis

In visual analysis – which Portney and Watkins (1993) consider to be the most commonly used method – the researcher looks for properties of the graph line which would indicate an effect of the intervention (Ottenbacher, 1986a). This might manifest itself in a change in *slope*, whereby the gradient of the graph line increases or decreases from one phase to the next (e.g. if a slight upward slope in the A phase became a steep ascending slope in the B phase). This is illustrated in the first A and B phases in Figure 16.4. A more striking effect would be a change in *trend*, whereby the direction of the graph line is reversed from one phase to the next (e.g. if a descending graph line in the A phase became an ascending line in the B phase). This is manifest in the second A and B phases in Figure 16.4. Another effect that may be discernible is a change in *level*. Here there is a shift in the value of datapoints from one phase to the next, such that the first one or two datapoints in one phase are noticeably higher or lower than the last one or two datapoints in the preceding phase. It should be noted that a change in slope or trend can occur without a change in level; although there is an obvious change in trend in the second

A and B phases in Figure 16.4, the values of the datapoints at the transition between phases do not differ very greatly. Equally, a change in level does not necessarily imply a change in trend or slope (Wampold and Furlong, 1981). Finally, a judgement can be made as to the *latency* of any between-phase changes. Thus, a change in slope may occur almost immediately after the transition from one phase to the next (low latency), or may not become obvious until midway through the second phase (high latency). The former is usually the more convincing evidence of an effect.

Further details on the principles and techniques of visual analysis can be found in Parsonson and Baer (1978), Ottenbacher (1986a), Johnston and Pennypacker (1993), and Franklin *et al.* (1996).

Statistical analysis

In statistical analysis, a wide variety of techniques may be used. Three of these will be described very briefly (See Box 16.3):

1. One might test for differences in the *mean values* of datapoints in consecutive phases by means of a procedure such as an unrelated *t* test or one-way analysis of variance (Kazdin, 1984; Wilson, 1995). The datapoints in each phase are treated as random samples from hypothetical populations of scores. If the statistical test determines that the samples come from distinct populations of scores with differing mean values, this is deemed to indicate a treatment effect. The drawback of this approach is that it takes no account of the time-related features of the graph line, such as trend or latency. Marked changes in trend may occur between phases with little variation in mean scores within each phase (e.g. the second A and B phases in Figure 16.4). Furthermore, the assumption of independence of datapoints required for such tests (Sections 14.2.4 and 18.1.2) may be hard to satisfy with data from single system studies (Ottenbacher, 1986a; Reboussin and Morgan, 1996; Backman and Harris, 1999).

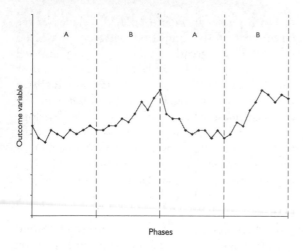

Figure 16.4   *Hypothetical data from an ABAB study to illustrate change in slope (between the first A and B phases) and change in trend (between the second A and B phases).*

Box 16.3   *Serial dependency*

Most of the statistical methods that may be applied to single system data will make certain assumptions about the nature and distribution of such data. A common such assumption is that the data are at an interval or ratio level of measurement. This can normally be satisfied by choosing an appropriate outcome measure. A potentially more troublesome assumption is that the datapoints are independent (see Section 13.1.3). However, when consecutive measurements are taken over time, the data often exhibit serial dependency. If data are serially dependent, the values of consecutive datapoints will be more similar than would be expected by chance; such data are not therefore statistically independent. The extent to which data are serially dependent is expressed by their *autocorrelation* (Matyas and Greenwood, 1996). Tests can be performed to determine whether data are serially dependent (though such tests are subject to a high Type II error rate if the number of datapoints is low), and if such tests are positive various transformations can be performed to reduce the autocorrelation of the data.

2. Statistical techniques can be used to test for changes in the *direction of the graph line*, such as trend or slope. For example, a 'linear celeration line' can be constructed for the data in the A phase, such that equal numbers of datapoints lie above and below it. This line is extended into the B phase, and according to the proportion of datapoints in the B phase that lie above (or below) it, a conclusion can be drawn as to whether there is a statistically significant difference in the rate of change of the outcome variable between phases (Wolery and Harris, 1982; Portney and Watkins, 1993).

3. A form of *time-series analysis* can be utilized. Many of these techniques – e.g. the autoregressive integrated moving average (McCain and McCleary, 1979) – are complex and require large numbers of datapoints. A simpler and less data-hungry procedure is the C statistic (Tryon, 1982). Briefly, this test first evaluates the data in the A phase to determine if there is a statistically discernible trend. If not, the test is then applied to the combined data of the A and B phase, again to test for a discernible trend. If such a trend is detected in the combined data, but not in the data for the A phase alone, it can be ascribed to the transition between phases.

Further details on these and other methods of statistical analysis can be found in Bloom and Fischer (1982), Kazdin (1982), Wolery and Harris (1982), Ottenbacher (1986a), Portney and Watkins (1993), Nourbakhsh and Ottenbacher (1994), Busk and Marascuilo (1992), and Gorman and Allison (1996).

As a rule of thumb, if some form of statistical analysis is anticipated, the following basic principles will increase its feasibility:

- Record as many datapoints as possible in each phase (bearing in mind the possible reactive effects of multiple measurements).
- Collect data at intervals that are as regular as possible (this normally requires collecting data at set times, seven days a week).

- Utilize outcome measures at an interval or ratio level of measurement (the range of techniques that can be applied to ordinal data is limited).
- Select outcome measures with high levels of reliability, so that random error does not obscure any systematic change in the data across phases.

Visual versus statistical analysis

There are various and conflicting arguments as to the relative merits of visual and statistical analysis of data from single system designs. The chief issues are as follows:

- According to some of its advocates, visual analysis of graphed single system data allows close, ongoing and responsive contact with the data, which 'allows those events and results that arouse interest and curiosity to be noticed and subsequently investigated systematically' (Parsonson and Baer, 1978, p. 109).
- Its detractors claim that visual analysis is not associated with a clear set of rules as to which types and magnitudes of effects should be judged significant, and may therefore be unreliable (DeProspero and Cohen, 1979; Kazdin, 1982).
- It is argued that, since visual analysis is inherently less sensitive than statistical analysis, the effects that emerge through visual analysis are likely to be of such a magnitude as to be clinically important (Baer, 1977; Payton, 1993; Newell, 1998).
- Against the preceding point, it is argued that seemingly minor effects, such as might be discernible on statistical but not on visual analysis, may be potentially important, and may produce clinically important effects once the intervention concerned has been further developed (Kazdin, 1982).

An increasing number of empirical studies are shedding light on some of the areas of dispute (Wampold and Furlong, 1981; Ottenbacher, 1986b; Hojem and Ottenbacher, 1988;

Bobrovitz and Ottenbacher, 1998; Bengali and Ottenbacher, 1998).

16.2.2 Ethical issues

The single system study has certain ethical advantages (Sim, 1994). Through its parsimonious use of patients, it clearly limits the number of participants that are at risk of experimental harm. Moreover, the intensive monitoring that occurs in the single system study suggests that any such harm will be identified promptly and effectively. The inherent flexibility of the single system study also makes it easier to optimize treatment for the patient than in a group study, and thus reduces the possibility of loss of therapeutic benefit.

Riolo-Quinn (1990, p. 31) argues that '[t]he ethical issue of withholding treatment from a large sample of control subjects is avoided when single-subject designs are used'. However, most single system designs involve no-treatment phases, and can claim only to avoid the *total* withdrawal of treatment. In a randomized controlled trial, on the other hand, it is often the case that all participants receive some form of treatment for the duration of the study, and the principle of equipoise ensures that no participant is knowingly disadvantaged with respect to any other (see Section 7.5.2). Appeals to the withdrawal of treatment that occurs routinely in clinical practice are sometimes made (French, 1993; Riddoch and Lennon, 1994), but are not necessarily relevant in the context of research (Sim, 1994). The single system study is not, therefore, immune to criticisms on the grounds of loss of therapeutic benefit. Designs that minimize the use of A phases are ethically superior from this point of view (see Box 16.2).

Further discussion of the ethical aspects of single system research can be found in Sim (1994).

16.3 THE CASE STUDY

A case study is an account of an individual person (e.g. a patient), a group (e.g. a cohort of students), a situation (e.g. a clinical case conference) or an institution (e.g. an inner-city health centre). In each of these, the unit of analysis is single. Hence, even if a group of people is studied, they are studied as a group, not as individuals. Similarly, if a case study focuses on an institution, individuals within it are studied as a means of elucidating the workings of the institution, not as primary objects of study themselves (Box 16.4).

Case studies address exploratory or descriptive research questions and adopt a non-experimental design. Hence, in clinical research, there is a clear distinction between the quasi-experimental single system study and the descriptive clinical case report. The former utilizes the principles of control and manipulation to draw inferences about treatment effectiveness, whereas the latter documents the process and outcome of a treatment programme without making a causal inference that the outcome was the consequence of the treatment administered (Rothstein, 1993b; Backman and Harris, 1999).

The purpose of a case study is *idiographic* rather than *nomothetic* (Smith *et al.*, 1995); that is, the case study is concerned with understanding the particular and the individual, rather than with seeking to produce generalizable statements (Box 16.5). 'We do not study a case primarily to understand other cases' (Stake, 1995, p. 4). The focus of the case study, in contrast to that of an approach such as the survey, is *intensive* rather than *extensive*. Thus, the criterion of representativeness that should be applied to the findings of case study research is that of theoretical, not statistical, representativeness (Mitchell, 1983; Sharp, 1998; see Section 8.2).

Box 16.4   *Multiple case studies*

A researcher may carry out two or more case studies on a similar theme. In their study of the experience of amyotrophic lateral sclerosis, Cobb and Hamera (1986) carried out case studies of two women with this condition, and Canelón (1995) performed case studies of three clients in relation to job site analysis. Similarly, a series of single system studies can be carried out as part of a replication strategy (Barlow and Hersen, 1984). Indeed, Yin (1984) emphasizes that the role of multiple case studies is one of replication, not one of sampling. In other words, the purpose of conducting more than one case study is not to build up an aggregate of cases (as when sampling for a survey or a group experiment). Rather, it is to produce a series of findings from individual cases, so as to draw comparison or contrast between these findings. The unit of analysis remains single. This said, it should be remembered that in any exploratory research based on a phenomenological perspective, the concern is with the individuality of each participant's account (Section 2.3.3). Hence, one should not draw too firm a dividing line between a phenomenological study based on a small group of participants and a series of case studies.

Box 16.5   *Case studies as 'anecdotal'*

The charge is sometimes levelled at case studies that they are anecdotal, on account of their single unit of analysis. However, evidence is anecdotal in terms of the way in which it is used, not on account of its individualized nature. In other words, to be anecdotal is to use a certain form of erroneous reasoning. Charlton and Walston (1998, p. 148) contend that 'the reason for the error has nothing to do with an inferiority of single cases to randomized groups; neither has it to do with the deficiencies of personal experience compared with the pooled experience of others'. They claim that '[w]hat is wrong with this kind of anecdote is that it privileges direct and recent experience even when such experience is poor in quality and unsupported or contradicted by other valid sources of relevant contextual knowledge'.

Table 16.2 *Hypothetical examples of case study research*

Type of study	Subject	Study objective	Principal sources of data
Clinical case report	A middle-aged man undergoing cardiac surgery	To document the patient's past medical history, the interventions presently being administered, and his response to these	Quantitative data, gathered retrospectively and prospectively, from case notes, clinical measurements, and structured observation
Clinical management case study	A neurological rehabilitation unit	To explore the decision-making processes and mechanisms used by the rehabilitation team in the management of patients in the unit	Qualitative and quantitative data gathered prospectively and retrospectively through interviews with staff and patients, analysis of case notes, and semi-structured observation of treatment and case conferences
Ethnographic case study	A woman with functional incapacitation due to multiple sclerosis	To explore the woman's perspective on her illness and its impact on her everyday life and social circumstances	Qualitative data gathered prospectively through a series of interviews with the woman and her family, and a reflective diary kept by the woman
Educational case study	A cohort of nursing students	To explore the formal and informal socialization processes occurring during the students' first semester of professional education	Qualitative data gathered prospectively and retrospectively by non-participant observation, interviews with students and educators, and content analysis of teaching materials and curriculum documents.

Through their focus on the individual case, case studies may serve as a useful counterbalance to the generalized conclusions of studies based on large samples, by highlighting an instance in which such claims do not hold true, or identifying the limits of application of a general theory (Stoecker, 1991). Accordingly, as well as their *intrinsic* interest in the individual, case studies may have an *instrumental* concern with the single instance, through the light that it sheds on a broader issue (Stake, 1994).

Characteristically, case studies are longitudinal; data may be gathered prospectively over a considerable span of time, and may also be gathered retrospectively. Thus, in her study of a woman with obsessive-compulsive disorder, O'Neill (1999) carried out interviews on two separate occasions, six weeks apart, and the interview process involved a considerable amount of reflection by the informant on events, feelings and perceptions that had occurred in the past. Multiple sources of data are often used, both qualitative and quantitative (Yin, 1984; Robson, 1993). Table 16.2 presents some hypothetical case studies to illustrate the variety of approaches that may be taken under the general heading of case study research. The various methods of data collection and analysis involved have been dealt with in previous chapters. Figure 16.5 illustrates the principal design features of a typical case study.

16.4 CONCLUSION

This chapter has outlined the principal features of single instance research. Case studies and single system studies can assist in answering certain exploratory, descriptive and explanatory questions in health care research. Although the strategy used in these approaches differs from that of other approaches such as surveys and randomized controlled trials, the specific methods utilized to collect and analyse data are much the same.

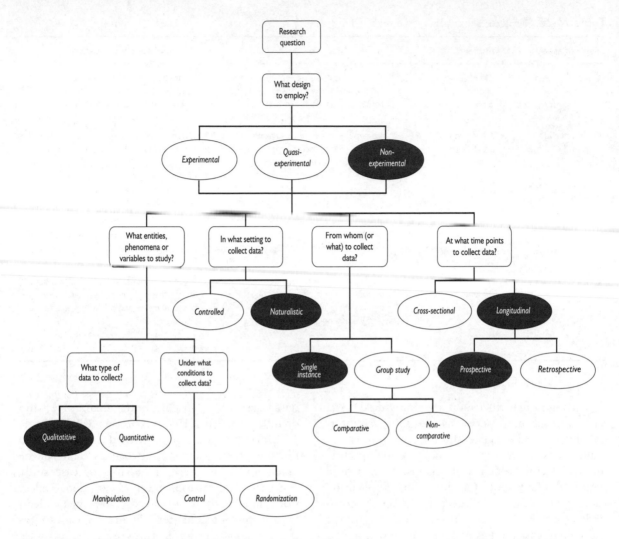

Figure 16.5   *Principal design features (shaded elements) of a typical case study.*

17 SYSTEMATIC REVIEWS, META-ANALYSIS AND MEASURES OF TREATMENT EFFECT

SUMMARY

This chapter explores the following topics:

- the nature and purpose of systematic reviews
- differences between systematic reviews and conventional narrative reviews
- the principal steps in conducting a systematic review
- the nature and purpose of meta-analysis
- approaches to data analysis in meta-analyses
- measures used to express the effect of an intervention

Most of the research designs and methods examined hitherto have concerned themselves with collecting first-hand data; as such they can be classified as forms of *primary analysis* (see Box 5.7). At times, it is appropriate to carry out *secondary analysis*. The defining characteristic of such research is that it involves the analysis of data that were recorded or gathered and analysed at an earlier time. Although a single study or a single dataset may sometimes be re-analysed in this way, it is more common to synthesize a number of studies or datasets and analyse them together, possibly after aggregating the data within them. This chapter will consider the systematic review as an example of secondary analysis. It will also examine the use of meta-analysis and will give an account of the various measures of treatment effect that are often utilized within systematic reviews and meta-analyses and are gaining increasing currency in the literature (Li Wan Po, 1998; Sackett *et al.*, 2000).

17.1 SYSTEMATIC REVIEWS

As part of the recent focus on evidence-based practice (see Section 2.1), there has been an increased awareness of the need for high-quality yet accessible evidence on which to base treatment decisions. This has in turn led to a fundamental reappraisal of the nature and role of the literature review. The traditional approach to reviewing the literature – sometimes referred to as the 'narrative' review (Crowley, 1996) – has been criticized on a number of counts. First, the coverage of the traditional review has been accused of being too narrow. The items included have tended largely to be those with which the author was familiar or those that the author had at his or her ready disposal. Rarely was a systematic process followed to ensure that a comprehensive trawl of literature was performed. Second, there has usually been neglect of unpublished items, or those that exist in the 'grey' literature (i.e. sources such as conference proceedings, dissertations, theses, reports with limited circulation, and the like).

Third, although the coverage of narrative reviews (i.e. the range of sources used) has been condemned for being too narrow, their scope (i.e. the aspects of a topic that they address) may be considered too broad. In other words, the narrative review can be criticized for failing to address a sufficiently precise question. A fourth problem is that authors of narrative reviews have often failed to assess the quality of their sources in a systematic way. In particular, this has been highlighted in respect of reviews of treatment effectiveness studies, such as randomized controlled trials. It is argued that unless the quality of such studies is evaluated, one cannot determine the credibility to be attached to their findings.

With considerations such as these in mind, a number of commentators have accused the traditional review article of lacking rigour and being prone to various subjective, and even idiosyncratic, influences (Collins *et al.*, 1987; Mulrow,

1987, 1994). In its place, the systematic review is now advocated as the approach of choice. Droogan and Cullum (1998, p. 16) are typical of many in arguing that '[s]ystematic reviews are the most reliable and valid means of summarising the available research findings in any given topic, and are therefore the foundation stones of evidence-based health care'.

The systematic review is conducted according to a strict set of objective methodological standards and procedures, analogous to those that would be used for a randomized controlled trial. Hence, just as patients are screened for their suitability for a trial, so individual studies are assessed for inclusion in a review. So, inclusion and exclusion criteria can be identified for studies in a systematic review just as they are for patients in a clinical trial. Similarly, just as the validity and reliability of outcome data are scrutinized in a trial, so the methodological strengths and weaknesses of individual studies are assessed according to a set of agreed criteria (Moher et al., 1995; de Vet et al., 1997; van Tulder et al., 1997).

In view of the fact that studies with statistically significant findings are more likely to be published, and to be published sooner, than those whose findings are non-significant (Easterbrook et al., 1991; Stern and Simes, 1997), rigorous and conscientious attempts are made to identify all relevant studies, both published and unpublished. It is important to bear in mind, however, that unpublished studies will not have been subjected to a process of peer review (Chalmers et al., 1987), and their quality should be scrutinized all the more carefully on this account. Mosteller and Colditz (1996, p. 16) suggest that 'we cannot regard peer-reviewed articles as coming from the same population as the unpublished articles', and suggest that the two categories of study should be handled separately.

Computerized bibliographic databases, such as Medline, CINAHL and EMBASE, are generally used for this purpose, but manual methods ('hand searching') are also employed to capture items that may have been indexed incorrectly or not indexed at all (Dickersin et al., 1994; Geddes et al., 1998). Where possible, relevant papers published in foreign languages should be sought (Greener and Grimshaw, 1996). Egger and Davey Smith (1998) note that 'positive' findings may be more likely to be published in an international journal in English, whereas 'negative' findings may appear in a national journal in the indigenous language. The inclusiveness of the review is crucial to its success. Failure to accomplish a comprehensive search of relevant sources will undermine the conclusions of an otherwise rigorous systematic review (Bjordal and Greve, 1998; Crombie and McQuay, 1998). The principal points of comparison between narrative and systematic reviews are shown in Table 17.1.

17.1.1 The process of systematic reviewing

Figure 17.1 shows the main stages in conducting a systematic review. More detailed discussions of the process are available elsewhere (e.g. Chalmers and Altman, 1995; NHSCRD, 1996). A few points are worthy of emphasis, however.

It is important to establish clearly the research question at the outset of the review. Otherwise, there may be a temptation to frame the question in the light of findings emerging from the review, with the potential for bias. The same applies to the inclusion and exclusion criteria used; these should not be established retrospectively, in the light of accruing findings.

The search process is generally two-stage. Initially, a wide trawl is made, usually by means of a computerized search of one or more databases. This will provide a working list of potentially eligible studies. It is unlikely, though, to have identified all the eligible studies relevant to the review. Some of these may be in the 'grey' literature, and are therefore unlikely to appear in a computerized search. Others may have been published in journals that are not indexed by the major databases, or may have been included only fairly recently. A supplementary search is therefore usually required in order to fill in the gaps.

Table 17.1 *Chief points of contrast between narrative reviews and systematic reviews; adapted from Cook et al. (1997)*

	Narrative review	Systematic review
Focus	Often addresses a broad range of issues, and brings these together in an overview	Usually focuses on a single specific question, without attempting to provide an overview of the topic
Research question	When present, is usually descriptive in nature	Usually explanatory
Search strategy	Often unstated or implicit	Explicit inclusion and exclusion criteria are used
Selection of sources	Selective and subject to conscious or unconscious selection bias	Comprehensive, with a deliberate avoidance of selection bias
Nature of sources	Mainly published sources, including both theoretical and empirical papers	Published and unpublished ('grey') sources; usually only empirical papers
Assessment of sources	Sometimes, and not usually according to specified criteria	Always, using specified criteria with the focus mainly on methodological issues
Conclusions	Summative	Cumulation or meta-analysis (meta-analysis)

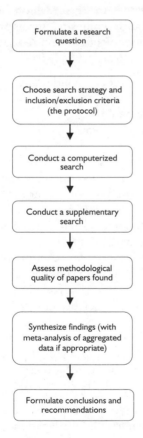

Figure 17.1 *Principal steps in conducting a systematic review.*

Direct contact with others working in the field is a potentially valuable exercise at this stage. They may be able to identify relevant trials that are as yet unpublished or that have eluded the search strategy used by the authors, and may also shed additional light on some of the studies already identified (Roberts and Schierhout, 1997).

It is important to try to establish whether two or more similar papers with authors in common describe separate studies or different elements of a single study (Droogan and Song, 1996; Vargas and Camilli, 1999). If the latter is the case, there is a danger that the results of a study will be at least 'double counted'. This may cause the effectiveness of an intervention to be overestimated (Tramèr *et al.*, 1997).

Assessment of the methodological quality of individual studies should be done by more than one assessor, using precisely the same criteria. Differences in ratings can then be settled by discussion, or through the involvement of an additional assessor. It is useful for the assessors to be blinded to the identity of the authors of the studies. It has also been suggested that the results of each study should be removed or concealed, so that these do not influence the quality score assigned (Jadad *et al.*, 1996; Cooper and Lindsay, 1998). Rosenthal (1991) suggests that ratings should be made twice: once with and once without knowledge of the study findings. In this way, the effect of awareness of the findings can be gauged.

When some studies receive low scores on methodological quality, a decision as to whether or not to include them should be made. One approach is simply to omit them, on the basis that poor-quality inputs to a review will produce poor-quality outputs (Bland *et al.*, 1995; Eysenck, 1995). Mosteller and Colditz (1996, p. 7) comment that '[n]o amount of careful combining of data from studies can overcome the inherent deficiencies in the original data'. This is to take an absolute view of their quality. Another approach is to include the studies if they constitute the best available evidence in the area concerned (Cooper and Lindsay, 1998), i.e. a relative view is taken of their quality.

17.2 META-ANALYTIC SYSTEMATIC REVIEWS

The process of meta-analysis plays an important role in systematic reviewing (Light, 1987; Egger and Davey Smith, 1997). The term 'meta-analysis' was coined by Glass (1976). It may be defined as 'the statistical analysis of results from a large number of individual research studies so as to integrate their findings' (Wood, 1995, p. 390).

A systematic review that incorporates meta-analysis does not merely assimilate the conclusions of individual studies, but aggregates the data on which these conclusions were based. In this way, it provides a more precise, and therefore more trustworthy, estimate of the true effect of a treatment (Beck, 1999). Individual trials that, taken individually, may have insufficient statistical power to provide credible information can contribute meaningfully to the conclusions derived from aggregated data. Furthermore, the findings of a meta-analysis are likely to have greater generalizability than those of individual studies, since the data on which they are based reflect a wider range of patients and treatment settings. Accordingly, a meta-analysis may provide a more credible indication

of the likely effects of therapeutic interventions, such that both clinicians and patients are better informed in their decision making (Antman *et al.*, 1992; Tickle-Degnen, 1998).

17.2.1 Approaches to meta-analysis

If a meta-analysis is performed on published randomized controlled trials, the data within each report can usually be extracted and pooled with those from other reports, providing that a minimum of information has been published (e.g. a mean between-group difference with its standard deviation or standard error). By using summary statistics in this way, the patients in the original studies are entered into the new analysis in groups.

Although a valid analysis can be conducted on data aggregated in this fashion, there are a number of shortcomings to this approach, which reflect the absence of data on individual patients (Clarke and Stewart, 1995, 1997):

- The researcher conducting the meta-analysis cannot check for the inclusion of ineligible patients.
- Analysis of subgroups can be performed only for those subgroups identified in the original reports, and only for those reports that have identified the same subgroups.
- Further analysis of subgroups is rarely possible, since this requires specific values of an outcome variable to be attributable to individual patients.
- Additional variables cannot be used to adjust the relationship between the principal intervention variable(s) and outcome variables(s), either because no information is provided on such variables, or if it does exist, because of the problem of attributing specific values to individual patients.
- Anomalies or inaccuracies in the data cannot normally be identified.

In the light of such issues, researchers may attempt to enter individual patient data into the meta-analysis. These raw data are rarely published, and the authors of the original studies must normally be contacted directly. This approach permits a far wider range of analyses to be carried out, and also provides a means of verifying the accuracy and completeness of the data to be used. If subgroup analyses are performed, these are not restricted to those subgroups identified in the published report, which may be subject to bias (Clarke and Stewart, 1995). Covariates can also be analysed, which may explain apparent heterogeneity among individual studies (Mosteller and Colditz, 1996). In addition, the dataset for a study can often be updated, since results accruing after the main results have been published can be obtained from the authors (Davey Smith and Egger, 1998).

17.2.2 Methods of analysis

A detailed consideration of the various methods of analysing aggregated data is beyond the scope of this chapter; details are provided in DerSimonian and Laird (1986), Rosenthal (1991), Thompson and Pocock (1991), Whitehead and Whitehead (1991), Olkin (1995), Cooper (1998), Elwood (1998), and Hedges and Vevea (1998). However, some of the central issues underlying the choice and conduct of the analysis will be considered. The basis of whatever strategy is chosen is twofold: to identify a measure of effect that is obtainable from, or calculable for, each study to be included; and to select a statistical model by which these can be aggregated.

The simplest form of analysis that can be performed within a meta-analysis is simply to tally the number of studies that have reported a result in favour of the intervention concerned. If there is a preponderance of studies supporting the intervention over those that do not, a statistical test such as a sign test or binomial test can be used to determine whether this is greater than would have been expected by chance. This is referred to as the *vote-counting* approach (Freemantle and Geddes, 1998). In many cases, deciding on whether a study supports an intervention is fairly straightforward, but it may be difficult when differences in a number of outcomes lie in opposite directions (Greener and

Grimshaw, 1996). A more serious problem with vote counting is that it treats all studies in the same way, irrespective of their size (and hence the likely precision of their estimates of effect) and the magnitude of the observed treatment effect. A further difficulty lies in deciding how to treat studies with effects that lie in a 'positive' direction but are statistically non-significant (Lancaster *et al.*, 1997). Should these be classified in the same category as studies that have shown a significant positive effect, or should they be omitted from the analysis? Mosteller and Colditz (1996) argue for the first of these positions, on the basis that potentially valuable information would otherwise be lost. A final drawback of the vote-counting approach is that it tends to be low in statistical power (Cooper, 1998).

Essentially, vote counting works by pooling the *results* of individual trials, rather than their data. A more rigorous approach to analysis incorporates the specific effect sizes reported by the studies (see Section 17.3.1 for a discussion of effect sizes). In order to reflect its precision as an estimate of the population effect, each effect may be weighted by multiplying it by the inverse of its standard deviation (i.e. 1 divided by the standard deviation). The smaller the standard deviation, the larger its inverse, and therefore the greater the weighting applied to the reported effect. In this way, studies that provide a more precise estimate of effect (which are usually the larger studies) will make a larger contribution to the overall estimate of effect when the data are aggregated.

In a similar manner, the effects reported by individual studies can also be weighted by a score based on the methodological quality of the individual studies. These scores are normally out of 100 (Table 17.2), so that, for example, an effect reported by a study with a quality score of 64/100 could be weighted by .64. However, Thompson and Pocock (1991) argue that such quality weightings are prone to a certain degree of arbitrariness – for example, in relation to the relative importance of different aspects of study design – and there is not yet agreement on their appropriateness (Mosteller and Colditz, 1996).

Table 17.2 *Quality scoring criteria used in a systematic review of randomized controlled trials of the treatment of fibromyalgia syndrome, modified from criteria published by van Tulder et al. (1997). The available scores sum to 100. The scoring shown is for studies in which patient blinding is feasible; where this is not an option, the points assigned to category K are transferred to category M, so that the total points assigned to blinding remain the same*

Criterion	Possible score	Calculation
A. Homogeneity	2	Description of inclusion and exclusion criteria (1 pt). Restriction to a homogeneous study population (1 pt)
B. Comparability of relevant baseline characteristics	5	Comparability for: duration of complaints, value of outcome measures, age, sex and distribution of symptoms (1 pt each)
C. Randomization procedure adequate	4	Randomization procedure described (2 pts). Randomization procedure that excludes bias (2 pts)
D. Dropouts described for each study group separately	3	Information from which group and with reason for withdrawal; no dropouts is 3 pts
E. Loss to follow-up	4	Loss to follow-up: all randomized patients minus the number of patients at main moment of effect measurement for the main outcome measure, divided by all randomized patients, times 100: <20%, 2 pts; <10%, 2 additional pts
F. Subjects in smallest group	17	Size of smallest group immediately after randomization: >50 patients, 8 pts; >100 patients, 9 additional pts
G. Interventions standardized and described	10	Experimental treatment explicitly described (5 pts). All other interventions explicitly described (5 pts)
H. Pragmatic study/control group adequate	5	Comparison with other treatments
I. Co-interventions avoided	5	Other medical interventions avoided in the design of the study (except analgesics, general advice, or use at home of heat, rest, or a routine exercise scheme)
J. Placebo controlled	5	Comparison with placebo therapy
K. Patients blinded	5	Attempted blinding of the patients with respect to the content of the interventions (3 pts). Blinding evaluated and fully successful (2 pts)
L. Outcome measures relevant	10	Outcome measures used and reported: pain (2 pts); sleep quality (1.5 pts); fatigue (1.5 pts); global measure of improvement (2 pts); functional status (ADL) (1 pt); return to work (or to normal activities) (1 pt); use of medication and/or medical services (1 pt)
M. Blinded outcome assessment	10	Effect measured by a blinded assessor (15 pts are possible if patient blinding is not feasible)
N. Follow-up period adequate	5	Including an effect measurement after 6 months or longer (5 pts)
O. Intention to treat analysis	5	When loss to follow-up is <10%: all randomized patients for most important outcome measures and on the most important moments of effect measurement minus missing values, irrespective of non-compliance and co-interventions. When loss to follow-up >10%: intention to treat as well as an alternative analysis that accounts for missing values
P. Frequencies of most important outcomes presented for each group	5	For most important outcome measures and on the most important moments of effect measurement; in the case of (semi-)continuous variables, presentation of the mean or median with standard error or percentiles

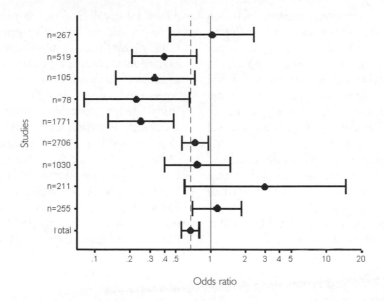

Figure 17.2 *A forest plot showing the odds ratios (and associated 95% confidence intervals) from nine studies of the use of diuretics for pre-eclampsia, using data provided by Thompson and Pocock (1991). An odds ratio of less than 1 favours diuretics over the control treatment. The solid vertical line marked at an odds ratio of 1 is the 'no effect' line. The dashed vertical line indicates the odds ratio for the aggregated data. So that the confidence intervals appear symmetrical on the plot, the horizontal scale is logarithmic.*

A study by Jüni *et al.* (1999) suggests that different scales may produce very divergent ratings of the quality of the same trial. Reflecting the controversy that surrounds methodological quality weighting, Olkin (1995) and LaValley (1997) suggest that an analysis should be done both with and without a quality weighting, so as to gauge its impact on the results of the analysis.

When individual patient data are used in a meta-analysis, the pooled dataset is analysed in much the same way as that resulting from a single primary study.

17.2.3 The issue of heterogeneity

When collating studies for a meta-analysis, it may become apparent that a few studies are heterogeneous with respect to the others. Such trials are usually apparent on a *forest plot*. A forest plot is a graph that displays the effect estimate – for example, the odds ratio (Section 17.3.2) – from a number of studies in a systematic review, along with their confidence intervals (Figure 17.2). The

larger studies tend to have narrower confidence intervals, and the confidence interval for the aggregated data from all of the studies is the narrowest. Any trial whose effect estimate lies on the other side of the 'no effect' line from most of the other studies, or whose confidence interval does not overlap at least some of those of the other studies, should immediately raise suspicions of heterogeneity. The eighth study from the top displayed in Figure 17.2 (*n* = 211) might raise such suspicion. A statistical test can be performed to determine whether the variation between the effects reported by individual studies is greater than could be expected by chance (Thompson and Pocock, 1991; Cooper, 1998). Unless the number of studies is large, these tests are liable to have low statistical power, and underlying heterogeneity may not be detected (Sánchez-Meca and Marín-Martínez, 1997; Blettner *et al.*, 1999).

If such statistical heterogeneity is found, attempts should be made to locate its source, which is likely to lie in some form of clinical heterogeneity – for example, different inclusion criteria, varying follow-up periods, different methods of treatment delivery, inconsistent methods of outcome assessment (Thompson, 1994). If necessary, heterogeneous studies should be placed into homogeneous groups which are then analysed separately. Alternatively, if one or two studies show evidence of genuine clinical heterogeneity, they can be omitted from the meta-analysis altogether. This should be done, however, only if the researcher is confident that these studies do not simply represent normal variation among studies that are in fact homogeneous. In any event, an analysis should probably be done with and without the studies, so as to quantify the effect of their removal.

17.2.4 Shortcomings and issues of controversy in meta-analysis

Meta-analysis has its critics. It tends, for example, to focus on a single outcome measure, whereas Eysenck (1995, p. 64) argues that 'effects are often multivariate rather than univariate'. Meta-analysis is hard to perform on studies of different design. It is not normally feasible to include data from quasi-experimental studies along with those from randomized controlled trials (RCTs), since the subsequent aggregate analysis will assume that *all* patients have been randomized to the interventions being tested. Moreover, although a meta-analysis will provide a more precise estimate of a treatment effect – as evidenced by a narrower confidence interval than that of any of the individual studies (Sim and Reid, 1999) – it cannot by itself detect bias or confounding arising from poor study design.

Because a meta-analysis is conducted retrospectively, the author is likely to be aware of the findings of the various studies he or she is gathering together. Consequently, there may be a tendency for the inclusion and exclusion criteria for the studies to be applied in such a way that only those trials likely to produce the anticipated outcome may be admitted to the analysis. West (1993) discusses specific examples that raise this suspicion.

Just as individual studies are assessed for their methodological quality, so meta-analyses themselves should be critically appraised. Sacks *et al.* (1987) examined 86 published meta-analyses of randomized controlled trials and judged only 24 of these to have addressed the six areas that they considered methodologically important (viz. study design, combinability, control of bias, statistical analysis, sensitivity analysis, application of results). More recently, Jadad *et al.* (2000) evaluated 50 systematic reviews and meta-analyses on asthma therapy. Of these, 40 were considered to have serious or extensive flaws. If a meta-analysis is based on a biased selection of studies, the meta-analysis itself is likely to be biased in its conclusions; Egger *et al.* (1997b) describe a graphical technique, the 'funnel plot', that can be used to detect such bias in a meta-analysis.

There is not yet consensus on a number of aspects of meta-analysis: the method of aggregate analysis to be used, whether to exclude some otherwise eligible studies, whether to use quality weightings, and so forth. In general, a *sensitivity analysis* should be performed as part of a meta-analysis (Egger *et al.*, 1997a). This involves conducting the analysis under more than one set of assumptions, or using more than one model of analysis, so that the effect of so doing on the findings of the meta-analysis can be gauged and any discrepancies investigated.

Finally, it should be noted that meta-analyses on the same topic may disagree with one another, and with the results of very large 'definitive' randomized controlled trials (Egger and Davey Smith, 1995; Moher and Olkin, 1995; Naylor, 1997). The findings of meta-analyses should not be accepted as the final word on a question, especially if there are shortcomings in the way that the meta-analysis concerned was conducted.

17.3 MEASURES OF EFFECT

There are a variety of measures used to quantify the effect of interventions. These are commonly used in systematic reviews and meta-analyses, and in the reporting of much epidemiological research. This section will review some of the most commonly used measures.

17.3.1 Effect size statistics

Health outcomes based on summated rating scales are measured in units that have no direct biological meaning. Examples include tools to measure mobility, ability to perform activities of daily living and satisfaction with life. The range of scores reflects the coding of the response options against individual items and the number of items in the scale. For such variables, the magnitude and direction of change can be expressed in terms of *effect size statistics*. Effect size statistics translate change over time, or change between subgroups, into a standard unit of measurement. This facilitates comparisons across different tools or across different studies (assuming that the studies do not differ on any important features such as design or accessible population). Effect sizes also enable a meaningful profile of change over several outcome variables to be presented in a study, and assist in statistical power calculations (Kraemer and Thiemann, 1987; Lipsey, 1998; Section 18.6).

Conventionally, effect sizes are described as small, medium or large (Cohen, 1992). The value associated with each descriptor depends upon whether change is measured in terms of independent means, medians, proportions or correlation coefficients (Ottenbacher and Barrett, 1989). For changes in means or medians, an effect size of 0.2 or less is designated as small, 0.5 as medium and 0.8 as large (Cohen, 1992). Common methods for computing effect sizes are given below; others can be found in Kazis et al. (1989) and Tatsuoka (1993).

$$\text{Effect size} = \frac{\text{mean outcome at time 2} - \text{mean outcome at time 1}}{\text{standard deviation of outcome measure at time 1}}$$

$$\text{Standardized effect size} = \frac{\text{mean outcome at time 2} - \text{mean outcome at time 1}}{\text{standard deviation of change scores over time}}$$

$$\text{Standardized comparison of change} = \frac{\text{mean change for treatment group} - \text{mean change for control group}}{\text{standard deviation of control group at time 1}}$$

For the last statistic, the denominator can be replaced by the pooled standard deviation of the two groups.

Median values replace the means when the distribution of the outcome measure is skewed. Effect size statistics are also useful to compare the responsiveness of tools to change, with respect to a particular health intervention, population and context (Thaney and Kristof, 1998).

17.3.2 Measures of relative likelihood of events

In much epidemiological research and some treatment effectiveness research, the researcher is interested in a dichotomous outcome, which may be either positive or negative; for example, whether a person contracts an illness or not, whether a patient recovers full independence or not, whether a patient experiences a recurrence of an injury or not (Box 17.1). In these cases, a measure is needed of the comparative likelihood of such an outcome. How much greater is the chance of contracting an illness among those

Box 17.1 *Positive outcomes and positive effects*

If an *outcome* of an intervention is desirable (e.g. greater functional independence), it is positive; if it gives rise to an undesirable state of affairs (e.g. readmission to hospital), this is a negative outcome. The positive *effect* of an intervention can either be to increase the likelihood of a positive outcome or decrease the likelihood of a negative outcome. Similarly, an intervention can have a negative effect either by increasing the likelihood of a negative outcome or by decreasing the likelihood of a positive outcome.

exposed to a potential causative factor than among those not exposed? How much more likely are patients managed under this treatment programme to have a recurrence than patients managed under an alternative programme?

Measures that express these comparative judgments are known as measures of relative likelihood. Two such measures will briefly be described – risk ratios and odds ratios.

Risk ratios

The risk of contracting an illness when exposed to a potential causative factor is given by:

$$\frac{\text{those exposed becoming ill}}{\text{those exposed becoming ill} + \text{those exposed remaining well}}$$

Similarly, the risk of contracting the illness when not exposed is:

$$\frac{\text{those unexposed becoming ill}}{\text{those unexposed becoming ill} + \text{those unexposed remaining well}}$$

Hence, if 66 out of 150 exposed individuals fall ill and 42 out of 240 unexposed individuals fall ill, we can calculate:

$$\text{risk of illness if exposed} = \frac{66}{150} = .440$$

$$\text{risk of illness if unexposed} = \frac{42}{240} = .175$$

The risk ratio (or relative risk) of the illness is simply the risk of those exposed divided by the risk of those unexposed:

$$\frac{.440}{.175} = 2.51$$

The risk of illness is thus 2½ times greater for those exposed than for those unexposed. If the risk of illness is the same for both exposed individuals and unexposed individuals, the risk ratio will be 1 (therefore a risk ratio of 1, not 0, would be the value expressed by a null hypothesis of no difference in risk). A risk ratio greater than 1 indicates that exposure carries a greater risk of illness than non-exposure. When used to

compare two methods of intervention that aim to prevent an undesirable outcome, the risk associated with the experimental (novel) treatment is divided by that associated with the control (standard) treatment. Consequently, a risk ratio of less than 1 shows the experimental treatment to be more effective than the control treatment, and a risk ratio of more than 1 shows the control treatment to be more effective than the experimental treatment.

Odds ratios

The odds of contracting an illness when exposed to a potential causative factor are:

$$\frac{\text{those becoming ill having been exposed}}{\text{those remaining well having been exposed}}$$

Similarly, the odds of contracting the illness when not exposed are:

$$\frac{\text{those becoming ill without having been exposed}}{\text{those remaining well without having been exposed}}$$

The odds ratio (or relative odds) is calculated in a similar way to the risk ratio: the odds of those exposed divided by the odds of those unexposed. As in the case of a risk ratio, an odds ratio of 1 indicates no difference in the odds of falling ill for exposed and unexposed individuals, and an odds ratio of more than 1 indicates a greater likelihood of falling ill among those exposed. Just as with a risk ratio, in treatment comparisons an odds ratio of less than 1 favours the experimental intervention and an odds ratio of more than 1 favours the control intervention (see Figure 17.2).

Using the same figures as when calculating the risk ratio, the odds ratio would be:

$$\text{odds of illness if exposed} = \frac{66}{84} = .786$$

$$\text{odds of illness if unexposed} = \frac{42}{198} = .212$$

$$\frac{.786}{.212} = 3.71$$

Thus, the odds of falling ill when exposed are between 3 and 4 times those of falling ill when not exposed.

It can be seen from the example above that the odds ratio differs from the risk ratio: for the same data, the risk ratio is 2.51 and the odds ratio is 3.71. This is because each measure uses different information. The *risk* of falling ill when exposed was the number of those who fell ill as a proportion of all those exposed, whereas the *odds* of falling ill when exposed was the number of those who fell ill following exposure as a proportion of those who remained well following exposure.

It follows that, in order to calculate a risk ratio, we need to know how many of those who were exposed fell ill. This information can be derived from a cohort study (see Figure 4.1 and Table 4.4), because the researcher knows how many individuals in the study sample were exposed to the causative factor (similarly, in a randomized controlled trial, the researcher knows how many participants were exposed to the treatment under scrutiny). A case-control study, on the other hand, shows how many people who are ill were previously exposed, but it does *not* indicate how many people who were originally exposed subsequently became ill. It therefore provides the information required to calculate an odds ratio, but not that required to calculate a risk ratio.

If a condition is rare, an odds ratio can be calculated from a risk ratio. In such a situation, the odds of the event will be very close to its risk, and the odds ratio will therefore approximate the risk ratio. Consequently, if a condition is uncommon (which is usually the situation in case-control studies), an odds ratio derived from a case-control study will closely approximate the corresponding risk ratio that would have been generated by a cohort study, had one been carried out instead (Dixon *et al.*, 1997). In the example used in this section, however, the risk ratio and the odds ratio differed appreciably (2.51 compared with 3.71), owing to the moderately high incidence of the illness.

The odds ratio and the risk ratio are useful measures for epidemiological or clinical effectiveness studies that have a dichotomous outcome. Despite some of its shortcomings, the statistical properties of the odds ratio make it more suitable than the risk ratio for statistical modelling of pooled data in meta-analysis (Laupacis *et al.*, 1988), and it is therefore more often seen in this context. A confidence interval can be calculated for either measure (Morris and Gardner, 1989). If a 95% confidence interval for either an odds ratio or a risk ratio excludes 1 (the null value), this is equivalent to rejecting the null hypothesis of no difference at the $p \leq .05$ level (see Table 13.4).

17.3.3 The number needed to be treated

A measure of outcome commonly used in treatment effectiveness studies – and which reflects baseline probabilities – is the *number needed to be treated* (Laupacis *et al.*, 1988). This is the number of patients to whom an intervention would need to be applied – or the number of patients who would need to be screened (Rembold, 1998) – in order either to achieve one positive patient outcome, or to prevent one negative patient outcome. The smaller the figure, the better. The number needed to be treated is often shortened to the grammatically inaccurate term 'number needed to treat', and is usually abbreviated to 'NNT'.

To calculate the NNT, either the *absolute risk reduction* or the *absolute benefit increase* must be determined (these can also be expressed in relative terms; see Box 17.2), depending on whether the intention of treatment is to reduce a negative outcome or to increase a positive outcome. These are calculated as the difference between the probability of an outcome when the treatment is given (the *experimental event rate*) and the probability of the outcome when the treatment is not applied (the *control event rate*).

The NNT is defined as the inverse of the absolute risk reduction or the absolute benefit increase (i.e. 1 divided by this measure). For example, a study might be undertaken of a counselling programme designed to help health professionals off work with stress to return to

Box 17.2   *Relative risk reduction*

As well as the absolute risk reduction, the relative risk reduction can be calculated. This is the absolute risk reduction divided by the control event rate. Because the relative risk reduction is expressed as a proportion of the control event rate, it is standardized. In other words, it does not reflect the absolute value of the control event rate. Suppose, for example, that a treatment were to reduce the probability of an undesirable outcome from .46 to .25. This would give a relative risk reduction of .46. If another treatment, applied to a different patient for a different condition, were to reduce the probability of an undesirable outcome from .11 to .06, this too would give a relative risk reduction of .46 (Table 17.3). In other words, the relative risk reduction does not discriminate between a situation in which a risk is reduced from 46% to 25% and one in which a risk is reduced from 11% to 6%, yet in terms of clinical importance there is a very marked difference between these two situations. When calculating risk reduction, the experimental control rate is subtracted from the control event rate; when calculating benefit increase, the control event rate is subtracted from the experimental event rate. This means that, in each case, a positive figure will favour the experimental condition and a negative figure will favour the control condition.

compared with 41 out of 185 who do not receive the programme, the following event rates would be calculated: experimental event rate = 30/114 = .263, control event rate = 41/185 = .222. The absolute benefit increase is .041 (.263 − .222) and the NNT is therefore:

$$\text{NNT} = \frac{1}{\text{absolute benefit increase}} = \frac{1}{.263 - .222}$$
$$= \frac{1}{.041} = 24.3$$

In order to gain one treatment success using the counselling programme (i.e. to return one member of staff to work who would not have returned if untreated), 25 clients need to pass through the programme (see Box 17.3). Figures for the number needed to be treated are always rounded up to the nearest whole number.

A confidence interval can be calculated for an NNT so as to express its precision as an estimate of the effect in the population (Altman, 1998). A further requirement is to assess the clinical importance of a particular NNT. Szatmari (1998, p. 40) suggests that this will be determined by 'the burden of suffering of the disorder as measured by prevalence, morbidity, and outcome; the economics and the difficulty of the treatment procedure; and, finally, the cost of not treating the disorder'.

Unlike the relative risk reduction (Box 17.2), the NNT is not standardized; it reflects the control, or baseline, risk. Table 17.3 shows measures of effect for the example given in Box 17.2. The baseline risk, as indicated by the control event rate, is very different for the two conditions, but the relative risk reduction does not reflect this, since it is a standardized measure. In contrast, the NNT (and the absolute

work. A successful outcome might be defined as the staff member's return to work within 6 weeks. If 30 out of 114 staff who undergo the programme return to work within 6 weeks,

Table 17.3   *Measures of effect for two hypothetical interventions applied to different conditions*

	Experimental event rate	Control event rate	Relative risk reduction	Absolute risk reduction	Number needed to be treated
Treatment A	.25	.46	.46	.21	5
Treatment B	.06	.11	.46	.05	20

Box 17.3   *Measuring negative treatment effects*

> Sometimes, the researcher's concern is with the negative, rather than the positive, effects of an intervention (i.e. its tendency either to promote negative outcomes or to impede positive outcomes). These are usually the side effects of the intervention. In such cases, the measure of effect is the *absolute risk increase* (logically, when a positive outcome is prevented one could also speak of the 'absolute benefit reduction', but this term seems not to be generally used). The measure of effect calculated from the absolute risk increase is the *number needed to harm*. This calculation uses the experimental and control event rates in the same way as the previous ones, with an event defined as the occurrence of the unwanted side effect. Sackett and Haynes (1997) provide further details.

risk reduction, from which it is derived) reflects the baseline risk. Working with a much lower baseline risk than Treatment A, Treatment B has to be applied to four times as many patients to gain one additional successful patient outcome.

The fact that the NNT is specific to a particular baseline risk makes it a useful measure of effect when an intervention is applied to a category of patients. However, although a category of patients will have a mean baseline risk, the baseline risk of individual patients is likely to vary. Cook and Sackett (1995) describe a simple method whereby the NNT can be divided by a factor that corresponds to the difference between the mean baseline risk for a category of patients and the specific baseline risk of an individual patient. If the patient is at twice the average risk, this factor would be 2; when divided by this factor, the NNT is reduced by half. This reflects the fact that when the baseline risk is higher, fewer patients have to be treated in order to record a successful patient outcome. Conversely, if the patient is at half the average risk, the factor is .5, and the NNT would increase twofold after being divided by this factor.

17.4 CONCLUSION

This chapter has provided an introduction to the nature, use and conduct of systematic reviews and meta-analysis. These forms of secondary analysis are playing an increasingly important part in evidence-based practice in health care, by virtue of their ability to provide precise and generalizable estimates of treatment effectiveness. An understanding of various means of treatment effect is also an important element within evidence-based practice, and this chapter has defined some of the main statistics used for this purpose.

18

ANALYSING DATA FROM DESCRIPTIVE AND EXPLANATORY STUDIES: FURTHER PRINCIPLES AND PROCEDURES

SUMMARY

This chapter explores the following topics:

- statistical methods for analysing differences between more than two sets of data on a single variable
- statistical procedures for assessing the reliability of an instrument
- prediction of a value for one variable from the values of one or more other variables
- statistical control for an extraneous variable
- procedures for determining minimum sample size

Most health professionals routinely compare outcome measures or characteristics of their patients across time or between subgroups. This process might be formalized in a research study through the use of inferential statistics, as seen in Chapter 14 with respect to two subgroups. In many instances, however, a research question involves a comparison across more than two time periods or more than two subgroups. The analysis of these situations will be considered in this chapter.

It is quite common for health care professionals to predict the time to recovery for a patient following a particular therapy or the expected level of performance on some physical indicator. Accordingly, this chapter will also introduce statistical methods that predict outcomes based on the relationships found in quantitative data. The methods are more complex and the information more technical than in previous chapters, but such predictions have significance for practical decision making, using resources efficiently, and providing information for consumers of health care. The focus

of the chapter will then shift to the role of intention-to-treat analysis within randomized controlled trials, and methods used to assess the reliability of measurement instruments. Finally, the issue of minimum sample size calculation will be addressed.

Specific procedures will be considered under a similar series of subheadings to those used in Chapter 14. More symbols and formulae are used in the present chapter than in Chapter 14; however, these can be skipped by readers who are not comfortable with them.

18.1 TESTING DIFFERENCES: MORE THAN TWO SETS OF DATA ON A SINGLE VARIABLE

Situations frequently arise in research that require comparisons across more than two sets of data. For example, muscle strength or ability to perform daily activities of living might be measured before and at 4 weeks, 12 weeks and 24 weeks following participation in a particular therapy regimen or educational intervention programme. Health status might be assessed under three different approaches to the management of arthritis, such as a goal-setting regimen dictated by a therapist, a goal-setting regimen that is mutually developed by the patient and the therapist, and a regimen comprising no formally set goals. The effectiveness of a rehabilitation programme for low back pain might be evaluated in terms of both its mode of delivery (i.e. on a group or an individual basis) and its duration (i.e. over 1, 2 or 3 weeks). Length of patient stay after a particular surgical procedure might be compared across different hospitals. Anxiety felt by parents of young children might be compared for parents with different long-term medical conditions such as arthritis, diabetes, multiple sclerosis and asthma.

When the collected data are quantitative in

nature, such comparisons might be analysed through a technique called 'analysis of variance'. This technique is introduced in this section.

18.1.1 Analysis of variance

Analysis of variance (ANOVA) is a technique by which the total variation associated with recorded values of an outcome variable is partitioned into separate components. The analysis tests the significance of the contribution of each of these components to the total variation. Depending upon what assumptions can be made, this is a hypothesis test about population means or population variances. This section is concerned with hypothesis tests about population means.

In a simple situation, the components of variation are assigned to specific sources plus a non-specific source (Figure 18.1). The specific sources represent the effects of variables in terms of which the data can be classified. These variables might be manipulated, such as intensity, duration and number of daily exercise sessions, or non-manipulated, such as medical condition and profession. The non-specific source represents the combined effects of random error, measurement error, variables not specifically identified, and uncontrolled variables that influence values of the outcome variable (for example, a patient's age, weight or attitude

towards a particular therapy). The aim is to design a study in such a way that random error is the major contribution to the non-specific source (i.e. other sources of non-specific information have been controlled as far as possible).

Statistical models for the various ANOVA techniques are given in Appendix II.

Uses of analysis of variance

ANOVA is used extensively to analyse data from explanatory studies. The chosen experimental design determines how the total variation can be partitioned into components and how the effects of different variables will be accounted for in the analysis. Hence, the design and the analysis are inextricably linked, and this requires the analysis to be considered carefully at the design stage. The researcher identifies all the variables that might be important sources of variation, in the light of the study objectives. This includes factors (where 'factor' is an equivalent term to 'intervention variable'; Table 4.1), variables whose effects might be confounded with those of the interventions (Section 7.2), and extraneous variables that might generate a lot of variation in the values of the outcome variable. A design is then selected that allows the effects of interest to be (1) estimable and (2) capable of being tested for significance in the analysis. Designs commonly used in health care research

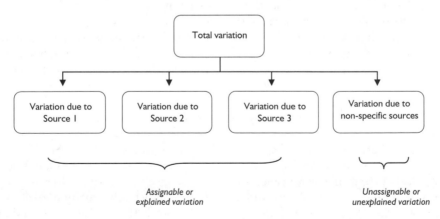

Figure 18.1 *Partitioning the total variation in the values of an outcome variable in a simple situation in which there are three sources of assignable variation.*

Table 18.1   *Some frequently used statistical methods for testing differences between more than two sets of data on one outcome variable. All methods require certain assumptions to be met if inferential tests are to be performed. See also Box 7.5*

| Number of factors | Relationship of sets of data | Level of measurement | |
		Ordinal	Interval/ratio
One	Unrelated: between-subjects measures	Kruskal–Wallis test	One-way ANOVA, Kruskal–Wallis test
	Repeated or within-subjects measures	Friedman test	One-way repeated measures ANOVA, Friedman test
	Cases put into blocks or matched	Friedman test	Randomized block analysis
Two	Both unrelated measures		Two-way ANOVA (factorial)
	Both repeated or within-subjects measures		Two-way repeated measures ANOVA
	One unrelated and one repeated measures		One between-subject and one within-subject measures ANOVA
Three or more	All unrelated measures		Factorial ANOVA
	All repeated measures		Factorial repeated measures ANOVA
	Combination of p unrelated and q repeated measures		p between-subjects and q within-subjects measures ANOVA

include one-way, factorial and repeated measures (Box 7.5 and Table 18.1). Simple examples of these will be presented a little later in this chapter. An understanding of the methods of analysis for these basic designs will provide a sound foundation from which to explore more complex designs. It will also enable students undertaking research projects to appraise their study objectives before collecting any data. It is not uncommon to find that initial objectives are too ambitious, resulting in impractical designs or analyses that are not feasible. With an understanding of design and data analysis, students might progressively modify their objectives until a feasible design is attained, while maintaining a worthwhile study.

ANOVA techniques are also employed as a convenient way to calculate reliability coefficients (Section 18.3), to test the significance of the contribution of individual variables towards the prediction of some specific attribute or performance indicator (Section 18.4), and to test the significance of differences between character- istics in more than two subgroups of data collected through surveys. In common with all inferential analyses, the use of ANOVA to test the significance of effects might lead to misleading inferences when its underlying assumptions are violated (Section 13.4.5). For this reason, assumptions accompany examples given in this chapter.

Different types of analysis of variance

The different ANOVA methods can be distinguished through key features. For explanatory studies, these include:

- the number of factors
- the assumptions that can be made about these factors (Box 18.1):
  - deliberately manipulated to take on specific settings, values or levels
  - deliberately manipulated to take on levels that are selected randomly from a population of interest (this situation is not discussed in this book)

Box 18.1 *Fixed and random effects*

The simplest experimental design comprises the deliberate manipulation of one factor (intervention variable) to create at least two distinct treatments. There are two possible situations here. First, the treatments might be specifically chosen by the researcher; for example, exercise sessions of duration 15 minutes, 30 minutes or 45 minutes. In such a situation, research hypotheses might be expressed in terms of differences in mean outcome values for the selected treatments, or in terms of estimating the effects of each treatment. An example hypothesis would be: the mean time to recover full functional ability is faster for exercise sessions lasting 30 minutes than for sessions lasting 15 minutes. Conclusions apply only to the selected treatments and are not generalizable to other similar treatments. The influence of a particular treatment is to increase or decrease values of the outcome variable by a fixed (or constant) amount compared with some overall mean value. This situation is called a *fixed effects model*.

Alternatively, the treatments might be a random sample from a large population; for example, five outpatient clinics randomly selected from all rehabilitation clinics in a large geographical region. In such a situation, research hypotheses might be expressed in terms of variability of treatment effects, or of estimating this variability, since knowledge about individual effects has no importance with regard to randomly selected treatments. An example hypothesis would be: the variance due to different clinics is larger than zero. In this case, conclusions are generalizable from the specific treatments considered in a study to the population from which they were randomly selected. The influence of a particular treatment is to generate variability in the outcome values. This situation is called a *random effects model or components of variance model*. In most studies, participants are represented by random effects.

Some studies involve more than one factor. The designation of effects as fixed or random has consequences for the calculations performed in hypothesis tests. A study might involve all fixed effects, all random effects, or a combination of fixed and random effects. The term *mixed model* does not refer to the presence of within-subject and between-subject factors but to the presence of both fixed and random effects (Box 7.5). Statistical computing packages have options that cater for these different models.

- the assignment of cases or participants to treatments (where 'treatments' comprise interventions identified by the levels of the factor in a study involving one factor only, and by the combinations of levels across all factors in a study involving two or more factors):
  - cases assigned completely at random to treatments
  - each case assigned to every treatment (i.e. cases are subjected to repeated measures)
  - blocks of cases set up so that cases *within* each block are similar with respect to important attributes but cases *across* blocks are different; cases within each block are randomly assigned to treatments
  - sets of cases set up so that cases within each set are matched with respect to important attributes; cases within each set are randomly assigned to treatments (i.e. cases are matched and the analysis is equivalent to using blocks of cases; see Section 18.1.7)
  - each case (or a block of cases) is assigned to every level of at least one factor, and then randomly assigned to the treatments identified by the levels of at least one other factor
- the level of measurement for the outcome variable(s)

- the assumptions, if any, that can be made about the distribution of sampling error.

These features will be evident in the examples that follow.

Use of statistical computing packages

The calculations required for ANOVA are laborious for all but the simplest design, and they are therefore usually performed using one of the readily available statistical computing packages. The requirements for entering the data may vary across packages and between designs within a package. Incorrect entry of the data is likely to result in the wrong analysis being performed. Similarly, details and layout of the output might vary between packages and designs, but the supplied information will include the separate components that are necessary for estimation or hypothesis testing.

18.1.2 One-way analysis of variance

One-way analysis of variance is the simplest of all ANOVAs, having only one factor, and hence only one specific source of variation. It is appropriate when comparing outcome measures across groups of independent cases. Such groups might be generated in two ways:

1. Several groups might be created by the random assignment of cases to levels of a single manipulated variable (the source of variation). For example, in a study investigating adherence to home exercise programmes, three groups are set up by randomly assigning patients (who satisfy certain inclusion and exclusion criteria) to a programme that is motivated by no goals, goals set by a therapist, or goals set collaboratively by a therapist and the patient. The random allocation of patients is equivalent to taking three random samples from the same population (Section 13.6), and is consistent, before the interventions, with an assumption that any differences in characteristics across the groups are due to sampling error. Other influences remaining the same, any post-inter-

vention differences in characteristics across the groups are ascribed to effects of the interventions.

2. Alternatively, several groups might arise from the selection of random samples from several populations or from some other sampling method that produces independent cases. The researcher's interest is in a comparison of characteristics across the populations. For example, in a study set up to investigate the influence that chronic disease has on perceived ability to fulfil a parenting role, random samples might be obtained from parents who have rheumatoid arthritis, diabetes, multiple sclerosis and asthma, thereby generating four groups of independent cases (assuming that persons with more than one of these conditions are excluded from the study).

In both situations, there might be different numbers of cases per group. Essentially, one-way ANOVA is used to determine whether observed differences in mean outcome values across the groups are greater than would be expected through sampling error. This is achieved by partitioning the total variation in outcome values into two components: variation between groups and variation within groups (Figure 18.2).

Research hypothesis

More than one research hypothesis might be stated when a study addresses three or more populations. In general, the hypotheses will refer to directional comparisons across at least two

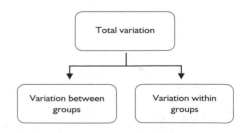

Figure 18.2 *Partitioning the total variation in outcome values for a simple one-way ANOVA.*

populations. These hypotheses will determine what a priori comparisons (Section 18.1.3) are performed during the analysis. For example, in the study on home exercise sessions, it is hypothesized that patients who set goals collaboratively with a therapist will have higher adherence levels with respect to their exercise sessions than those who either have no goals or have the goals imposed by a therapist.

Data

The data comprise values associated with independent cases in three or more groups. In the present example, percentage adherence values for exercise sessions were obtained using diaries kept by 75 patients randomly assigned to a home exercise programme that entailed no goals, goals set by a therapist, or goals set collaboratively by a therapist and the patient. These data are summarized in Table 18.2 and depicted in a scatter plot in Figure 18.3.

Model

In the home exercise example, the study was designed to test the effects of three different approaches to goal setting upon adherence to home exercise sessions. In words, the percentage adherence for a particular patient could be described thus:

percentage adherence value for one patient	= mean value unique to the particular approach to goal setting + error

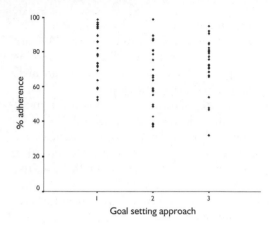

Figure 18.3 *Percentage adherence values for performing home exercise sessions under different goal-setting approaches (n = 25 for each approach). 1 = none; 2 = therapist; 3 = collaborative.*

and the mean value unique to the particular approach to goal setting could be expressed thus:

mean adherence value for one approach	= mean value common to all approaches + effect unique to the particular approach to goal setting

When the data have been collected, the percentage adherence values are sample statistics, i.e. *known* quantities. In contrast, the mean value unique to the particular approach to goal setting, the mean value common to all approaches, and the effect unique to the particular approach to goal setting are population parameters, i.e. *unknown* quantities that are estimable from the collected data. The model can be written more explicitly in terms of symbols (see Appendix II).

This statistical model is called an *additive* model, since it describes individual values of percentage adherence by taking a common mean percentage adherence and adding the effect of the influence from the manipulated (or controlled) variable, and then adding a component for error. The error term is referred to as *experimental error* and combines the effects from all uncontrolled influences on individual percentage adherence values.

Table 18.2 *Percentage adherence values for performing home exercise sessions under different goal-setting approaches*

Goal-setting approach	n	Mean (s.d.)	Minimum	Maximum
None set	25	79.1 (15.2)	52.6	99.0
Therapist set	25	65.6 (17.7)	37.2	99.0
Collaboratively set	25	73.3 (14.9)	32.3	95.0

s.d. = standard deviation.

Assumptions

The assumptions for the one-way ANOVA are:

- The data constitute values from random samples from two or more normally distributed populations.
- These populations have unknown means (μ_i) and unknown variances (σ_i^2).
- The unknown population variances are equal ($\sigma_i^2 = \sigma^2$), this is referred to as 'homogeneity of variance' or 'homoscedasticity' (Section 13.4.5).
- The underlying random variable of interest is continuous.
- The data are measured on an interval or ratio scale.

In terms of the model, these assumptions can be written as follows:

- The model is additive.
- The experimental error terms are identically and independently distributed, on a normal distribution, with mean zero and constant variance.
- There is independence between the cases: thus, the value of the outcome variable for one case does not affect, and is not affected by, the value of the outcome variable for any other case (Section 13.1.3).
- The effects of the different interventions (τ_i) are unknown constants and, for convenience, the effects are assumed to sum to zero; i.e. the effect of one approach might be to consistently increase the percentage adherence to a particular value higher than the common mean percentage adherence, whereas the effect of another approach might be to consistently decrease the percentage adherence to a particular value lower than the common percentage mean adherence.

Checking the assumptions

The assumptions are checked by reference to the sampling method or method of assignment of cases to groups, details of the measurement tool, and any recognized methods for checking normality, outliers and homogeneity (Sections 13.4.5 and 13.4.11; Box 14.3). In the home exercise example,

- the patients were randomly assigned to three different goal setting approaches; hence, post-intervention the data effectively constitute random samples from three populations
- percentage adherence is a ratio level of measurement (and, in theory, can take any value between 0 and 100)
- percentage adherence for one patient should not influence or be influenced by percentage adherence for any other patient in the study
- Levene's test on homogeneity of population variances indicated no reason to doubt the assumption of equal population variances ($F = 0.940$, p value $= .40$)
- normal probability plots of percentage adherence for each group cast no serious doubt on the assumption of normally distributed populations (see point 5 under 'Other comments' below) and indicated no extreme values.

Statistical hypotheses

The general null hypothesis states equality of the population mean values; that is, no difference in the mean values of the populations from which cases in the groups are sampled. The alternative hypothesis is that a difference exists between at least two of the population mean values. The null hypothesis might be: there is no difference in the mean percentage adherence values for patients motivated by no goals, goals set by a therapist, and goals set collaboratively by a therapist and the patient. The alternative hypothesis might be that the mean percentage adherence is different for at least one of the approaches. These hypotheses are often written as:

$$H_0: \mu_1 = \mu_2 = \mu_3 = \mu$$
$$H_1: \mu_i \neq \mu_j \text{ for some } i,j$$

Equivalently, the null hypothesis could be worded as: the three approaches to goal setting have no effect on percentage adherence to home exercise sessions. The alternative hypothesis might be that at least one approach to goal setting has an effect on percentage adherence to home exercise sessions. In symbols, these hypotheses are:

$$H_0: \tau_1 = \tau_2 = \tau_3 = 0$$
$$H_1: \tau_i \neq 0 \text{ for at least one } i$$

Note that, although the research hypothesis may well be directional, the statistical hypotheses are non-directional (Section 13.4.4).

Rationale for test

The rationale for a one-way ANOVA is presented in terms of the example on adherence to home exercises in which patients are randomly assigned to three goal-setting approaches, creating three groups. The total variation in percentage adherence values is partitioned into two components that are termed 'variation between groups' and 'variation within groups' (Figure 18.2).

Patients within a group are subject to the same approach, and variation within a group is therefore due to differences between the patients assigned to that approach and unassignable sources of error. Under the assumption of equal population variances, variation within each of the three groups can be combined to form one estimate of the variation due to error.

Patients in different groups are subject to different approaches, and variation between groups is therefore due to differences between the effects of the three approaches, differences between the patients assigned to the different groups, and unassignable sources of error. When the null hypothesis is true, the effects are all zero and variation between groups is due to error. When the null hypothesis is false, at least one effect is non-zero and variation between groups is due to effects of the approaches plus error.

A comparison of between-groups and within-groups variation can be used as a basis for a test on the null hypothesis. The magnitudes of these two components of variation are related to the number of groups and the number of patients, respectively. Hence, a ratio of mean components is used to test the null hypothesis:

$$\text{Ratio} = \frac{\text{variance between groups}}{\text{variance within groups}}$$

The variance within groups is an estimate of the variance due to error (σ^2). When the null hypothesis is true, the variance between groups is also an estimate of the variance due to error and the expected value of the ratio is 1. However, when the null hypothesis is false, the variance between groups is an estimate of variance due to error plus a non-zero, positive systematic error due to the effects of the approaches. In this situation, the expected value of the ratio is greater than 1.

The calculated value of the ratio is subject to sampling error and might, therefore, be greater than 1 by chance. Under the assumptions stated earlier, the sampling distribution of the calculated ratio follows a theoretical distribution called Fisher's F. The F distribution is used to calculate the probability of getting a ratio of the obtained magnitude or greater when random samples are drawn from populations having equal mean values. When this probability is sufficiently small (e.g. $p \leqslant .05$), the F ratio is considered to be statistically significant.

Results and their interpretation

It is usual to present summaries of the data for each group. Table 18.3 presents the number of observations, mean and standard deviation of the outcome values, and confidence intervals for the population mean outcome value for each group. The confidence intervals for mean percentage adherence scores are depicted in Figure 18.4.

The results of the ANOVA are usually reported in an 'analysis of variance table' (Table 18.4). A brief explanation of the components in this table is given under 'Analysis of variance table and statistical testing of effects' in Section 18.1.9.

The p value is used to make a statistical decision about the null hypothesis, with a

Table 18.3 *Summary and 95% confidence intervals for mean percentage adherence values for performing home exercise sessions under different goal-setting approaches*

Goal-setting approach	n	Mean (s.d.)	95% confidence interval for mean percentage adherence
None set	25	79.1 (15.2)	72.8 to 85.4
Therapist set	25	65.6 (17.7)	58.2 to 72.9
Collaborative	25	73.3 (14.9)	67.2 to 79.5

s.d. = standard deviation.

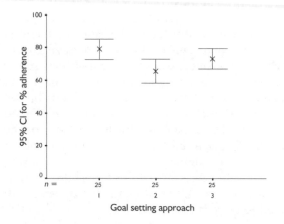

Figure 18.4 *95% confidence intervals for the mean percentage adherence values for performing home exercise sessions under different goal-setting approaches. X indicates the sample mean and the bars indicate the confidence interval. 1 = none; 2 = therapist; 3 = collaborative.*

Table 18.4 *ANOVA table for percentage adherence values*

Source of variation	Degrees of freedom	Sum of squares	Mean square	Variance ratio	p value
Between groups	2	2305.38	1152.69	4.50	.014
Within groups	72	18432.62	256.01		
Total	74	20738.00			

decision to reject being made for p values less than or equal to the chosen significance level. From the results in Table 18.4 and using a significance level of .05, the null hypothesis is rejected ($F = 4.50$, p value = .014). Based on this study, there is evidence to doubt the assumption of no difference in the effect of no goal setting, therapist-set goals, or collaboratively set goals on mean percentage adherence scores for home exercise sessions.

Further analyses or statistics

An obvious question to ask at this point is what approach produces a different effect? This is pursued through further analyses. *A posteriori* or *post hoc contrasts* (Section 18.1.4) are usually performed when the variance ratio in the ANOVA table is statistically significant. They enable groupings of mean values to be formed in which differences between groupings are greater than expected by chance and differences within groupings are consistent with sampling error. Options for methods such as Bonferroni, Tukey, Duncan, Scheffé and Newman–Keuls are available in most statistical computing packages. Findings from these a posteriori tests might be reported in terms of groupings with significantly different mean values, or groupings for which the mean values are not significantly different. The clinical importance of the findings might be considered through confidence intervals of the differences (Sections 13.3 and 13.5) or, where outcome can be expressed in terms of a dichotomy, the number needed to be treated (Section 17.3.3).

In the present example, Bonferroni tests (Table 18.5) indicate no statistically significant differences (at a significance level of .05) between the mean percentage adherence values for (1) therapist-set and collaboratively set goals, and (2) no goals and collaboratively set goals. There is, however, evidence of a significantly lower mean percentage adherence value for therapist-set goals compared with no goals (the 95% confidence interval for the difference being 2.4% to 24.6%).

A priori contrasts (Section 18.1.3) can be

Table 18.5 Results from Bonferroni tests on group means

Group A	Group B	Mean difference (Group A – Group B)	p value	95% confidence interval for difference in means
No goals set	Therapist set	13.53	.011	2.44 to 24.63
No goals set	Collaboratively set	5.77	.618	−5.32 to 16.87
Therapist set	Collaboratively set	−7.76	.272	−18.85 to 3.34

tested for statistical significance whether or not the variance ratio in the ANOVA table is statistically significant. Options for pre-planned specific contrasts and for general contrasts (using methods such as Bonferroni) are available in most statistical computing packages.

Other comments

1. An unrelated *t* test is a special case of a one-way ANOVA on two groups, with unrelated cases (in fact, the value of the *F* ratio equals the square of the value of the *t* statistic).

2. A one-way design is an example of a completely randomized design: cases are assigned completely at random to specifically chosen levels of a manipulated variable to determine the effects of that manipulation on a particular outcome measure.

3. In a completely randomized design, each treatment is assigned to a number of different cases (or participants). Comparisons across different treatment effects involve comparisons across different cases and, hence, the design is often referred to as a *between-subjects* design.

4. Completely randomized designs provide a standard against which the efficiency of other types of experimental design is measured.

5. ANOVA is robust to moderate departures from the assumptions of normality and homogeneity (Portney and Watkins, 1993; Howell, 1997), except when the groups contain unequal numbers of cases.

6. In this section, it has been assumed that the levels of the factor included in a study are the only ones of interest to the researcher, i.e. a *fixed effects* model (Box 18.1).

7. One-way ANOVA is commonly used to analyse data collected through surveys involving random selection of participants. Comparisons are made on some chosen variable (e.g. a measure of physical functioning) across identifiable groups of participants (e.g. different types of arthritis).

8. Different assumptions can be made about the distribution of the random error term in a statistical model, for example in *generalized linear models* (Krebs, 1993; Armitage and Berry, 1994). These situations are not considered in this book.

18.1.3 Multiple testing

In many studies, analysis of the data involves multiple hypothesis testing; that is, the testing of more than one planned statistical hypothesis. These tests are called *a priori*, since they are formulated at the design stage before any data are collected. Such a priori comparisons might be conducted in the context of various research designs and situations, for example:

- A survey involving one group of participants, in which it is planned to perform pairwise comparisons across more than two subgroups (defined according to, for example, different diagnoses, types of arthritis, sources of referral, severity of condition, or specific age groups).
- Similarly, an experiment involving more than two treatment groups in which it is planned to compare each pair of groups, e.g. treatment A versus treatment B, treat-

ment A versus treatment C, and, treatment B versus treatment C (essentially the situation in the exercise adherence study used as an example in the previous section).

- An experiment or a survey in which multiple outcome variables are measured on every participant and each variable is to be subjected to a hypothesis test. In the Low Back Pain Study, the effectiveness of two different management approaches was assessed by pain intensity, pain affect, self-rated symptomatic change, and a condition-specific measure of the effect of low back pain on health status (Table 7.1). The use of questionnaires within a survey commonly leads to multiple statistical testing of associations between study variables; e.g. self-report measures of physical ability, depression, anxiety, pain, fatigue, coping, and duration of illness.

- An experiment or clinical trial involving more than one factor in which it is planned to test all main effects and all interaction effects with respect to a specified outcome variable (factorial experiments are considered in Section 18.1.9).

- An experiment or quasi-experiment in which values of an outcome variable are measured on every participant at several points in time (repeated measures are discussed in Section 18.1.6).

When one hypothesis test is performed, there is a chance (equal to the selected significance level, α) that a true null hypothesis is rejected; that is, a significant result is found when in fact no effect exists in the population. When multiple hypothesis tests are performed, each at a significance level of α, the probability of finding at least one erroneous significant result can then be much greater than α (Box 18.2). For example, for four independent tests, each performed at a significance level of .05, there is a probability of .19 that at least one erroneous significant result is found. This might have

serious consequences for the conclusions when taken as a whole.

For independent tests, we can use the simple Bonferroni method to adjust the significance level of individual tests so that the probability of a Type I error over the multiple tests is equal to α (Campbell and Machin, 1993; Bland and Altman, 1995). With k independent tests, an overall significance level of α is maintained if each test is performed at a significance level of α/k. Four issues arise with regard to this method of adjustment. The first concerns large k, or, equivalently, a small level of significance for each individual test. The selected significance level and power directly influence the required sample size, with tests performed at smaller significance levels needing larger sample sizes to achieve the same power. Hence, Bonferroni's method can lead to unrealistically large sample sizes to maintain the power of multiple tests. Several alternative procedures have been suggested in the literature; for example, Bonferroni–Holm's, Hochberg's (Shaffer, 1995).

A second issue is that Bonferroni's method is based on the assumption of independent tests, and is not therefore applicable in many studies where the hypothesis tests are not independent. Questionnaires, for instance, result in data representing study variables that are measured on the same participants and that might or might not be independent. Individual hypothesis tests performed at a significance level of α/k, on k correlated variables, will produce a significance level smaller than α over all the tests and have reduced power (Bland and Altman, 1995). Such tests are called *conservative*, because they stand an increased risk of not statistically detecting effects in the population. Everitt (1998) suggests that the Bonferroni adjustment is acceptable for up to five simultaneous tests, after which it is liable to be unduly conservative. Modified methods allowing for logically related hypotheses are discussed by Shaffer (1995).

The third issue is that the Bonferroni method is concerned with the general assumption that all null hypotheses are true simultaneously. Epidemiologists argue that this situation is rarely of

Box 18.2   *Type I error in multiple hypothesis testing*

When a null hypothesis (H_0) is tested at a significance level of .05, the probability of rejecting a true H_0 is .05, which is the chance of finding a significant result when H_0 is true. The probability of not rejecting a true hypothesis is .95 (= 1 − .05), which is the chance of finding a non-significant result when H_0 is true. When two independent null hypotheses are individually tested at a significance level of .05, the probability of retaining both null hypotheses when they are both true is $.95^2 = .90$. Therefore, the probability of rejecting at least one true null hypothesis is .10. Probabilities for other numbers of independent tests are given in the table below. In general, when k independent null hypotheses are individually tested at a significance level of s, the probability of finding no significant result when all H_0 are true is $(1 − s)^k$ and, hence, the probability of finding at least one significant result when all H_0 are true is $1 − (1 − s)^k$, which for small s is equal to ks. Hence, to contain the Type I error to α over all tests, we set $\alpha = ks$, or $s = \alpha/k$. This adjustment to the individual significance levels is called *Bonferroni's method*.

Probability of rejecting at least one true H_0 given different Type I errors

No. of tests k	Significance level for individual tests	Probability of retaining all H_0 (given that all H_0 are true)	Probability of rejecting at least one true H_0
1	.05	.95	.05
2	.05	.90	.10
5	.05	.77	.23
10	.05	.60	.40
15	.05	.46	.54
20	.05	.36	.64
The general situation is given by:			
k	s	$(1 − s)^k$	$1 − (1 − s)^k$

either interest or use to researchers (Perneger, 1998). Further, it might produce a different interpretation from the same data depending upon how many other tests were performed. Another concern raised is that the increased Type II error might lead to important effects being deemed non-significant, which could result in the denial of appropriate care to patients. Proponents of these arguments recommend describing and justifying the performed statistical hypothesis tests as the best approach. This provides sufficient information for a reader to reach a reasonable conclusion for himself or herself about the findings.

The final issue is that when α has been adjusted by the Bonferroni method – e.g. from .05 to .0125 – a statistically significant compar-

ison is significant in terms of the original (.05), not the adjusted (.0125) significance level. The purpose of the adjustment is to maintain the original significance level in the face of multiple comparisons, not to substitute a different significance level.

This section has dealt with some of the issues surrounding planned multiple hypothesis testing. There are also situations in which multiple tests might be performed following an initial appraisal of the data; these are discussed in the next section.

18.1.4 Further analyses

Even when multiple hypothesis tests are not planned at the design stage, it is quite common to perform unplanned (*a posteriori*) tests after initial tests have been performed on the data and a decision has been reached to reject a null hypothesis. This situation leads naturally to further investigation of the data. Questions that might be considered include: Where does frequency of use differ across the types of therapy for patients with rheumatoid arthritis? Which therapy produces a different mean effect? Which method leads to the largest change in median pain intensity?

When the initial statistical comparison is across two groups (or two time periods) a consideration of the corresponding means, medians or proportions of outcome values will automatically reveal the existence and direction of any difference. When three or more groups are studied, further analyses are required to reveal what statistically significant differences exist. There might be a significant difference between every pairing of the mean values, or between one mean value and the rest. The further analyses require multiple comparisons to be made between the mean values. A study involving four groups would require six comparisons to compare the mean values across all pairs of groups. If each comparison were performed at a significance level of .05, the achieved probability of a Type I error over all the multiple comparisons would be .26 (see Box 18.2). That is, the probability of finding at least one statistically significant difference between two mean values just by chance would be much greater than .05. Several methods exist that control the overall Type I error rate in a posteriori tests. These include Fisher's least significant difference, Tukey's honestly significant difference, Duncan's multiple range, Scheffé and Newman–Keuls. Zwick (1993) and Sato (1996) present a comparison of the various procedures in terms of their emphasis on Type I and Type II errors. A selection of these methods is offered in most statistical computing packages.

18.1.5 Kruskal–Wallis test

The Kruskal–Wallis is a nonparametric test that compares groups of unrelated cases (as defined in Section 18.1.2). It is appropriate when the outcome variable has an ordinal level of measurement, or when the assumptions underlying the one-way ANOVA are not met (that is, the data do not constitute values from random samples from normally distributed populations with equal variances). The Kruskal–Wallis test is used to determine whether observed differences in median outcome values are greater than would be expected by chance (Box 18.3).

Box 18.3   *The Kruskal–Wallis test and 'analysis of variance'*

The Kruskal–Wallis test is sometimes described as a 'one-way analysis of variance by ranks'. Similarly, the Friedman test, discussed in Section 18.1.8, is sometimes referred to as a 'two-way analysis of variance by ranks' (Siegel and Castellan, 1988). However, we will reserve the term 'analysis of variance' for the parametric procedures (ANOVA) to which it is most commonly applied. This is for four reasons. First, the assumptions underlying ANOVA procedures are very different from those of their non-parametric counterparts; this may be overlooked if these two types of procedure are given a common description. Second, the notion of variance applies to mean values (Section 12.4.3). However, the Kruskal–Wallis and Friedman tests operate on sample medians, not sample means. Third, the test statistic in ANOVA procedures is a variance ratio (hence 'analysis of variance'). This is not the basis on which the test statistic of either the Kruskal–Wallis or the Friedman test is generated. Finally, it is theoretically possible to carry out a one-way ANOVA or a repeated measures ANOVA on data that have previously been converted to ranks. Such procedures, which would not be equivalent to the Kruskal–Wallis and Friedman tests, would more properly merit the description 'analysis of variance by ranks'.

Research hypothesis

A possible research hypothesis is that patients who set goals collaboratively with a therapist will be more compliant with respect to their home exercise sessions than those who either have no goals or have the goals imposed by a therapist. In this example, adherence is measured on an ordinal scale, rather than on an interval scale in terms of percentage adherence (as was the case in Section 18.1.2).

Data

The data comprise values associated with unrelated cases in three or more groups. For example, scores from 1 to 5 might be obtained that reflect patients' adherence to home exercise sessions (with 1 denoting 'very poor adherence',

through to 5 denoting 'very good adherence') for 75 patients randomly assigned to three goal-setting approaches. These data are summarized in Table 18.6 and depicted in a bar chart in Figure 18.5.

Assumptions

The assumptions for the Kruskal–Wallis test are:

- The data constitute values of cases in three or more groups independently drawn from their respective populations; or the data constitute values of cases independently drawn from one population

Table 18.6 *Adherence scores for performing home exercise sessions under different goal setting approaches. Figures are numbers of patients (%) in each group*

| Goal-setting approach | Adherence score | | | | |
	1 (very poor)	2 (poor)	3 (moderate)	4 (good)	5 (very good)
None set	0 (0)	0 (0)	7 (28)	10 (40)	8 (32)
Therapist set	0 (0)	6 (24)	10 (40)	8 (32)	1 (4)
Collaboratively set	0 (0)	3 (12)	4 (16)	15 (60)	3 (12)

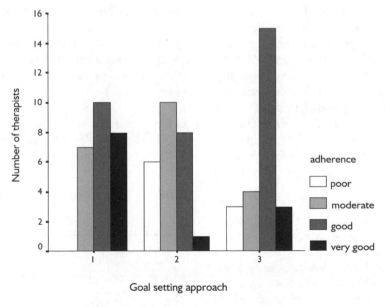

Figure 18.5 *Adherence scores for home exercise sessions under different goal-setting approaches. 1 = none; 2 = therapist; 3 = collaborative.*

with random assignment to three or more groups.
- The data are measured on at least an ordinal scale.

Checking the assumptions

The assumptions are checked by reference to the sampling method and details of the employed measurement tool. In the home exercise example, patients were randomly assigned to groups and adherence was measured on an ordinal scale of 1 to 5.

Statistical hypotheses

The null hypothesis states that the populations have equal median values, whereas the alternative hypothesis states that the populations have different medians. In the home exercise example, the null hypothesis might be that there is no difference in population median adherence scores for patients motivated by no goals, goals set by a therapist, and goals set collaboratively. The alternative hypothesis is that the median score is different for at least one of the approaches.

Rationale for test

Interest is centred on the comparisons of median scores across three or more groups. Data from the groups are jointly ordered from smallest to largest and the values are assigned ranks without regard to group membership – the smallest value is assigned a rank of 1, the next smallest a rank of 2, and so forth. There is a slight modification to the rank assigned to equal values (ties) but this does not affect the rationale of the test. When the population median values are equal, each group will contain a mixture of low through to high ranks. When there is a difference in the population median values, at least one group will be associated with more than its fair share of low ranks or high ranks. The Kruskal–Wallis test determines whether the observed disparity in ranks across groups is unlikely to have occurred by chance, when the populations have equal median values.

Results and their interpretation

For each group, the sample size, median, minimum and maximum outcome values are reported. The p value and test statistic (H or χ^2) are also reported (see Note 4 under 'Other comments' below).

The p value is used to make a statistical decision, with values less than or equal to the chosen significance level leading to rejection of the null hypothesis (Section 13.4.7) and a conclusion that there is evidence to doubt the assumption of equal median values in the populations.

From the results in Table 18.7 and using a significance level of .05, a p value of .0026 indicates rejection of the null hypothesis. Based on this study, there is evidence to doubt the assumption that the median adherence scores are the same for the three goal-setting approaches. Further analysis is necessary to determine more about these differences.

Further analyses

Most statistical computing packages do not provide options for nonparametric multiple comparisons. Siegel and Castellan (1988), Portney and Watkins (1993), Pett (1997) and Conover (1999) discuss methods that can be performed manually. Alternatively, if the significance level is adjusted for multiple testing (Box 18.2), a series of Wilcoxon rank sum tests (Section 14.2.6) can be performed on every pair of groups.

Other comments

1. The Kruskal–Wallis test is equivalent to the Wilcoxon rank sum test and the Mann–

Table 18.7 *Comparison of adherence scores when home exercise is motivated by different goal-setting approaches*

Goal-setting approach	Median (min, max)
None set	4.0 (3.0, 5.0)
Therapist set	3.0 (2.0, 5.0)
Collaboratively set	4.0 (2.0, 5.0)

$\chi^2 = 11.9$; $p = .0026$.

Whitney U test (Section 14.2.6) when there are two groups.

2. The test is fairly insensitive to a few tied ranks (more than one case with the same value). However, the power of the test diminishes as the number of ties increases, and so a modified statistic is recommended (Siegel and Castellan, 1988; Conover, 1999). Most statistical computing packages automatically compute a modified or adjusted statistic.

3. In theory, the test is appropriate for ordinal scales containing two or more options. However, a chi-square test (Section 14.1.1) might be considered when the number of response options is two or three.

4. The H statistic is reported when there are three groups and five or fewer cases per group. The χ^2 statistic is usually reported when there are more than five cases in any group, or more than three groups (Siegel and Castellan, 1988; Conover, 1999).

5. When the assumptions are met for the one-way ANOVA, the relative efficiency of Kruskal-Wallis is about 95% and is always at least 86% (Conover, 1999). Under certain circumstances, the relative efficiency is vastly higher than 100% (Conover, 1999).

6. The *Jonckheere test* for ordered alternatives (also referred to as the 'Jonkheere-Terpstra' or 'Terpstra-Jonkheere' test) is applicable when the alternative hypothesis refers to a unidirectional association between population median values; for example, median performance values might progressively decrease as the dosage of a particular drug increases. This test, unlike the Kruskal–Wallis test, requires there to be an equal number of cases in each group. Details are given in Neave and Worthington (1988), Siegel and Castellan (1988), and Hicks (1999).

18.1.6 One-way repeated measures analysis of variance

Most research in health care involves studying people. In a one-way between-subjects design (Section 18.1.2), participants are allocated randomly to treatments so that each person is allocated to one treatment only and each treatment is assigned to several participants. This feature leads to a potential disadvantage of the design. People are individuals, with different physiology, psychological characteristics, experiences and training, which means that responses to the same treatment might show a large variability by virtue of these differences across individuals. This variability contributes to the experimental error against which differences between treatment effects are judged. An inflated experimental error leads to an insensitive test on the treatment effects.

One method of controlling for the variability between people is to observe every person under each of the treatments or different conditions. Each person acts as his or her own control and has repeated measurements recorded. In this type of design, responses across the different treatments can be compared for each person and, hence, the variability across people is eliminated from the experimental error. This is called a *repeated measures* or *within-subjects* design. Figure 18.6 shows the partitioning of the total variation in outcome values.

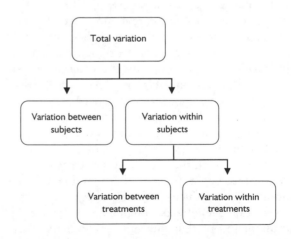

Figure 18.6 *Partitioning of the total variation in outcome values for a repeated measures design with one within-subjects factor.*

The repeated measures design is particularly useful for investigating the impact of a treatment over time. For example, short-term and longer-term effects of a hospital-based self-management programme might be investigated through scores on an arthritis self-efficacy scale recorded, say, prior to, 4 weeks after, 1 year after and 2 years after completion of a programme. Similarly, in the Low Back Pain Study, scores on the Aberdeen Back Pain Scale were recorded for a group of patients prior to, 1 week after and 12 weeks after completion of an individual-based cognitive-behavioural approach to the management of low back pain.

A repeated measures design is also used to investigate how people respond under different conditions, where each person is exposed to every condition. For example, levels and duration of pain experienced by women with benign breast cancer might be studied under different drug regimens; the effects of different stimulation parameters might be compared in a study of transcutaneous nerve stimulation for individuals with chronic back pain; or three different wrist splints might be assessed in terms of their ability to permit pain-free functional activity of the hand. Since repeated measures designs typically require far fewer participants, they are also useful when investigating treatments for rare conditions or when there is a scarcity of potential participants.

However, there are some problems associated with this type of design (see the discussion of crossover trials in Section 7.3.2). Successive outcome values might be influenced by fatigue, memory, boredom, practice effects (Table 7.2), carry-over effects, or order effects (Section 7.3.2). In many applications, careful choice of the time interval between different treatments or conditions might prevent these problems from occurring or reduce their effects to a negligible level. Practice effects, might be overcome by training the participants in a preliminary phase of the study. In other situations, it might be feasible to choose a design (for example, a crossover design; Section 7.3.2) that permits these nuisance effects to be separated from the

treatment effects during the data analysis; more details are given in Winer *et al.* (1991). The choice of a strategy requires these aspects to be considered thoroughly during the early stages of the study.

Research hypothesis
Typical research hypotheses address comparisons between the effects of different conditions, or changes on some measure of ability or performance over time. For example, self-reported impact of low back pain on health is reduced following participation in a particular rehabilitation programme and, as a separate secondary hypothesis, this reduction is maintained for at least three months.

Data
The data comprise repeated values for every participant, with measurements recorded under at least three different conditions or treatments, or on at least three successive time intervals. For example, scores on the Aberdeen Back Pain Scale were recorded for participants prior to, 1 week after and 12 weeks after completion of a particular rehabilitation programme. These data are summarized in Table 18.8 and depicted in Figure 18.7.

Model
For the rehabilitation example, the model can be expressed as follows (see also Appendix II):

Table 18.8 *Summary of Aberdeen Back Pain Scale scores for participants who responded before, 1 week after and 12 weeks after the rehabilitation programme*

Time	*n*	Mean (s.d.)	Minimum	Maximum
Before the programme	62	40.91 (2.09)	36.1	46.3
1 week after the programme	53	39.49 (2.34)	33.0	47.0
12 weeks after the programme	48	39.64 (2.46)	33.3	45.9

s.d. = standard deviation.

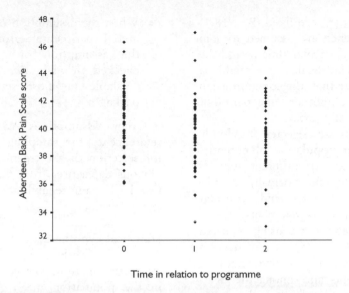

Figure 18.7 *Aberdeen Back Pain Scale scores for participants allocated to an individual-based rehabilitation programme. 0 = Before the programme (n = 62); 1 = 1 week post-programme (n = 53); 2 = 12 weeks post-programme (n = 48).*

Aberdeen Back Pain = mean value unique to the
Scale score   particular time period
                  before/after rehabilitation
                + an effect unique to the
                  individual participant
                + an effect unique to the
                  combination of that
                  individual and that
                  particular time period
                + error

and

mean value   = a mean value common
unique to particular   to all time periods (and
time period before/   participants)
after rehabilitation   + an effect unique to the
                  particular time period
                  before/after rehabilita-
                  tion

The interested reader may wish to refer to Winer *et al.* (1991) or Howell (1997) for a more complete discussion of this model. The term 'an effect unique to the combination of that individual and that particular time period' is called an *interaction* and reflects the inconsistency of indi-

viduals' scores across the different time periods. Interactions are discussed in more detail in Section 18.1.9. The important point here is that the interaction term is indistinguishable from the experimental error term. This does not change the statistical test on differences between treatment effects, but no test can be made concerning interaction effects; this leads to the first of the assumptions given below. This assumption is worth remembering when choosing this design and when interpreting results following its use.

Assumptions
The usual assumptions for the one-way repeated measures ANOVA are:

• There is no interaction between subjects and treatments; i.e. there is a consistent pattern of Aberdeen Back Pain Scale scores across time for all participants.
• The experimental error terms are independently and normally distributed, with mean zero and constant variance with respect to treatments.

- Treatment effects (τ_j) are fixed (Box 18.1) and for convenience are assumed to sum to zero; i.e. at a particular time period the Aberdeen Back Pain Scale score might be consistently higher than the common mean score, whereas at another time period it might be consistently lower.
- The participants are selected randomly from some larger population of potential subjects; the effects of different subjects are independently and normally distributed, with mean zero and constant variance with respect to treatments.
- Circularity (or sphericity): using repeated measures on each participant introduces a dependency among the outcome values for different treatments and among the treatment populations; circularity is the necessary (and sufficient) assumption about these dependencies for the statistical tests to be valid. Further details can be found in Hays (1988) and Winer *et al.* (1991).
- The data are measured on an interval or ratio scale.

Checking the assumptions

Many of the assumptions are routinely checked using graphs:

- A visual check (albeit somewhat crude) on the assumption of no interaction is provided by plotting outcome values against each condition or time point for each participant; if the patterns across conditions or time points are similar for all participants the assumption of no interaction appears tenable – what constitutes 'similar' is open to debate. More formal tests are described in Winer *et al.* (1991).
- Most statistical computing packages provide estimates of the experimental error terms, called 'residuals'. A straight line appearance to a normal probability plot of the residuals casts no doubt on the assumption of normally distributed experimental errors (Box 14.3). Normal probability plots are commonly available in statistical computing packages.

- When the assumption of normally distributed experimental errors is not doubted, the assumption of circularity can be checked through *Mauchly's test*. This is available in most statistical computing packages.

Other assumptions can be checked by reference to the sampling method and criteria for selection of the treatments. There were no obvious departures from the assumptions in the low back pain rehabilitation example, and no extreme values.

Statistical hypotheses

The null hypothesis states that the treatment effects are all zero, that is, there is no difference in the population mean Aberdeen Back Pain Scale score (μ_k) at the three time periods before and after the rehabilitation programme. The alternative hypothesis is that at least one effect is non-zero, or a difference exists between the population mean Aberdeen Back Pain Scale scores for at least two of the time periods. In terms of symbols, these might be written as:

$$H_0: \tau_1 = \tau_2 = \tau_3 = 0$$
$$H_1: \tau_j \neq 0 \text{ for at least one } j$$

or

$$H_0: \mu_1 = \mu_2 = \mu_3 = \mu$$
$$H_1: \mu_k \neq \mu_j \text{ for some } k, j$$

Since primary interest is on testing treatment or time effects, it is very unusual to perform a statistical test on the differences *between* subjects. In fact, these are expected to be large – hence the use of a repeated measures design to eliminate variability due to subjects from the experimental error.

Rationale for test

The rationale follows a similar argument to that for one-way ANOVA, but acknowledges that variation between treatments and variation within treatments are components of the variation within subjects (Figure 18.6). For example, comparisons of the effect of a rehabilitation programme can be made across three time periods for each participant who completed all three assessments on the Aberdeen Back Pain Scale.

Assuming no interaction exists between subjects and treatments, variation between treatments is due to differences between the effects of the different treatments and unassignable sources of error. Variation within treatments is due to unassignable sources of error. Hence, a ratio of mean square between-treatments variance to mean square within-treatments variance provides a test on the null hypothesis of no treatment effects. This ratio follows a Fisher's F distribution when the specified assumptions are met.

Results and their interpretation

It is usual to present summaries of the data for each treatment, condition or point in time. Table 18.9 shows the number of participants, mean and standard deviation of Aberdeen Back Pain Scale scores at the three time points and 95% confidence intervals for the population mean Aberdeen Back Pain Scale score at each time point. These are displayed in Figure 18.8. The confidence intervals might be useful when gauging the importance of any observed differences.

The results of the ANOVA are reported in the customary ANOVA table (Table 18.10). A brief explanation of components of an ANOVA table is given in Section 18.1.9.

The p value is used to make a statistical

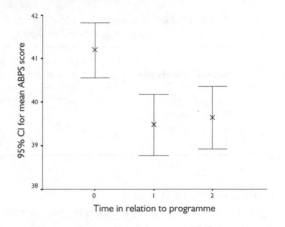

Figure 18.8 Estimates for the mean (X) and 95% confidence intervals (bars) for the Aberdeen Back Pain Scale (ABPS) score for those participants allocated to an individual-based rehabilitation programme who completed assessment at all three time points (n = 48). 0 = Before the programme; 1 = 1 week post-programme; 2 = 12 weeks post-programme.

decision about the null hypothesis, with a decision to reject being made for p values less than or equal to the chosen significance level. From the results in Table 18.10 and using a significance level of .05, the null hypothesis is rejected ($F = 33.83$, p value $< .0005$). Based on this study, there is evidence to doubt the assumption that mean Aberdeen Back Pain Scale scores are the same before, 1 week after and 12 weeks after a rehabilitation programme. These differences are explored through further analyses.

Table 18.9 Summary and 95% confidence intervals for mean Aberdeen Back Pain Scale score before, 1 week after and 12 weeks after a rehabilitation programme, for participants who completed assessment at all three time points

Time point	n	Mean (s.d.)	95% confidence interval for mean Aberdeen Back Pain Scale score
Before rehabilitation	48	41.20 (2.20)	40.56 to 41.84
1 week after rehabilitation	48	39.47 (2.42)	38.77 to 40.18
12 weeks after rehabilitation	48	39.64 (2.46)	38.92 to 40.35

s.d. = standard deviation.

Table 18.10 ANOVA table for Aberdeen Back Pain Scale scores (one-way repeated measures ANOVA)

Source of variation	Degrees of freedom	Sum of squares	Mean square	Variance ratio	p value
Between subjects	47	669.27	–	–	–
Between time points	2	86.88	43.44	33.83	< .0005
Within time points	94	120.69	1.28		
Total	143	876.84			

Further analyses or statistics

A posteriori contrasts are usually performed when the variance ratio in the ANOVA table is statistically significant. Some authors (Hays, 1988; Portney and Watkins, 1993; Howell, 1997) recommend using a modified version of Tukey's honestly significant difference procedure for determining groupings of mean outcomes for which differences within groupings are consistent with chance expectancies, and differences between groupings are greater than expected by chance. This modification uses the feature of correlated outcomes to produce more powerful tests. It involves computing separate estimates of the variation owing to experimental error for every pair of treatments, conditions or time points of interest. Examples are given in Hays (1988), Portney and Watkins (1993) and Howell (1997).

Other contrasts that might be available in statistical computing packages include Helmert and reverse Helmert (SPSS, 1999). In Helmert contrasts, successive comparisons are formed with subsequent mean effects, defined according to the specified ordering of the factor levels. For example, in a study involving repeated measures at four points in time with associated effects denoted by T1, T2, T3 and T4, Helmert contrasts would represent:

- T1 compared with the mean of (T2, T3 and T4)
- T2 compared with the mean of (T3 and T4)
- T3 compared with T4

Reverse Helmert forms successive comparisons with previous mean effects, for example:

- T1 compared with T2
- Mean of (T1 and T2) compared with T3
- Mean of (T1, T2 and T3) compared with T4

Such comparisons may not be meaningful from a practical perspective and need to be interpreted with care.

In the rehabilitation example, Helmert contrasts indicated that the mean Aberdeen Back Pain Scale score averaged over 1 week and 12 weeks following the programme was significantly lower than the mean Aberdeen Back Pain Scale score before the programme ($p < .0005$; $n = 48$; 95% confidence interval for the mean decrease 1.21 to 2.07). However, no significant difference was found between mean Aberdeen Back Pain Scale score at 1 week and at 12 weeks after the programme ($p = .46$; $n = 48$; 95% confidence interval for the mean difference -0.60 to 0.39). Hence, there is evidence that Aberdeen Back Pain Scale score is lowered by the programme and that this lower level is maintained up to 12 weeks after the programme.

Other comments

1. Unless the nature of the conditions or treatments dictates a specific ordering, the treatments are administered in a random order, with a separate randomization for each participant (Winer et al., 1991).
2. Violation of the assumption of homogeneity of variance does not seriously bias results from the F test for between-subject designs (e.g. completely randomized designs).

However, in a repeated measures design, violation of circularity (homogeneity of variance and of covariance) generally leads to biased results and a higher chance of statistical significance. An adjustment factor is used to correct for the bias. It is applied to the degrees of freedom ascribed to the variance ratio for the purpose of making the statistical decision (Hays, 1988; Portney and Watkins 1993; Howell, 1997).

3. In general, no statistical test is performed on differences between subjects in a one-way repeated measures design, although many statistical computing packages include them in the printed ANOVA table. Such tests rarely provide useful information, since a large between-subjects difference is anticipated anyway. Further, the validity of the test is dependent upon the assumption of no interaction between subjects and treatments and, therefore, its interpretation might be questionable.

4. Repeated measures analyses face problems when sample sizes are unequal across treatments, conditions or times.

5. This section has considered a one-way repeated measures ANOVA involving three points in time. Data from participants who did not complete the Aberdeen Back Pain Scale on all three occasions were excluded from the analysis. This is called a *per protocol* analysis and it might have introduced a bias in the results. Alternative analyses are considered in Section 18.2.

6. The statistical test on treatment effects represents a comparison of mean outcome values across the treatments and is valid whether or not an interaction effect exists between the subjects and the treatments. In the simple one-way repeated measures design analysed in this section, the interaction effects are confounded with experimental error and, therefore, cannot be tested for statistical significance. However, a non-zero interaction indicates an inconsistency across subjects for outcome values associated with each treatment. Hence, inferences drawn from the statistical test on treatment effects might be misleading when a strong interaction actually exists (Section 18.1.9).

Alternative procedures

1. A technique called *multivariate analysis of variance* (MANOVA) is used to analyse data from a repeated measures design when the assumption of sphericity is doubted. This analyses multiple outcome measures (i.e. more than one) simultaneously. The reader is referred to Tabachnik and Fidell (1996) for details.

2. The Friedman test might be used when the assumptions of a one-way repeated measures ANOVA are not met (Section 18.1.8).

3. A repeated measures design is inappropriate when, for example, carry-over or practice effects are important and cannot be eliminated. A randomized block design or a matched-subject design might be a suitable alternative in these situations (Section 18.1.7).

4. Between-subject variability might be reduced by introducing into the model (and hence the analysis) variables that represent measured characteristics that are known to influence the outcome values and are different across the participants. This is called *analysis of covariance* (ANCOVA; Section 18.5).

18.1.7 Randomized block design and matched-subjects design

The analysis of one-way completely randomized designs was considered in Section 18.1.2. In these designs, comparisons are made across groups of participants; each participant is randomly allocated to one group and each treatment is allotted to one group. Routinely, each group contains the same number of participants. To some extent, outcome values are dependent upon which participants are assigned to which treatment. However, the process of random allocation tries to ensure that there are no systematic differences in characteristics of participants between the groups, so that differences across participants are not confounded with any systematic variation due to the imposed treatments. In this way, any statistically significant between-group differences found in the analysis may be ascribed to treatment effects. However, the statistical test is performed by comparing between-group variance to within-group variance (Section 18.1.2), and the latter might be inflated by the effects of individual participant differences. A one-way repeated measures design tries to control for differences across participants by observing every participant under each of the treatments or conditions. This has the advantage that comparisons between treatment effects can be made for each participant; i.e. a within-subjects analysis (Section 18.1.6). The statistical test is performed by comparing between-treatment variance to within-treatment variance. If the individual characteristics of participants have a large influence on outcome values, the one-way repeated measures design will provide a more powerful test on treatment effects than a completely randomized design.

There are, however, many situations in which it is impractical to measure outcomes on one person under several treatments or conditions (Sections 7.3.2 and 18.1.6). The randomized block design and the matched-subjects design are alternative designs that control between-subject variability when outcomes are measured under one treatment or condition for each participant.

Randomized block designs

A randomized block design uses groupings of participants who are similar in each grouping on characteristics that influence outcome values. Such groupings are usually called *blocks*, which derives from the original use of this design in agriculture, where 'blocks' refer to plots of land. Participants within each block are randomly allocated to treatment groups in equal numbers (Section 7.2.2). Usually, the number of participants in a block equals the number of treatments. Assuming that the important characteristics have been correctly identified and are measurable at the recruitment stage, this

strategy should result in small within-block variability and large between-block variability. Further, comparisons between treatment effects can be made within each block. Therefore, total variation in outcome values can be partitioned into between-block variation and within-block variation. In addition, variation within blocks comprises variation between treatments and variation within treatments (Figure 18.9). Hence, the statistical test on treatment effects is performed by comparing between-treatment variance to within-treatment variance. This is comparable with the procedure discussed for a one-way repeated measures design.

Data from a randomized block design are frequently analysed by making use of the calculations within a two-way ANOVA (Section 18.1.9), with the added assumptions of no interaction between blocks and treatments, and fixed effects for the blocks. This suggested approach to the analysis produces a valid test of differences between the treatment effects and valid estimates, when the between-block differences are a nuisance rather than a prime interest in a study (Daniel, 1991; Winer *et al.*, 1991; Armitage and Berry, 1994). No test is performed on block effects.

The randomized block design provides a more powerful test on differences between treatment

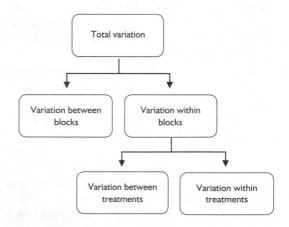

Figure 18.9 *Partitioning of the total variation in outcome values for a randomized block design, and for a matched-subject design, with 'block' taken to denote 'set'.*

effects than a completely randomized design when characteristics are chosen appropriately (Montgomery, 1991).

The design and analysis are expressed in the following model for outcome values (see also Appendix II):

outcome value = mean outcome value unique to a particular treatment (or condition)
+ a unique effect of a particular block
+ experimental error

and

mean outcome value unique to a particular treatment (or condition) = mean outcome value common to all treatments
+ a unique effect of the particular treatment

Matched-subject designs

Matched-subject designs attempt to control between-subject differences by using sets of participants who are matched, in each set, on characteristics that influence outcome values (Section 7.2.2). Although matching implies a greater degree of equivalence than blocking (Section 7.2.2), these sets of matched participants are analogous to the blocks of participants used in a randomized block design. The number of participants in a set equals the number of treatments or conditions. Participants within a set are randomly allocated to a treatment group, so that each treatment is used once in each set. The discussion of the rationale for the randomized block design holds for the matched-subject design. Similarly, Figure 18.9 illustrates the logic of the analysis, with the term 'block' read as 'set'.

Unfortunately, finding matches even on one characteristic might prove to be laborious, time consuming and expensive (Hays, 1988). Further, many potential participants might be excluded from the study if insufficient matched subjects are available or willing to participate. Although the within-block variability in a randomized block design is likely to be larger than the within-set variability for a corresponding matched-subjects design, the randomized block is a more realistic design as it allows groupings on similar characteristics.

Other comments

1. Some researchers use the term 'matched-subjects' to describe studies that match important characteristics across *all* participants (Keppel and Saufley, 1980). In general, such studies constitute a completely randomized design and use a set of potential participants who satisfy very select inclusion criteria – thereby greatly restricting any generalization of findings (this is essentially the process of *specification* referred to in Section 7.2.2). In general, this design might not be of practical use.
2. Other techniques exist to account for differences between subjects. Analysis of covariance is one such frequently used technique, and is briefly discussed in Section 18.5.

18.1.8 Friedman test

The Friedman test is a nonparametric equivalent to one-way repeated measures, randomized blocks or matched-subjects ANOVA (discussed in Sections 18.1.6 and 18.1.7). It is used when the assumptions underlying the parametric statistical tests are not met, or when the outcome variable has an ordinal level of measurement. The Friedman test is sometimes called a 'two-way analysis of variance by ranks' (but see Box 18.3). Basically, the test determines whether differences between median outcome values measured under different treatments or conditions are greater than would be expected by chance. The sets of data compared might arise in one of three situations:

1. One group of subjects might be measured on one outcome variable under three or more conditions.
2. Three or more groups of subjects who had been randomly allocated from blocks might be measured on one outcome variable.
3. Three or more groups of matched subjects might be measured on one outcome variable.

The design might be represented by a two-way table with different conditions in the columns and different subjects, blocks or matched sets in the rows.

Discussion of the technique is based on data from the survey in the Rheumatoid Arthritis Study. In one of the questions, therapists were asked to indicate their level of endorsement of several statements concerning the management of these patients. A five-point Likert scale was used, ranging from 1 ('strongly disagree') through to 5 ('strongly agree'). This exemplifies the first of the situations described in the preceding paragraph.

Research question

In this example, the researcher wishes to know: does the therapists' level of endorsement differ across these statements? Note that the comparison is between the statements (conditions), not between the therapists (cases).

Data

The data are classified according to two variables: (1) cases (therapists), and (2) conditions under which the measurement was taken (statements). Data from 117 therapists are summarized in Table 18.11 and depicted in Figure 18.10. The bar chart clearly indicates differences in ratings between the statements.

Assumptions

The assumptions for the Friedman test are:

- Data from a particular case are independent of the data within any other case.
- The data are measured on at least an ordinal scale.

Checking the assumptions

The assumptions are checked by reference to the measurement tool employed and the two variables with respect to which the data are classified (cases and conditions). In this example from the Rheumatoid Arthritis Study, use of a Likert scale produces data at an ordinal level of measurement. The data are classified by therapist (case) and statement (condition) – each respondent rated every statement. The therapists represent a random sample of therapists who treat or manage patients with rheumatoid arthritis; hence, the first assumption is met.

Statistical hypotheses

The null hypothesis might be worded in terms of median values. In the Rheumatoid Arthritis Study example, the null hypothesis is that the median agreement rating is the same for each of the four attitude statements. The alternative hypothesis is that the median rating is different for at least one statement.

Table 18.11 *Therapists' ratings on four statements with respect to patients with rheumatoid arthritis (n = 117). Data in the table are number of therapists (with percentages in parentheses)*

| Statement | Rating | | | | |
	Strongly disagree	Disagree	Neither	Agree	Strongly agree
1 Restoring function is more important than treating pain	4 (3)	13 (11)	27 (23)	64 (55)	9 (8)
2 Treatment must not aggravate the patient's pain	0 (0)	1 (1)	22 (19)	55 (47)	39 (33)
3 These patients are generally well informed on their condition	3 (3)	62 (53)	34 (29)	18 (15)	0 (0)
4 In general, these patients need a lot of encouragement to participate in therapy	2 (2)	9 (8)	82 (70)	19 (16)	5 (4)

Rationale

The objective is to compare median scores across conditions. Ranks are assigned to the data from each case: the smallest value from each case is assigned a rank of 1, the next smallest value from each case is assigned a rank of 2, and so forth. There is a modification to the rank assigned to equal values (ties) but this does not affect the rationale of the test. If the population under each condition has the same median value, then approximately equal numbers of each rank will appear against each condition. If there is a difference in the median values, then at least one condition will be associated with more than its fair share of low ranks (e.g. 1's or 2's) or high ranks (e.g. 4's or 5's). The Friedman test determines whether the disparity in ranks between the conditions is unlikely to have occurred by chance when the population has the same median value against each condition.

Results and their interpretation

The median, minimum and maximum outcome values are reported for each condition. The sample size, χ^2 value and p value are also reported.

The p value is used to make a statistical decision about the null hypothesis, with a decision to reject being made for p values less than or equal to the chosen significance level. From the results in Table 18.12 and using a significance level of .05, the null hypothesis is rejected (p value $< .0005$). There is evidence to doubt the assumption that therapists equally rate the four statements. Further analysis is needed to identify where most disagreement exists.

Further analyses or statistics

The bar chart in Figure 18.10 provides quite a clear picture of the differences in opinion across the statements for these data, but comparisons will not always be so simple. By using multiple comparisons, it is possible to identify groupings with significantly different median values, or groupings for which the median values are not significantly different. Techniques for these comparisons are given in Siegel and Castellan (1988), Portney and Watkins (1993), Pett (1997), Sheldon *et al.* (1996), and Conover (1999), but these are not available in most statistical computing packages.

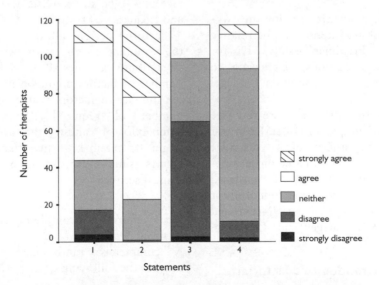

Figure 18.10 *Therapists' ratings on four statements with respect to patients with rheumatoid arthritis (n = 117). Statements are: (1) 'Restoring function is more important than treating pain'; (2) 'Treatment must not aggravate the patient's pain'; (3) 'These patients are generally well informed on their condition'; and (4) 'In general, these patients need a lot of encouragement to participate in therapy'.*

Table 18.12 *Comparison of therapist ratings on four statements with respect to patients with rheumatoid arthritis (n = 117)*

Statement	Median (min, max)
1 Restoring function is more important than treating pain	4 (1, 5)
2 Treatment must not aggravate the patient's pain	4 (2, 5)
3 These patients are generally well informed on their condition	2 (1, 4)
4 In general, these patients need a lot of encouragement to participate in therapy	3 (1, 5)

min = minimum value; max = maximum value;
$\chi^2 = 146.0$; p < .0005.

Other comments

1. The Friedman test is appropriate for comparing median values across two groups when the paired cases within each group are measured on an ordinal scale.
2. Most statistical computing packages compute a modified statistic when there are ties in the data (more than one case with the same value).
3. When the assumptions are met for the two-way ANOVA with no interaction, the relative efficiency of the Friedman test is 64% for two groups (or conditions), increasing to 91% for 20 groups (or conditions) (Siegel and Castellan, 1988).
4. In the same way that the Jonkheere test (see 'Other comments' in Section 18.1.5) can test the alternative hypothesis of a particular order in the medians of three or more independent sets of data, *Page's test* for ordered alternatives performs the same function for matched or repeated sets of data (Neave and Worthington, 1988; Siegel and Castellan, 1988; Hicks, 1999).

18.1.9 Completely randomized factorial designs

The designs discussed in previous sections of this chapter involved one factor with two or more levels. These simple designs are appropriate when

a researcher wishes to investigate the effects of treatments created by the manipulation of one variable; for example, the effect of type of exercise on adherence to the exercise regimen. Similarly, a researcher might wish to determine whether respondents in a survey differ with respect to subgroups classified in terms of one attribute; for example, difference in self-reported anxiety levels according to type of arthritis. However, a number of important research questions concern the combined influence of more than one factor or attribute. Factorial designs have an important role here. In Section 7.3.1, it was suggested that, in the Low Back Pain Study, Dr Buckley might have wished to investigate two questions: (1) Is group or individual cognitive-behavioural therapy more effective? (2) Should the duration of the treatment programme be 1, 2 or 3 weeks? Such a study is investigating two factors – mode of delivery of the programme and duration of the programme (see Table 7.3). To take another example, a researcher might wish to investigate how type of exercise, the length of each session, and number of sessions per week affect adherence. This involves three factors – type of exercise, duration of session, and frequency of session.

Factorial designs allow a researcher to study the simultaneous effects of two or more factors or attribute variables (Box 18.4). In theory, any number of factors might be investigated, but as the number of factors is increased so too is the number of required participants and the complexity of running the study. Typically, it might be feasible to investigate two or three factors simultaneously in a study within a clinical setting.

Basic features of a completely randomized factorial design

A completely randomized factorial design satisfies the following characteristics:

- It studies the simultaneous effects of two or more factors.
- The treatments comprise all combinations of levels of the factors:

Box 18.4 *The Solomon four-group design*

A specific application of the factorial design that can be used to investigate testing effects (Table 7.2) is the *Solomon four-group design* (Spector, 1981). Here, one factor is the intervention being tested (e.g. treatment A versus treatment B), and the other factor is the presence or absence of a pre-test. Two of the study groups receive treatment A, one with a pre-test and one without a pre-test. The other two groups receive treatment B, again one with and one without a pre-test. All groups receive a post-test. Using this design, the researcher can determine whether a testing effect is present, and if so whether it interacts with the interventions being evaluated.

- every level of a factor is associated (*crossed*) with every combination of levels of all other factors
- each treatment is unique (i.e. the content of each treatment is distinct from that of all others).
- Participants are randomly allocated to groups:
  - the groups comprise equal numbers of participants
  - the number of groups is equal to the number of treatments.
- Treatments are randomly allocated to groups; there are equal numbers of replicates on every treatment.

A completely randomized factorial design can be described according to:

1. The number of factors; for example, a two-way or two-factor design involves two factors and a three-way or three-factor design involves three factors, and so forth.
2. The number of levels associated with each factor; for example, a 2 × 3 design includes a factor with two levels and a factor with three levels, a 2 × 3 × 4 includes a factor with two levels, a factor with three levels and a factor with four levels. A 2 × 2 × 3 design is sometimes written as a $2^2 \times 3$ design (Graziano and Raulin, 1993).

Since the treatments comprise all combinations of levels of the factors, the second descriptor also provides the number of treatments considered. For example, a 2 × 3 design involves six treatments.

Main effects

The following simple, hypothetical study will serve to illustrate the information obtained through use of a factorial design. A small study was performed in a child psychiatry unit to investigate whether anxiety was affected by the size and wall colour of a room in which clinical assessment interviews were conducted. Anxiety levels were measured following participation in a standardized interview and are given below (Table 18.13). Participants were randomly allocated to rooms of varying size (small or medium) and wall colour (yellow, green or blue). There were 18 participants, of whom six were interviewed in a room with each wall colour, nine were interviewed in a room of each size, and three were interviewed in a room of each combination of colour and size. As there are six possible combinations of room size and wall colour, this is the total number of interventions tested in the design. This demonstrates a feature of two-way completely randomized factorial designs; the levels of one factor (room

Table 18.13 *Anxiety levels in a hypothetical study involving a 2 × 3 design. Data in the table are anxiety scores for individual children, where 3 children were interviewed in a room of each combination of colour and size*

| | | Wall colour | | |
		Yellow	Green	Blue
	Small	10	7	4
		11	9	3
Room		9	11	8
size	Medium	11	5	8
		13	4	8
		12	6	5

size) are completely crossed with all levels of the second factor (wall colour). Hence, these designs are often called *crossed* designs (which should not be confused with *crossover* designs, as defined in Section 7.3.2).

The 18 anxiety values allow separate estimation of the effects of (1) wall colour and (2) room size. These are called *main effects* (Boniface, 1995). The main effect of room size involves a comparison of mean anxiety values for a small room (mean 8, $n = 9$) and a medium sized room (mean 8, $n = 9$). No main effect of room size is apparent in this study. The main effect of wall colour involves comparisons across mean anxiety values for rooms with yellow walls (mean 11, $n = 6$), green walls (mean 7, $n = 6$) and blue walls (mean 6, $n = 6$). Some differences are apparent across these mean values; ANOVA would determine whether such observed differences are larger than expected by chance when there are no population effects due to wall colour.

The separate main effects are estimated with precision equivalent to that which would be obtained from two separate one-way designs; a first involving 18 participants randomly allocated to the two room sizes, and a second involving 18 participants randomly allocated to the three wall colours. This approach would have required 36 participants, demonstrating a saving on time and number of required participants by employing a two-way design.

Simple effects

There is a potential difficulty when interpreting main effects. The main effect of room size entails computing a mean from the anxiety values of nine children interviewed in a small room and of nine different children interviewed in a medium-sized room. However, for each room size, three of the participants encountered yellow walls, three encountered green walls and three encountered blue walls. This balance of numbers, together with a complete crossing of factor levels, ensures that any effects due to wall colour do not affect the main effect of room size, and vice versa (a property called *orthogon-*

ality). Moreover, the main effect of room size is equivalent to a mean anxiety value computed from the three comparisons of (1) small to medium-sized yellow rooms, (2) small to medium-sized green rooms, and (3) small to medium-sized blue rooms. These separate comparisons are called *simple effects* (Boniface, 1995). When these simple effects are identical, the main effect is the same as each simple effect. A difficulty exists, however, when the simple effects are different, since main effects might not provide a complete picture of the data in this situation.

Interaction effects

We shall consider the simple effects of room size in this hypothetical study. The simple effects are given by the differences in mean anxiety values for children interviewed in rooms of different sizes but of the same wall colour. Using the information in Table 18.14, the simple effects are:

$$12 - 10 = 2 \quad \text{for yellow walls}$$
$$5 - 9 = -4 \quad \text{for green walls}$$
$$7 - 5 = 2 \quad \text{for blue walls}$$

There is an increase in mean anxiety of two units when an interview takes place in a medium compared with a small room, when the walls are yellow or blue. The effect of a change in room size is the same for yellow and blue wall colours, i.e. the changes are consistent. However, there is a decrease of four units when an interview takes place in a medium compared with a small room when the wall colour is green. The effect of a change in room size is different for green walls.

Table 18.14 *Anxiety values for wall colour, room size, and combinations of wall colour and room size. Data in the table are mean values*

Room size	Wall colour			Room means
	Yellow	Green	Blue	
Small	10	9	5	8
Medium	12	5	7	8
Colour means	11	7	6	

This inconsistency in the simple effects is called *interaction*. An interaction occurs when the difference in outcome value between the levels of one factor is not the same at all levels of the other factor(s). ANOVA would determine whether such observed differences are larger than expected by chance when there are no interaction effects (in the population) due to room size and wall colour.

Using graphs to consider interactions

Plots of mean outcome values are a useful way of visualizing interaction effects. The interaction between room size and wall colour is drawn

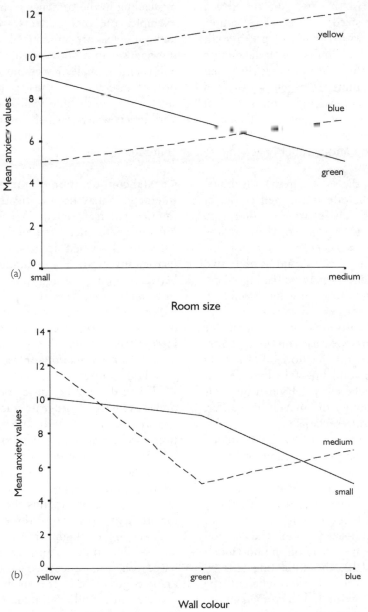

Figure 18.11   *Two plots (a and b) showing the interaction of room size and wall colour.*

from two perspectives in Figure 18.11(a) and (b).

In the previous section it was seen that the simple effects of room size with respect to yellow and blue walls were identical, with each simple effect having value = 2. This is indicated in Figure 18.11(a) by the corresponding two parallel lines that rise by two units between small and medium-sized rooms. The simple effect of room size with respect to green walls was a decrease of four units, as indicated in Figure 18.11(a) by the corresponding line that decreases by four units between small and medium-sized rooms. This line crosses (is not parallel with) the lines representing yellow and blue wall colours. In general, non parallel lines indicate an interaction and parallel lines indicate no interaction.

Figure 18.11(b) is the same interaction drawn with respect to simple effects for wall colour at different room sizes. There are two points to note here. The first is that the ordering of the colours is irrelevant, since colour is a nominal level of measurement. The second is that two types of interaction effects may be distinguished. The simple effect between yellow and green wall colours is a decrease in mean anxiety of one unit for small rooms and a decrease of seven units for medium sized rooms (i.e. as you read across from yellow to green on the horizontal axis in Figure 18.11(b), the solid line falls by one unit on the vertical axis whereas the broken line falls by seven units). Although the magnitudes differ, the direction of the difference is consistent. This is called an *ordinal* interaction. Ordinal interactions do not contradict the direction of differences given by main effects.

However, the simple effect between green and blue wall colours is a decrease in mean anxiety of four units for small rooms but an increase of two units for medium-sized rooms (i.e. as you read across from green to blue on the horizontal axis in Figure 18.11(b), the solid line falls by four units on the vertical axis whereas the broken line rises by two units). The magnitudes differ, but, more importantly, the direction of differences is contradictory. This is called a

disordinal interaction. Disordinal interactions might contradict the direction of differences given by main effects.

For either type, interactions might support a recommended treatment in a way that is not apparent from the main effects. That is, the interpretation of main effects might be very misleading in the presence of interactions. In this example, the main effects would suggest that anxiety levels are minimized when children are interviewed in a room with blue or green walls and is either small or medium in size. Consideration of interactions leads us to choose either a small room with blue walls or a medium room with green walls. A small room with green walls appears not to be so conducive to interviewing children.

General consideration of interactions

Interactions may be investigated in a completely randomized factorial design when two or more outcomes are measured under each treatment. They are described according to the number of factors involved. For example, the interaction between room size and wall colour is called a *two-factor interaction* or a *first-order interaction* (since at least two factors are required before combinations of levels have any meaning). An interaction involving three factors is called a *three-factor interaction* or *second-order interaction*, and so forth.

Hence, the number of factors in a study determines the highest-order interaction that might be considered in that study and how many interactions are possible at each lower order (Table 18.15). The estimation and testing of high-order interactions requires large sample sizes (Table 18.16), which, along with complexity of interpretation, largely explains the popular choice of including at most two or three factors in a study.

A researcher might choose not to investigate all possible interactions. A choice should be based on theoretical considerations or prior knowledge of the treatments and conditions involved in a study. Soundness of the interpretation of findings must also be considered. For example, a second-order interaction is effectively

Table 18.15 *Identification of the interactions in designs with two, three or four factors. Capital letters are used as a representation for factor names*

Number of factors	Names of factors	Order of interaction	Interactions	Total number of interactions
2	A B	First	AB	1
3	A B C	First	AB AC BC	4
		Second	ABC	
4	A B C D	First	AB AC AD BC BD CD	11
		Second	ABC ABD ACD BCD	
		Third	ABCD	

Table 18.16 *Sample size required to estimate and to test all interactions in studies with varying numbers of factors and levels per factor*

Number of levels per factor	Minimum sample size required to *estimate* all interaction effects			Minimum sample size required to *test* all interaction effects		
	Number of factors			Number of factors		
	2	3	4	2	3	4
2	4	8	16	8	16	32
3	9	27	81	18	54	162
4	16	64	256	32	128	512

a comparison across first-order interactions between two factors (e.g. A, B) computed at each level of a third factor (e.g. C). As such, the second-order interaction (ABC) comprises a systematic shift from the mean response common to all treatments additional to that explained by the first-order interactions and main effects. Hence, ABC has no meaning when all first-order interactions are excluded from the model on which the analysis is based.

Model

Data analyses are dependent upon the manner in which the data were collected and the nature of each variable in the study – i.e. the study design. A statistical model symbolizes the study design. It identifies the population parameters that can be estimated and statistically tested from data collected according to that design, subject to certain assumptions. Hence, it relates to the partitioning of the total variation (Figure 18.12

and Section 18.1.1). It also enables predictions to be made for values of the outcome variable.

For non-standard or complex designs, formulation of the statistical model at the design stage helps to prevent individual effects from being overlooked, and provides a check on the capability of the study to produce estimates of those effects germane to its aims (Daniel, 1991; Winer *et al.*, 1991).

As an example of a two-factor design, we can return to the elaboration of the Low Back Pain Study referred to in the introduction to this section. Patients with low back pain were allotted randomly to one of six exercise programmes comprising all combinations of a group-based or an individual-based programme and durations of 1, 2 or 3 weeks. Health status was recorded on the Aberdeen Back Pain Scale (ABPS) after completion of a programme.

In words, the ABPS score for a particular patient could be described as:

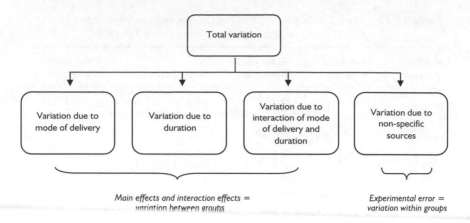

Figure 18.12 *Partitioning of variability in a completely randomized two-factor design involving different modes of delivery and different durations of a therapy programme.*

ABPS score = a mean value common to all
exercise programmes
+ effect unique to the
particular mode of delivery
+ effect unique to the
particular duration
+ effect unique to the
particular combination of
mode and duration
+ experimental error

and in symbols as given in Appendix II.

In this model, individual ABPS scores are described in terms of overall mean ABPS score, plus the effects of different influences from the controlled variables (namely, the main effects and interaction effects of mode of delivery and duration of programme), plus a component for experimental error.

Experimental error does not imply errors on the part of the experimenter. Rather, it comprises the effects from all uncontrolled influences on ABPS score, including random error, measurement error, extraneous variables and variables not specifically identified in the model. The variance due to error is central to testing effects for statistical significance and signifies how closely the model can predict ABPS score for an individual patient. Larger variances produce less sensitive tests and poorer predictions.

Partitioning of the total variability in a completely randomized factorial design

ANOVA is used to analyse the data from a factorial design. The total variability in outcome values is partitioned into between-groups and within-groups variation (Figure 18.2). The between-group variation is further partitioned into separate components reflecting each main effect and each interaction effect that the study is designed to estimate. Figure 18.12 illustrates the two-factor study elaboration of the Low Back Pain Study. Here, it will be recalled, Dr Buckley sought to test both the mode of delivery of the therapy programme (group or individual cognitive-behavioural therapy) and the duration of the programme (1, 2 or 3 weeks), as evaluated by scores on the Aberdeen Back Pain Scale (ABPS).

Assumptions required to perform valid statistical tests

The assumptions for a one-way design were specified in Section 18.1.2 and are appropriate when each population is interpreted as referring to a treatment. More generally, assumptions are made about individual effects in the model. Assumptions for the two-factor exercise study are as follows:

- The experimental error terms are identically and independently distributed, and follow a normal distribution, with mean zero and constant variance.

- There is independence between ABPS scores; i.e. an ABPS score for a participant does not affect and is not affected by the score of any other participant.
- The effects of different modes of delivery are unknown constants, and, for convenience, are assumed to sum to zero; i.e. the effect of one mode of delivery might be to consistently increase the ABPS scores to a particular value higher than the common mean ABPS score, whereas the effect of another mode of delivery might be to consistently decrease the ABPS score to a particular value lower than the common mean ABPS score.
- The effects of different duration of the programme are unknown constants, and, for convenience, are assumed to sum to zero; i.e. the effect of one duration might be to consistently increase the ABPS scores to a particular value higher than the common mean score, whereas the effect of another duration might be to consistently decrease the ABPS score to a particular value lower than the common mean ABPS score.
- The effects of different combinations of mode of delivery and duration are unknown constants, and, for convenience,

the effects are assumed to sum to zero; i.e. the effect of one combination of mode of delivery and duration might be to consistently increase the ABPS score to a particular value higher than that expected from the common mean score and the main effects of mode of delivery and duration, whereas the effect of another combination of mode of delivery and duration might be to consistently decrease the ABPS score to a particular value lower than expected from the common mean ABPS score and main effects of mode of delivery and duration.

- The underlying random phenomenon of interest (ABPS score) is continuous.
- The data are measured on an interval or ratio scale.

Analysis of variance table and statistical testing of effects

Each component in the partitioning of the total variation represents a 'source of variation' in the ANOVA table (Table 18.17). The corresponding measure of variation is called a 'sum of squares'. For example, the sum of squares due to mode of delivery is the variation of mean ABPS score associated with each mode of delivery about the common mean ABPS score across both modes of delivery. This quantity is small when there are no differences between the effects due to the different modes of delivery. The error sum of

Table 18.17 An outline ANOVA table for a two-factor design involving two different modes of delivery and three different durations of a therapy programme, and in which each intervention is assigned to r participants. The circled numbers denote the calculations that would be performed. The asterisks indicate those cells in which p values would appear

Source of variation	Degrees of freedom	Sum of squares	Mean square	Variance ratio	p value
Between modes of delivery	$2 - 1 = 1$	①	⑥ = ①/1	⑥/⑨	*
Between types of duration	$3 - 1 = 2$	②	⑦ = ②/2	⑦/⑨	*
Due to interaction between mode of delivery and duration	$1 \times 2 = 2$	③	⑧ = ③/2	⑧/⑨	*
Experimental error	$6(r - 1)$	④	⑨ = ④/(6(r − 1))		
Total	$6r - 1$	⑤			

squares is the sum of variations within each treatment; hence, the need for an assumption of homogeneity of population variances.

A parallel partitioning exists on the degrees of freedom. The degrees of freedom of a sum of squares is equal to the number of independent elements in that sum of squares (Montgomery, 1991). For example, degrees of freedom associated with the sum of squares due to mode of delivery is 1, which is 2 (the number of different modes of delivery) minus 1.

Mean squares are estimates of variance and are computed by dividing a sum of squares by its degrees of freedom. Variance ratios are computed by dividing each mean square due to a particular source by the experimental error mean square, assuming a fixed effects model (Box 18.1).

The statistical hypotheses for our two-way example are:

1. H_0: Mode of delivery of the programme does not affect ABPS score (i.e. both mode of delivery effects are zero).
   H_1: Mode of delivery affects ABPS score.
   H_0: Duration of the programme does not affect ABPS score (i.e. all effects due to different durations are zero).
   H_1: At least one of the durations of the programme affects ABPS score.
2. H_0: Particular combinations of mode of delivery and duration do not affect ABPS score (i.e. all interaction effects are zero).
   H_1: At least one combination of mode of delivery and duration affects ABPS score (i.e. at least one interaction effect is non-zero).

Each null hypothesis is tested using the corresponding variance ratio, which follows a Fisher's F distribution when the specified assumptions are met and when the population effects are zero. The rationale for these tests follows a similar reasoning to that given for one-way designs (Section 18.1.2).

Each separate p value is used to make a decision to reject or not reject the corresponding null hypothesis. As usual, a null hypothesis is rejected when the associated p value is less than or equal to the chosen significance level. The p values in an ANOVA table are influenced by sample size and magnitude of population effects (Section 13.5). It is common to present 95% confidence intervals for mean outcomes at each level of each factor and for each treatment when interaction effects are statistically significant.

Further analyses

Further analyses (Section 18.1.4) are performed when at least one null hypothesis is rejected. Groupings of homogeneous means are set up. Differences between groupings are larger than expected by sampling error and differences within a grouping are consistent with sampling error. There are two situations with respect to this two-way example:

1. The null hypothesis of zero interaction effects is retained

Separate further analyses might be performed on mean ABPS score across levels of each factor associated with a statistically significant variance ratio. The interaction term can be omitted from the model and the ABPS score is predicted from main effects and the mean value common to all exercise programmes. This is often referred to as *additivity* of main effects. Further, since mode of delivery has only two levels, a significant main effect for this factor would imply a significant difference in mean ABPS scores across the two modes.

2. The null hypothesis of zero interaction effects is rejected

Further analyses are performed on the mean values for each treatment or combination of levels of mode of delivery and duration. The ABPS score is predicted from main effects, interaction effects and the mean value common to all exercise programmes.

Mean square due to experimental error

The mean square for the total variation is not included in an ANOVA table (e.g. Table 18.17) because we are interested in finding important contributions to this variance, not in the variance itself. The mean square corresponding to the 'Total' line would be the variance of ABPS scores, ignoring all information about mode of delivery and duration. This is equivalent to assuming the model:

ABPS score value = a mean value common to all exercise programmes
+ experimental error

This is the appropriate model when all effects are zero and therefore is useful for predicting an ABPS score when it is not affected by mode of delivery, duration, or the combined influence of mode of delivery and duration. A study would not be performed if a researcher held the a priori belief that this model represented reality.

One occurrence of each treatment

When each treatment occurs once in a study, the inherent degrees of freedom associated with experimental error are zero (for example, Table 18.17 with $r = 1$). In this situation, experimental error is confounded with the variation due to the highest-order interaction. Tests of hypotheses on main effects and lower-order interactions can be performed if an assumption of zero highest-order interaction effects in the population is tenable.

In contrast, tests on main effects in randomized block and matched-subjects designs are valid in the presence of interaction effects between blocks and treatments. It is, however, convenient and more usual to assume zero interaction effects in these designs and fixed factor effects: the interaction term can then be omitted from the model and from the ANOVA table.

18.1.10 Other designs

The simple designs discussed in this book form the basis for many other useful designs. Partitioning total variability into its separate components provides a basis for constructing a model, understanding features of these designs, and analysing the resulting data. Figures 18.13 and 18.14 show, respectively, the partitioning for a two-way repeated measures design and a one-between-subjects and one-within-subjects design, which are two commonly used designs.

The Low Back Pain Study in its original form

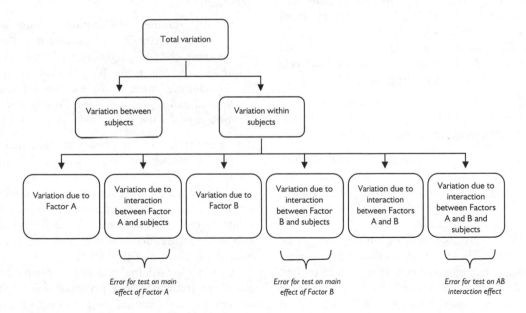

Figure 18.13 *Partitioning of the total variation in outcome values for a repeated measures design with two within-subjects factors (A and B).*

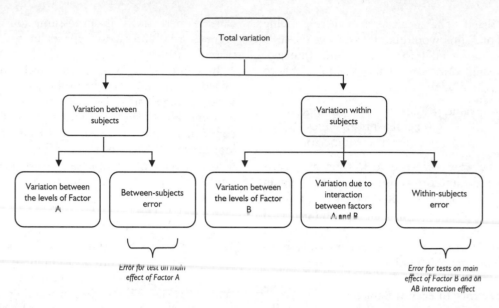

Figure 18.14 *Partitioning of the total variation in outcome values for one between-subjects factor (A) and one within-subjects factor (B).*

– i.e. without the factorial modification described in the preceding section – involved one between-subjects factor (mode of delivery of therapy: individual or group based) and one within-subjects factor (time: measures repeated at three points in time), as schematized in Figure 18.14. With the factorial modification, it would have involved an additional between-subjects factor (duration of the programme: 1, 2 or 3 weeks).

18.2 INTENTION-TO-TREAT ANALYSIS

The data in most clinical trials are incomplete or contain some cases for whom things have not gone as originally planned. This might be due to participants' dropping out of the study, or switching to a treatment other than that to which they were assigned, or turning out to be ineligible for the treatment allocated to them. Data might be missing because no measurement was recorded. In an *intention-to-treat* analysis, the data from each participant are analysed in accordance with the treatment to which he or she was randomized, regardless of whether or

not that participant actually received that treatment (Newell, 1992a; Lewis and Machin, 1993). Bland (1995, p. 15) explains the basis for this approach:

> [T]he random allocation procedure produces comparable groups and it is these we must compare, whatever selection may be made within them. We therefore analyse the data according to the way we intended to treat subjects, not the way in which they were actually treated.

The more traditional approach to data analysis is a *per protocol* or *on-randomized-treatment* analysis. In this approach, data are analysed in accordance with the treatment received, whether or not that was the treatment to which participants were randomized. A comparison of features of intention-to-treat and per protocol analyses is given in Table 18.18.

A discussion of the possible consequences of the more traditional per protocol approach will illustrate the merits of intention-to-treat analysis. In the Low Back Pain Study, it may be that slightly more patients dropped out from,

Table 18.18 *Features of intention-to-treat and per protocol analyses*

Intention-to-treat approach	Per protocol approach
Tests the policy of assigning participants to particular treatments.	Tests the result of participants' receiving a particular treatment.
Retains cases with incomplete data in the analysis – missing values are estimated (or imputed; Tabachnick and Fidell, 1996).	Excludes cases with incomplete data from the analysis; hence, effectively reduces sample size.
Might be considered unrealistic, since it ignores issues of switching treatment.	Might be considered unrealistic, since it ignores issues of dropout and non-adherence.
Some debate exists concerning appropriate methods for imputation and the maximum number of cases for whom values ought to be imputed.	Analysis is performed on data that contain a potential bias – excluded cases might share some common attributes.
Precision of estimates (e.g. on means) might be overestimated.	Analyses on different outcome variables might contain data from different cases and different numbers of cases.
Attenuates differences between groups, making it harder to demonstrate statistical significance in a comparative study.	The reduced replication reduces the power of statistical tests.
Attenuation of between group differences might make it easier to demonstrate no statistical significance in an equivalence study that seeks to show that two interventions are of equal effect and therefore interchangeable (Jones et al., 1996).	Produces unequal replication across treatments, resulting in statistical tests (e.g. ANOVA) being less robust to departures from the assumption of homogeneity of variance.

or did not comply with, treatment delivered through individual-based therapy than with group-based therapy. Moreover, the reasons for dropout or non-compliance may have been rather different ('may have been' because the researcher can often only surmise the exact reasons for dropout). In the individual-based approach, perhaps dropout was greatest among those patients whose back pain was of below-average severity, whereas there was no particular pattern in dropout from the group-based approach. Alternatively, it may be that patients with certain psychological characteristics found individual-based therapy somewhat unacceptable and as a result tended not to attend after a certain point; no such effect occurred in group-based therapy. The disproportionate loss from individual-based therapy of patients with low severity pain or with specific psychological characteristics has created a systematic difference between the two groups of participants in terms of these factors. The two interventions are no longer being tested on comparable groups of participants. Furthermore, if analysis is to be restricted to those participants who have main-

tained themselves on the treatment to which they were randomized, this may involve some rather subjective decisions as to who should or should not be classified in this category (Altman, 1991a).

In a per protocol analysis, participants for whom data are incomplete are excluded from analysis. There is, as yet, no clear agreement on the policy to adopt for cases with incomplete data in an intention-to-treat analysis (Hollis and Campbell, 1999). However, we would argue that it is in keeping with the logic of this type of analysis to retain such cases in the analysis. Hence, missing values might be replaced by estimated or 'imputed' values (Tabachnick and Fidell, 1996). Commonly used imputation methods are described in Table 18.19.

A recommended procedure is to conduct both an intention-to-treat and a per protocol analysis, since this will reveal the effect of dropouts or other protocol deviations (Bradford Hill and Hill, 1991; Lewis and Machin, 1993). On some occasions, an analysis of the pattern (e.g. characteristics of cases, treatment group) of missing values might reveal useful information. On other

Table 18.19 *Some commonly used methods of imputation*

Method	Details
Assuming no change	Carry forward a value for the participant concerned from an earlier measurement of that variable: • magnitude of effects are reduced, making it more difficult to demonstrate statistical significance of change.
Imputing a mean value	Use the common mean: • mean of all available values for that variable at the time of measurement • this is a conservative estimate as the common mean remains unchanged • however, it produces a reduced variance associated with that variable. Use the group mean: • mean of available values for that variable at the time of measurement for participants possessing some common characteristic (such as being allocated the same treatment) • not as conservative as using an overall mean; the common mean might be changed. Use the case mean: • mean of available values for that variable across all measurement occasions for the participant concerned or matched participants • might change the values of group means and the common mean.
Imputing a predicted value	Predicted from a regression of the variable concerned on one or more other variables using cases with complete data: • requires data to be available on variables that are known to be closely related to the variable concerned • might produce unrealistic values • increases the degree of correlation between variables • reduces the variance of values on the variable concerned.

occasions, it might be possible to classify cases with incomplete data so that they constitute a separate group. An analysis is then performed including this additional group.

18.3 MEASURES OF RELIABILITY

Most data collected in explanatory and descriptive studies are subject to measurement errors, which can affect the appropriateness and interpretation of results from statistical analyses performed on those data. Large measurement errors might obscure the nature of relationships between variables or important differences between treatment effects. It is, therefore, important to assess the amount of measurement error that is assignable to the use of a particular instrument.

In Section 9.3, reliability was considered in terms of the consistency or reproducibility of data. Three forms of reliability were defined: *equivalence* (the degree to which an instrument produces consistent measurements for a given entity, when used by two or more investigators, or in two different forms), *stability* (the extent to which an instrument performs consistently when used by one investigator to measure the same entity on repeated occasions) and *internal consistency* (a measure of the homogeneity of a multi-item instrument). The analysis of internal consistency reliability was considered in Section 15.3. Here we will consider appropriate methods for assessing equivalence and stability, and highlight some inappropriate methods that might initially appear to be applicable.

Assessment of the reliability of data obtained using particular measurement tools is important in most areas of research dealing with quantitative data (see Section 9.4 for a discussion of reliability in relation to qualitative data). Hence, the literature on methods of assessment contains many different terms to denote measurement, rater and subject. Some alternatives are given in Table 18.20.

Table 18.20 *Alternative terminology employed in descriptions of reliability indices*

Term	Alternative terms
Measurement	Observation, outcome value, rating, score
Rater	Researcher, investigator, examiner, assessor, judge, method
Subject	Entity, item, target, patient, participant

18.3.1 Inappropriate methods for assessing reliability

Use of correlation coefficients

It was pointed out earlier that equivalence and stability should normally be analysed in terms of agreement rather than association (Box 9.2). A measure of association such as Pearson's product moment correlation coefficient (Section 14.1.3) may not, therefore, be appropriate (Rose, 1991). A hypothetical situation in which two raters use the same instrument to take measurements (at an interval level) on a number of subjects will illustrate this. If the raters concur precisely for each pair of measurements, the value of Pearson's correlation coefficient will be 1. If measurements made by rater A are two scale points higher for each subject than those made by rater B, then the value of Pearson's correlation coefficient will also be 1. In this second situation, the sets of measurements made by the two raters have a perfect positive correlation, even though the raters do not agree on a single subject. The same phenomenon would occur with any constant additive or multiplicative adjustment to the measurements made by one of the raters (Bartko, 1976). Thus, Pearson's correlation coefficient provides a measure of association, but not of agreement.

A similar situation exists for rank-order correlation coefficients such as Spearman's rho or Kendall's tau (Section 14.1.4), since perfect agreement on the *rankings* of pairs of measurements does not equate with agreement of the paired measurements themselves (Bartko and Carpenter, 1976).

Use of t tests

A related *t* test was considered in Section 14.2.2 as an appropriate test on the effect of an intervention, or on the difference between two population mean values. An important feature of a related *t* test is that it assesses the chance occurrence of an observed mean difference (assuming random sampling) when the population mean difference is zero. This might appear to be a suitable method for assessing reliability. However, testing an assumption about a zero mean difference is not equivalent to testing for zero differences between individual pairs of measurements.

The result from a related *t* test depends, in part, upon the amount of variability between the individual differences in paired sample measurements. A statistically non-significant result (i.e. retaining the hypothesis of a zero population mean difference) is likely to occur when this variability is high, but a high variability indicates substantial differences in paired measurements, which reflects low reliability (Maher, 1993). A statistically significant result (i.e. rejecting the hypothesis of a zero population mean difference) is more likely to occur, for the same mean difference in paired sample measurements, when the variability is low than when it is high (Haas, 1991a). A low variability is indicative of higher consistency in differences between paired measurements, which is one aspect of reliability. Thus, almost paradoxically, if a non-significant result from a related *t* test were taken to be an index of reliability, this would occur most readily when the variability in measurements is high. Further, hypothesis tests in general do not quantify the extent of agreement in paired measurements. Thus, the role of the related *t* test is limited to testing for bias, not variability, in paired measurements.

It is worth noting that when paired measurements come from the same rater using the same measuring instrument (i.e. intra-rater reliability), bias is usually zero, unless there is a testing effect whereby the first set of measurements influences the second set (Table 7.2). In contrast, when paired measurements come from separate raters (inter-rater reliability) or from different instruments (alternative forms reliability), between-rater or between-instrument bias is usually non-zero.

18.3.2 Intraclass correlation coefficients

An alternative, and more appropriate, statistic to assess agreement is the intraclass correlation coefficient, usually abbreviated to 'ICC'. There are several forms of ICC that can produce different indices when applied to the same data. The different forms are identified according to how raters are chosen (i.e. a random selection of raters or particular raters of interest) and how raters are assigned to subjects (random assignment of a set of raters to a subject or every rater assigned to every subject). An ICC is calculated using variance estimates derived from analysis of variance (ANOVA) and may be viewed as a ratio of the 'variance of interest' over the sum of the 'variance of interest plus error' (Shrout and Fleiss, 1979).

Inter-rater reliability

There are three frequently used models of ICC for assessing inter-rater reliability and alternative forms reliability (two types of equivalence). The models and forms of the ICC are defined in Box 18.5. An instrument with established ICC(2,1) inter-rater reliability provides the ability to generalize measurements to other raters who might use the tool. This index is examined in more detail below.

The statistical model that underlies the calculation of an ICC(2,1) might be written as:

measurement = 'true' value for a subject (using that instrument)
+ component of measurement error unique to a rater
+ a random error component of measurement error

where an assumption of no subject-by-rater interaction (Section 18.1.9) has been made. The

Box 18.5 *Types of intraclass correlation coefficients used to assess inter-rater reliability*

There are three models of ICC (Shrout and Fleiss, 1979). Model 1 is used when measurement is made for each subject by a different set of raters, randomly selected from a larger population of raters. In Model 2, measurement is carried out on each subject by the same set of raters, randomly selected from a larger population of raters. Model 3 is similar to Model 2, except that the raters concerned are the only ones of interest; i.e. they are not considered to be a random sample from a larger population of raters (in other words, raters are fixed rather than random effects; Box 18.1). Within each model, there are two forms: a rater might make either one measurement or several measurements on a subject. In the latter situation, the mean of k measurements is used in the calculation of an ICC. Hence, there are six types of ICC (given in the table below). The type used should be indicated when the value of an ICC is quoted. These methods are also suitable for assessing alternative forms reliability.

Choice of raters	Assignment of raters to subjects	Measurements from each rater on a subject	
		Single	Mean of k
Randomly selected	Different set of raters assigned to each subject	Model 1, 1	Model 1, k
Randomly selected	Every rater assigned to each subject	Model 2, 1	Model 2, k
Not randomly selected	Every rater assigned to each subject	Model 3, 1	Model 3, k

subject effects, rater effects and random error are assumed to be normally distributed and the corresponding components of variance are estimated through mean squares from a two-way ANOVA with repeated measures on raters and subjects (Shrout and Fleiss, 1979; Haas, 1995). Under these assumptions (Rankin and Stokes, 1998):

$$ICC\ (2,1) = \frac{\text{subject variability}}{\text{subject variability + rater variability}\\ \text{+ random error variability}}$$

The ICC(2,1) ranges from 0 to 1. A value of 0 indicates that subject variability is negligible compared with measurement error (comprising rater variability plus variability due to random error) and subjects cannot be distinguished from each other in terms of the measurement of interest. When ICC(2,1) is 1, measurement error is negligible compared with subject variability and the instrument enables subjects to be clearly distinguished on the basis of the measurement of interest. However, the magnitude of subject variability is influenced by the choice of subjects included in a reliability study. When the subject population is fairly homogeneous with respect to the measurement of interest, subject variability is very small and an acceptable level of reliability will be achieved for relatively small measurement errors. When the subject population is heterogeneous with respect to the measurement of interest, subject variability is large and an acceptable level of reliability might be achieved for much larger measurement errors. That is, the value of an ICC is influenced by the between-subject variability (Mitchell, 1979; Keating and Matyas, 1998). It is, therefore, important that intraclass correlation coefficients are evaluated in a reliability study that involves subjects for whom the range of measurements is representative of those expected in future use of the instrument. Further, it should be noted that symptomatic and asymptomatic subjects might lead to very different values for the ICC (Haas, 1991b), as might raters with different levels of skill.

The inclusion of rater variability in the denominator ensures that an ICC (2,1) index reflects rater agreement rather than rater consistency (Shrout and Fleiss, 1979). A p value may be calculated for a test on the hypothesis that the population ICC is 0. A 95% confidence interval may also be calculated – except for ICC(3,1) or ICC(3,k), since an inference to a population of raters is not intended. Details of the calculation of ICCs are given by Shrout and Fleiss (1979), Krebs (1984), Portney and Watkins (1993) and Rankin and Stokes (1998).

Intra-rater reliability
Studies designed to consider stability are called intra-rater reliability or test-retest reliability studies. An instrument with established intra-rater reliability provides the ability to detect change over time. An estimate of intra-rater reliability is obtained by replacing 'rater' by 'time' (or trial) in the calculation for an ICC(2,1).

Inter-rater and intra-rater reliability from the same study
Inter-rater and intra-rater reliability can be assessed in the same study by having each rater take one measurement from several subjects (Haas, 1995). This saves resources and avoids problems such as 'blinding' raters to their previous measurements, bias of second measurements, subject reactivity to repeated measurements, and subject inconvenience. Formulae are given in Box 18.6.

18.3.3 Precision
An ICC is a dimensionless index of reliability; low values give poor subject differentiation and high values give good subject differentiation. However, it does not convey the expected magnitude of measurement error. Precision of intra-rater and inter-rater measurements may be estimated through repeatability and reproducibility limits, respectively (Mason et al., 1989; Altman, 1991a). These limits are obtained by analogy with confidence interval estimation of the difference between two means (Section 14.3). Formulae for calculation of approximate limits are given in Box 18.6.

335

Box 18.6   *Using a two-way ANOVA with repeated measures on raters and subjects to calculate inter-rater and intra-rater reliability indices, and repeatability and reproducibility limits*

The following ANOVA table shows the notation used to represent components of variation for a two-way ANOVA with repeated measures on raters and subjects (each rater taking one measurement on each subject).

Source of variation	Degrees of freedom	Mean square
Between subjects	$n - 1$	MSB
Within subjects	$n(r - 1)$	MSW
Between raters	$r - 1$	MSR
Experimental error	$(n - 1)(r - 1)$	MSE
Total	$nr - 1$	

Here, n = number of subjects, r = number of raters. Using this notation, inter-rater and intra-rater reliability indices may be calculated using:

$$\text{ICC}(2,1) = \frac{\text{MSB} - \text{MSE}}{\text{MSB} + (r - 1)\text{MSE} + r(\text{MSR} - \text{MSE})/n}$$

and

$$\text{intra-rater ICC} = \frac{\text{MSB} - \text{MSE}}{\text{MSB} + (r - 1)\text{MSE}}$$

Repeatability limits express the limits of variability that can be expected on the difference between repeated, independent measurements made on a subject by the *same* rater (Mason et al., 1989). Approximate 95% repeatability limits for the difference in two mean values each based on m independent measurements taken by one rater on the same subject are:

$$\text{obs diff} - 2.77 \, (\text{MSE}/m)^{1/2} \text{ to obs diff} + 2.77 \, (\text{MSE}/m)^{1/2}$$

where 'obs diff' denotes the observed difference between the two mean values. In many practical situations, practitioners might take a mean of three measurements (i.e. $m = 3$) rather than relying solely on one measurement (i.e. $m = 1$) from a subject. This has the effect of improving the ability to discriminate between subjects with the same instrument.

Reproducibility limits express the limits of variability that can be expected on the difference in independent measurements made on a subject by *different* raters. Approximate 95% reproducibility limits for the difference in measurements independently made by two different raters on the same subject are given by:

$$\text{diff} - 2.77 \, (\text{MSW})^{1/2} \text{ to diff} + 2.77 \, (\text{MSW})^{1/2}$$

where each rater takes one measurement, and 'diff' denotes the difference between these two measurements. When each rater takes m independent measurements, approximate 95% reproducibility limits are given by:

$$\text{diff} - 2.77\{\text{MSW} - (m - 1)\text{MSE}/m\}^{1/2} \text{ to diff} + 2.77\{\text{MSW} - (m - 1)\text{MSE}/m\}^{1/2}$$

where 'diff' denotes the observed difference between the two mean values.

Haas (1991b) recommends that both reliability and precision should be reported for a study, noting that an instrument might produce good reliability but poor precision and vice versa. Their relative importance within a particular study needs to be weighed by the researcher.

18.3.4 Bias and limits of agreement

Altman and Bland have developed a visual and clinically meaningful representation of agreement between paired measurements on an interval scale (Altman and Bland, 1983; Bland and Altman, 1986). The paired measurements might be values recorded on a set of subjects by two different raters or by one rater using two different instruments. Lack of agreement is summarized through two measures: *bias* and *95% limits of agreement* – these indicate systematic and random differences in raters' measurements, respectively. Bias is the mean difference between the paired measurements, and 95% limits of agreement represent two values within which approximately 95% of the differences between paired measurements will lie

(assuming that the differences are normally distributed). Figure 18.15 illustrates the bias and limits of agreement for two raters on measurements from 25 subjects on a 1–100 interval scale. The vertical axis represents the difference between the paired measurements, and the solid reference line indicates the mean difference (or bias, – .48 in our example). The dashed reference lines indicate two standard deviations above and below the mean difference, and represent the 95% limits of agreement (–16.91 and 15.95 in our example). These statistics are estimates of the values that apply to all paired measurements. Hence, we could calculate 95% confidence intervals for the bias and for the upper and lower limits of agreement, to assess the precision of our estimates (Bland and Altman, 1986). It is important, however, not to confuse the 95% limits of agreement themselves and any 95% confidence intervals calculated on them (Chinn, 1991b).

The horizontal axis represents the mean of each of the paired measurements. This allows us to judge whether the magnitude of the difference between paired measurements is related to the

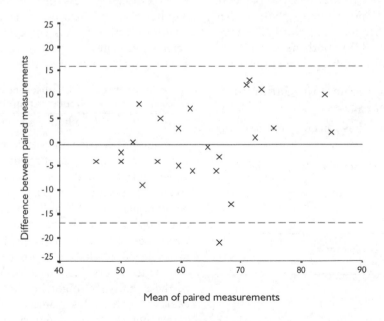

Figure 18.15 *Bias and 95% limits of agreement for measurements of two raters on a 1–100 scale.*

absolute value of the measurements (Nevill and Atkinson, 1997; see Box 9.2). When such a relationship exists, it is usual to analyse the data on a transformed scale (Altman, 1991a). Independence of the means of the paired ratings and the differences between the paired measurements can be judged visually, or by a hypothesis test on the correlation between them (Altman and Bland, 1983).

It can be seen that this graphical representation is highly informative. The magnitude and range of between-rater differences, their degree of homoscedasticity, and any aberrant measurements are readily apparent. Furthermore, it is useful to identify the bias and the variability of the measurements separately, since they are conceptually distinct and have different implications. For example, it can be seen in Figure 18.15 that the bias is small but the variability is moderate (a situation that we discussed in Section 18.3.1 with reference to the *t* test). These raters' measurements display quite a moderate degree of random variability but little systematic difference.

The relative merits of the ICC and the limits of agreement have been extensively debated in the literature (Bland and Altman, 1990; Müller and Büttner, 1994; Streiner and Norman, 1995; Rankin and Stokes, 1998). Both have a role to play in the investigation of measurement error.

18.3.5 Assessing agreement in relation to nominal and ordinal scales

The focus hitherto has been on assessing

agreement on an interval or ratio scale and the methods, based on means and variances of the measurements, are clearly inappropriate for nominal or ordinal data.

A common situation in which a researcher may wish to assess agreement on a nominal scale is in relation to diagnoses. Table 18.21 shows judgements from two clinicians who have assessed 100 patients in relation to a diagnosis of chronic fatigue syndrome. One way of trying to gauge the agreement between the two clinicians is to calculate the *overall percentage agreement* (calculated on all paired ratings) or *effective percentage agreement* (calculated on those paired ratings where at least one clinician agrees on the presence of the disease). In this example, there is 77% overall agreement and 42.5% effective agreement. However, these data do not take into account the agreement that would be expected by chance alone. Chance agreement will vary depending on the incidence of the disease in question; if it is either very common or very rare, chance agreement will be high. Effective percentage agreement has the merit of minimizing the chance agreement that would occur when a disease is very rare. Nonetheless, what is required is a measure of agreement that separates out, and thus corrects for, this chance agreement. The kappa (κ) coefficient (Cohen, 1960) is such a measure:

$$\kappa = \frac{\text{proportion of observer agreement} - \text{chance agreement}}{1 - \text{chance agreement}}$$

A kappa coefficient of 1 indicates perfect agreement, and a coefficient of 0 indicates agreement no better than that expected by chance. A negative kappa, which is unlikely to be obtained, would indicate agreement worse than that expected by chance (Bartko and Carpenter, 1976; Altman, 1991a). For the data in Table 18.21, kappa is .44 ($p < .0005$; 95% confidence interval .24 to .63). An interpretation of these statistics might be: for these two clinicians and for this sample of 100 patients, agreement about the diagnosis of chronic fatigue syndrome, corrected for chance agreement, was

Table 18.21 *Diagnostic assessments in relation to chronic fatigue syndrome from two clinicians for 100 patients. The main diagonal cells represent agreement, and the off-diagonal cells represent disagreement*

		Clinician 2		Total
		Present	**Absent**	
Clinician 1	Present	17	14	31
	Absent	9	60	69
Total		26	74	100

estimated as being greater than .24 and less than .63, with a mean of .44 ($n = 100$).

When dealing with ratings on an ordinal scale, it is important to retain the hierarchical nature of the categories. Suppose that two clinicians were assessing a sample of patients in terms of the severity of their locomotor disability, on a three-point scale ('mild', 'moderate', 'severe'). Here, disagreement by one scale point (i.e. mild/moderate, or moderate/severe) is less serious than disagreement by two scale points (i.e. mild/severe). To reflect this, the kappa coefficient can be weighted, so that it attaches greater weight to large disagreements than to small disagreements (Cohen, 1968). There are a number of methods of weighting that can be used, but quadratic weighting is common. This involves weighting each disagreement by a factor equal to the square of the difference between the position of two ratings (see Table 18.22).

Formulae for the calculation of kappa are provided by Altman (1991a), Portney and Watkins (1993) and Armitage and Berry (1994). Many statistical computing packages have commands to calculate kappa. The coefficient can be adapted for more than one rating per patient from each clinician (Conger, 1980; Haley and Osberg, 1989), or for situations in which clinicians may not each rate all of the same patients (Fleiss, 1971).

The kappa coefficient provides a measure of agreement across all categories in a scale; ratings for each category should be inspected to determine whether or not the magnitude of agreement is consistent across the scale (Portney and Watkins, 1993). Furthermore, the kappa coefficient does not by itself indicate whether disagreement is due to random or systematic differences between the clinicians' ratings (Hartmann, 1977).

18.3.6 Standards for agreement

Boundaries for describing ICC reliability indices are given by Portney and Watkins (1993) as follows:

below .75   poor to moderate reliability
.75 to .90   good reliability
.91 to 1   adequate reliability for clinical measurements.

Landis and Koch (1977) have proposed the following as standards for strength of agreement using the kappa coefficient:

0	poor
.01 to .20	slight
.21 to .40	fair
.41 to .60	moderate
.61 to .80	substantial
.81 to 1	almost perfect

Altman (1991a) proposes a similar formulation, but with slightly different descriptors. The choice of such benchmarks is inevitably arbitrary; Dunn (1989), for example, believes that Landis and Koch's standards are too generous.

Many writers (Dunn, 1989; Brennan and Silman, 1992; Streiner and Norman, 1995; Keating and Matyas, 1998) urge caution with respect to the use of benchmarks such as these. At the root of such concern is the fact that correlation coefficients and the like are specific to a particular context. The range of measurements used to calculate an ICC will influence its magnitude, independently of the actual agreement between paired measurements. Hence, for two raters using the same measuring instrument, a lower ICC is likely to result from a sample of homogeneous subjects than from a more varied sample, even though the true

Table 18.22 *Assessments of locomotor disability by two clinicians in relation to 100 patients, on a three-point ordinal scale. Figures in parentheses are quadratic kappa weightings*

		Clinician 2			Total
		Mild	Moderate	Severe	
Clinician 1	Mild	20 (0)	6 (1)	2 (4)	28
	Moderate	12 (1)	28 (0)	4 (1)	44
	Severe	2 (4)	10 (1)	16 (0)	28
Total		34	44	22	100

Unweighted $\kappa = .45$; weighted $\kappa = .57$.

concordance of their assessments is unlikely to be different. It is unwise, therefore, to make comparisons of ICCs across samples from different populations (Chinn, 1991b). In a similar way, the number of raters and the number of measurements per subject from each rater will also affect the size of an ICC. Therefore, ICCs should not be compared across studies that involve different numbers of raters, or different numbers of measurements from each rater (Müller and Büttner, 1994).

The kappa coefficient is influenced by the prevalence of the attribute in the population, i.e. where prevalence is either very high or very low, chance agreement is also high and kappa is reduced accordingly (Brennan and Silman, 1992). The weighted kappa coefficient is also influenced by such factors as the number of categories and the choice of weightings (Dunn, 1989; Haas, 1991a). Dunn (1989) suggests that interpretation of the kappa coefficient is assisted if the researcher calculates the maximum value it could attain, given the marginal totals (for the data displayed in Table 18.21, the maximum attainable $\kappa = .88$).

These coefficients are hard, therefore, to interpret out of context and cannot readily be compared across different contexts. It is generally preferable to express the strength of agreement between raters in a way that is immediately transferable to the context in which the measurements were made. Hence, when assessing agreement on an interval or ratio scale, repeatability or reproducibility limits, or 95% limits of agreement should be presented in addition to, or possibly instead of, an ICC.

18.4 PREDICTIVE RELATIONSHIPS BETWEEN VARIABLES

Determining the nature of the relationship between two or more variables is an objective in many descriptive and explanatory studies. Sometimes, the relationship in question is one of difference (e.g. the mean difference between two or more sets of data; Sections 14.2, 18.1), or of association (e.g. the correlation between two

sets of data; Section 14.1.2). On other occasions, researchers wish to examine predictive relationships, i.e. to determine whether values of one variable can be predicted from those of one or more other variables. For example, a researcher might wish to know if anxiety level can be predicted from heart rate, or blood pressure can be predicted from age, sex and body weight.

In certain situations, relationships of this sort between variables may be described by mathematical expressions. *Regression analysis* provides a method for predicting values of one variable from a knowledge of values on one or more other variables when the relationship between these variables may be expressed in terms of a mathematical model. Simple linear regression is the basic form of regression analysis and is applicable when the relationship between two variables may be represented by a straight line. This simple relationship is often used as an initial model in the absence of prior information about the nature of the variables of interest.

Regression is closely linked with correlation. However, the two procedures provide information on different aspects of an associative relationship between sets of data. Correlation provides information on two aspects of an association between variables: its *direction* (whether the coefficient is positive or negative) and its *strength* (the magnitude of the coefficient). The *form* (whether the correlation is linear, curvilinear, etc.) is not directly indicated by a correlation coefficient (See Section 14.1.3). Regression analysis assesses the *nature* of a linear association between variables (what specific value of one variable is related with what specific value of another variable). This enables a predictive relationship to be determined.

18.4.1 A straight line
Properties of a straight line
A straight line represents the simplest relationship between two variables that are measured on an interval or ratio scale. The variables are generally labeled X and Y. Data for a case comprise a pair of values, which mark one point

when drawn on a graph with the value of X plotted on the horizontal axis (X axis) and that of Y on the vertical axis (Y axis). Figures 18.16(a) and (b) show data that satisfy perfect straight line relationships; all data in each graph fall exactly on a straight line.

Every straight line may be completely defined by two characteristics or parameters, an *intercept* and a *slope* (also referred to as 'gradient'). The intercept is the value of Y when X equals zero; this might be a positive or negative quantity depending on the variables involved. In Figure 18.16, the intercept is 2 for the line in plot (a) and 10 for the line in plot (b).

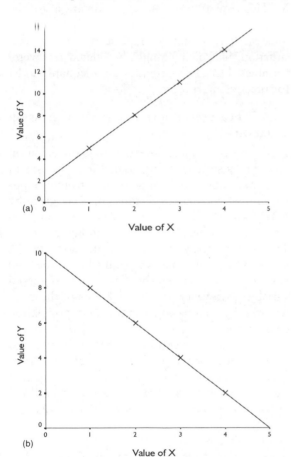

Figure 18.16 *Examples of a perfect straight line with (a) positive slope, Y = 2 + 3X, and (b) negative slope, Y = 10 – 2X.*

The slope is defined as the change in Y per unit increase in X. Figure 18.16(a) depicts a line with a positive slope; values of Y increase as values of X increase. The line moves up 3 units towards higher Y values for each step of one unit towards higher X values. That is, Y increases by 3 units per unit increase in X, or the slope of this line is 3. Figure 18.16(b) depicts a line with a negative slope; values of Y decrease as values of X increase. The line moves down 2 units towards lower Y values for each step of one unit towards higher X values. That is, Y decreases by 2 units per unit increase in X, or the slope of this line is –2.

Formula for a straight line

The intercept and the slope define a unique line, which can be stated mathematically as:

$$Y = \text{intercept} + \text{slope} \times X$$

or, in terms of symbols:

$$Y = a + bX$$

where a = intercept and b = slope.

The mathematical representations for the two example lines are: $Y = 2 + 3X$ in Figure 18.16(a); $Y = 10 - 2X$ in Figure 18.16(b). Each equation enables a value of Y to be calculated at a given value of X. For example, using the first equation, when $X = 4$, $Y = 2 + (3 \times 4) = 14$. This is identical to one of the observed pairs of data (4, 14). When $X = 1.5$, $Y = 2 + (3 \times 1.5) = 6.5$, which does not represent an observed pair of data, but is a point (1.5, 6.5) that nonetheless lies on the straight line. The straight line equation enables Y to be predicted at a value of X, irrespective of whether or not that value occurred in the data.

18.4.2 Simple linear regression

Unfortunately, the examples considered above are idealized. Data collected in a real study comprise a random sample from a population of interest and are subject to measurement, sampling and other sources of random error. These errors cause some values to be larger and others smaller than those predicted from a math-

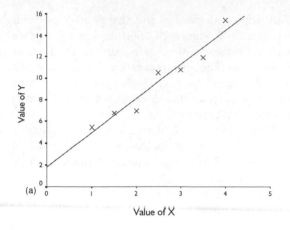

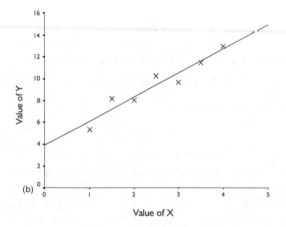

Figure 18.17   *Scatter plots of data (X, Y) in two random samples of size 7 from a population in which expected values of Y = 2 + 3X. Ŷ = predicted values of Y; and the line on each plot is the regression line of best fit. (a) Regression equation Ŷ = 1.80 + 3.16X; standard error = 0.93. (b) Regression equation Ŷ = 3.91 + 2.21X; standard error = 0.78.*

ematical model. For example, we expect some data points to lie above a straight line and others below it, even when we know that there is a linear relationship between two variables (Figure 18.17).

Simple linear regression analysis takes account of variation by determining a line of 'best fit' to the data, such that an observed value of Y (at a specified value of X) is predicted with minimum error. The fitted line is 'best' in the sense that the sum of squared differences between observed

and predicted values of Y is smaller than the corresponding sum of squared differences for any other line. This method is often referred to as the method of 'least-squares' and the resultant line as the 'least-squares line of best fit for Y on X'. The term 'Y on X' indicates that minimization involves squared deviations in the Y direction only (i.e. vertical distances of observed values from the fitted line) and implies that negligible error is present in the X values.

The line of best fit to a specific set of data (such as depicted in Figure 18.17) is called a *regression line* and is described by an equation called a *simple linear regression equation* of Y on X. This equation is an approximation to the model relating Y to X in the population of interest. It is usually a simplification of the real situation, in which Y might be related to several variables, but often provides an adequate model for practical purposes.

18.4.3 Features of a simple linear regression equation

Features of a simple linear regression equation are demonstrated using data in two small, random samples ($n = 7$) generated from a population in which expected values of Y are given by $E[Y/X] = 2 + 3X$ (Box 18.7). The data and associated lines of best fit are shown in Figure 18.17. This is, admittedly, an artificial situation, since it is highly unlikely that we would know the true nature of a relationship between observed variables. However, it will enable us to illustrate features by comparing sample and population characteristics.

The usual convention is that Y is used to denote values of the *predicted* variable and X for values of the *predictor* variable. For example, if age were used to predict blood pressure, blood pressure would be labeled as Y and age as X.

Data

A regression equation is computed using data collected from a random sample drawn from the population of interest. The data might be collected through a survey or a clinical trial (in which X is controlled at values specified by the

Box 18.7   *Simple linear regression model and assumptions*

Regression analysis is based on a model of the true relationship between variables in a population of interest. A simple linear regression model is represented by:

$$Y = \alpha + \beta X + \varepsilon \qquad (1)$$
$$E[Y/X] = \alpha + \beta X \qquad (2)$$

where:

Y is the value of the outcome (predicted) variable;

X is the value of the predictor variable;

α is the intercept of the line (expected value of Y when $X = 0$); α is a parameter;

β is the slope of the line (expected change in Y per unit increase in X); β is a parameter;

$E[Y/X]$ is the expected value of Y at a specified value of X (= mean value of Y at a specified value of X);

ε is the error term associated with a value of Y.

The assumptions that underlie this model are:

1. Each value of X is observed without error (in practice this implies negligible measurement error).
2. The linear model is a correct representation of the relationship between X and Y.
3. A subpopulation of Y values exists at each value of X, and the mean Y values for these subpopulations lie on the same line (as stated by equation (2)); equivalently, the mean of the error terms is zero at each value of X.
4. The variances of the subpopulations of Y are all equal; equivalently, the variance of the error terms is the same at every value of X.
5. The error terms are serially independent; i.e. one error term does not affect and is not affected by other error terms.

An additional assumption is required when the model is used for interval estimation or hypothesis testing:

6. The error terms are normally distributed at each value of X.

When assumptions 1 to 5 are met, the parameters α and β may be estimated using data from a random sample drawn from the population of interest. The line of best fit to the data may be represented by the regression equation:

$$\hat{Y} = a + bX$$

where:

$\hat{Y}$ is the predicted value of Y at a given value of X (= value of Y on the fitted line at a given value of X, or mean value of Y);

X is the value of the predictor variable;

a is the regression constant, which is the predicted value of Y when $X = 0$; it is an estimate of the intercept α;

b is the slope, or regression coefficient, which is the mean change in Y for a unit increase in X, other factors remaining the same; it is an estimate of the true slope β.

This is called a 'least-squares line of best fit' of Y on X. The statistics a and b are calculated to minimize the sum of squared differences between Y and $\hat{Y}$.

researcher), and comprise pairs of values measured on two variables (X, Y) for every participant in the study. A scatter diagram (Section 14.1.2) of the data provides a visual representation of a predictive relationship between two variables.

Constant

The constant in a regression equation is a point estimate of the intercept in the population. It is the predicted value of Y when $X = 0$. For example, using data from the sample in Figure 18.17(a), the constant is 1.80.

A constant may not have a practical interpretation, because $X = 0$ is often an unrealistic value and/or might be outside the region of sampled X values. For example, it is nonsensical to consider the weight of a person with zero height, or the forced vital lung capacity for a person aged 20 years when the sample comprises persons aged 65 to 85 years of age.

Slope

The slope of a regression line is an estimate of the slope of the linear relationship in the population. The equivalent statistic in a regression equation is called a *regression coefficient* and is a point estimate of the change in Y per unit increase in X. Using the data in Figure 18.17(a), the slope is 3.16.

The difference between the estimated slope and the true slope (0.16 in our example) is due to the influence of different sources of error such as measurement error, sampling error and other sources of random error. A second random sample drawn from the same population is likely to produce a regression equation with a different slope. For example, a slope of 2.21 was obtained from a second random sample drawn from our hypothetical population (Figure 18.17(b)).

The regression coefficient usually has a practical interpretation. For example, in healthy adult males between the ages of 65 and 85 years, there is an estimated reduction of 0.12 percentage points in the ratio of forced expiratory volume in one second to forced vital lung capacity (FEV_1/FVC), for every year older than 65 years of age (Coggon, 1995). Strictly speaking, we should add, 'for people with characteristics similar to those in the present study and assuming that all other factors affecting forced vital lung capacity remain constant (i.e. behave in the same way as in the present study)'.

Predicting Y at a given value of X

Predicted values of Y (denoted by $\hat{Y}$) lie on the regression line and may be calculated from the regression equation (Box 18.7). Using the data in Figure 18.17(a), the regression equation is $\hat{Y} = 1.80 + 3.16X$ and, for example, the predicted

value of Y when $X = 2$ is 8.12 ($\hat{Y} = 1.80 + (3.16 \times 2) = 8.12$), which is 1.13 units higher than the observed value of 6.99. The observed point (2, 6.99) lies below the fitted line.

The difference between an observed and predicted Y value (in our example, $6.99 - 8.12 = -1.13$) is called a *residual* and is due to the influences of different sources of error. Hence, residuals reflect the lack of fit of the regression line to the data as a consequence of the combined effects of different sources of error. Larger residuals (ignoring their sign) denote observed Y values that are farther away from the fitted line.

The standard deviation of the residuals for all the observed data provides one measure of the goodness-of-fit of a regression line to those data. This statistic is called the *standard error of the estimate* (or just 'standard error' when the context precludes ambiguity). A small standard error indicates that the observed Y values are close to a regression line and a large standard error that observed data are scattered within a wide band around a regression line. In general, 'small' and 'large' may be assessed against the range of Y values. In our example, Y values range from 5 to 15 and the standard error is 0.93, which is moderately small, as displayed by the closeness of the data points to the fitted line in Figure 18.17(a).

Interval estimates

When certain assumptions are met (Box 18.7), interval estimates may be computed for predicted values of Y given X. Such intervals are based around point estimates obtained from the regression line and use the standard error of the estimate to take account of unassignable sources of error. Larger standard errors lead to wider intervals. The necessary assumptions are frequently checked through graphical analyses of the residuals. Details are given in Altman (1991a) and Armitage and Berry (1994).

In this section, we have referred to 'predicted value of Y' as being that value of Y calculated from the regression equation when we substitute a specific value for X. This is often called the 'fitted value of Y', since it lies on the fitted line. It

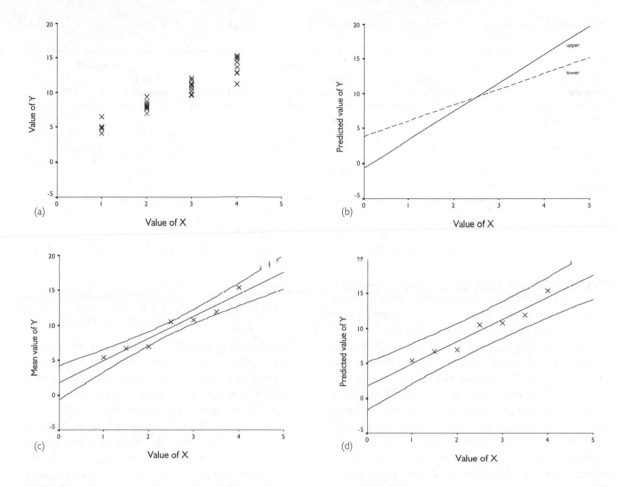

Figure 18.18 *Features of interval estimates, based on random samples from a population in which predicted values of Y = 2 + 3X. (a) Different values of Y that might be observed at given values of X. Interval estimates are based on the assumption that values of Y are normally distributed, with equal variances, at each value of X. (b) The lines depict the limits in a 95% confidence interval for the true slope. They cross at the mean Y value and mean X value, since a least-squares line of best fit always passes through this point. (c) the outer curves represent 95% confidence intervals for a mean value of Y at given values of X. The line represents the regression equation $\hat{Y} = 1.80 + 3.16X$. (d) The outer curves represent 95% prediction intervals for an individual value of Y at given values of X. The line represents the regression equation $\hat{Y} = 1.80 + 3.16X$.*

is an estimate for two different situations: (1) a mean value of Y for all cases that might occur at the specific X value, and (2) a value of Y for an individual case at the specific X value. For example, if we were to consider the ratio of forced expiratory volume in one second to forced vital capacity (FEV_1/FVC), we might be interested in estimating the mean FEV_1/FVC value for all 70-year-old males, or the FEV_1/FVC value for an individual male who was 70 years of age. Uncer-

tainty in the latter would be much larger than in the former and this is reflected in the width of interval estimates (Sections 13.3 and 13.5).

An interval estimate for a mean value of Y at a specific value of X is called a *confidence interval for the mean*, and that for an individual case a *prediction interval*. Plots (c) and (d) in Figure 18.18 show interval estimates based on the simple example depicted in Figure 18.17(a).

Confidence intervals might also be computed

Table 18.23   *Comparison of population and sample characteristics for two random samples (n = 7) drawn from that population*

| | | Sample 1 | | Sample 2 | |
Feature	Population parameter	Point estimate	95% CI	Point estimate	95% CI
Intercept (constant)	2	1.80	−0.65 to 4.24	3.91	1.87 to 5.94
Slope	3	3.16	2.26 to 4.07	2.21	1.45 to 2.96
Expected Y at X = 2	8	–		–	
Predicted Y at X = 2	–	8.12		10.03	
Observed Y at X = 2	–	6.99		8.08	
Standard error	1.00	0.93		0.77	

CI = confidence interval.

for the true slope (or for the intercept when this is meaningful). The upper and lower limits of an interval might be used to perform a statistical test on the hypothesis that the true slope is some pre-specified value. Table 18.23 contains point estimates and corresponding confidence intervals for the true slope and intercept for our simple regression equations based on two random samples ($n = 7$) from a population in which predicted Y values are $2 + 3X$. Data from sample 1 would not cast doubt on the assumption that the true slope was 3, at a significance level of .05. This confidence interval is depicted in Figure 18.18(b). Data in sample 2, however, would result in a rejection of the assumption, which, in this hypothetical situation, we know would be a Type I error (Section 13.4.8).

Other comments

1. The width of interval estimates depends upon the sample size, the observed range of X values, and the magnitude of the error terms (which in part is due to adequacy of the assumed model).
2. The width of interval estimates conveys information about the usefulness of a regression equation in a particular situation. This can be illustrated through data based on an example given in Coggon (1995). Data on age, forced expiratory volume in one second (FEV_1) and forced vital capacity (FVC) were collected for a random sample of 100 males, aged from 60 to 85 years, attending a well-person clinic.

Based on these data, a ratio of FEV_1/FVC (which is expressed as a percentage) might be predicted from age, using:

$$\text{predicted } (FEV_1/FVC) = 78.07 - 0.210(\text{age})$$

A 70-year-old male is predicted to have a FEV_1/FVC ratio higher than 47.9 percentage points and lower than 78.8 percentage points (95% prediction interval). This interval is almost certainly too wide to be useful in practice for the purposes of screening or clinical decision making. This wide prediction interval may be due to a very high variability from one male to another, or it may indicate that variables other than age affect values of FEV_1/FVC, and that these variables were not controlled for in the sample.

3. The choice of variables in a model may be based on previous research findings, experience or theoretical considerations.
4. Goodness-of-fit of the line to the data may be expressed in a statistic called the *coefficient of determination* (introduced in Section 14.1.3). This is the proportion of variation in the Y values that may be accounted for by predicting Y from a least-squares line of best fit on X. It is equivalent to the square of Pearson's product moment correlation coefficient (Section 14.1.3).
5. Goodness-of-fit of a regression line may be tested using ANOVA techniques. Details are given by Armitage and Berry (1994).

6. A regression equation represents a line of best fit to a given set of data, with a particular range of X values. It is dangerous to predict Y at values of X outside this range, since the assumed model might be inappropriate. For example, the relationship between height (cm) and age (years) may be represented by:

$$\text{predicted height} = 45 + 9(\text{age})$$

for children between the ages of 1 and 12 years. Using this equation, a person aged 25 years would be predicted to be 270 cm tall.

7. A scatter diagram is a useful first step in any regression analysis. It provides a visual check on the presence of extreme values, gaps in the observed data set, and non-linear relationships (Figure 18.19).

8. A linear relationship often provides an inadequate representation of the relationship

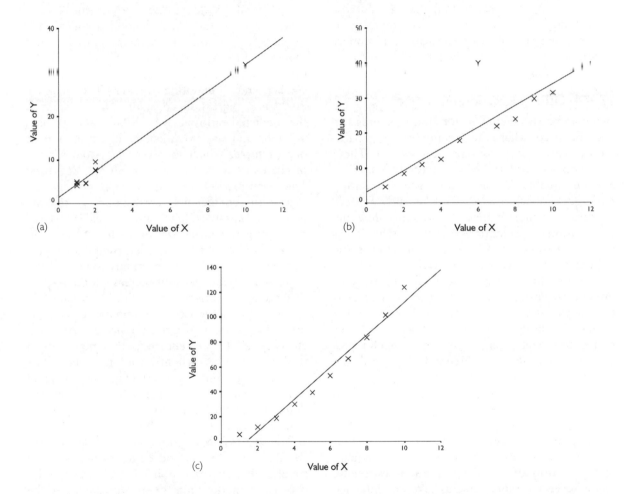

Figure 18.19 *Examples of the influence of extreme values, outliers and non-linear relationships on the regression line; r^2 = coefficient of determination. (a) $r^2 = .99$. A false impression of the goodness-of-fit caused by a few data points at high X values. There is no indication of what form the relationship might take between $X = 2$ and $X = 10$. (b) $r^2 = .67$. The regression line is shifted towards the outlier at $X = 6$. (c) $r^2 = .95$. The data points fall in a regular pattern around the regression line. A curve might provide a better fit to the data. r^2 = coefficient of determination.*

between two variables. This might be indicated by a plot of standardized residuals against X. Some non-linear relationships may be transformed to satisfy the requirements of linear regression. Other non-linear relationships may be adequately modelled by a polynomial, i.e. where the X term is raised to a power greater than one (Allison, 1999).

9. When the outcome variable is dichotomous, for example, presence or absence of some condition, then *logistic regression* (or multiple linear logistic regression) is a suitable technique. Logistic regression is often used in the analysis of case-control and cohort studies (Figure 4.1). Details are given in Schlesselman (1982) and Altman (1991a).

18.4.4 Other regression techniques

Nonparametric methods for linear regression may be used when the assumptions for parametric regression techniques are not met. These are discussed in detail in Conover (1999). They are unavailable in most statistical computing packages and, hence, infrequently used. Moreover, although these techniques allow the distributional assumptions of parametric linear regression to be set aside, they still require the data to be at interval or ratio level.

Multiple linear regression, modelling of non-linear relationships, and using regression analysis to analyse data from clinical trials are three frequently used extensions to simple linear regression. Brief descriptions of these techniques are given here. Further discussion is beyond the scope of this book.

Multiple linear regression

In simple linear regression, values of one variable are predicted from values of a second variable. This often provides an inadequate representation of the true situation, especially when several variables might have an influence upon the predicted variable. For example, a person's weight might be related to his or her height, age, number of calories consumed per day, occupation and gender. The ratio of forced expiratory volume in one second to forced vital capacity might be related to age, number of cigarettes smoked per day, and gender. Multiple regression enables values of one variable to be predicted from values of several other variables (Nick and Hardin, 1999).

An example multiple linear regression equation involving two predictor variables is:

$$\hat{Y} = 80.09 - 0.147(\text{age}) - 13.18(\text{smoke})$$

where $\hat{Y}$ is a predicted value of the ratio of forced expiratory volume in one second to forced vital capacity; 'age' and 'smoke' are predictor variables. 'Age' denotes a client's age in years and 'smoke' is a dummy variable that represents the smoking status of a client at the time of data collection – a value 0 denoting non-smoker and 1 denoting smoker. The quantity 80.09 is a regression constant. The constant is the predicted ratio when both 'age' and 'smoke' are zero and has no practical interpretation in our example, which involves a random sample of clients between the ages of 60 and 85 years. The quantities –0.147 and –13.18 are partial regression coefficients corresponding to the predictor variables 'age' and 'smoke', respectively. In general, they are estimates of the mean change (increase when a coefficient has a plus sign and decrease for a minus sign) in the predicted variable per unit increase in the respective predictor variable, assuming that values of all other predictor variables remain constant or fixed. In our example, the predicted ratio for a client is 0.147 percentage points higher than that for another client who has the same smoking status but is 1 year older. The predicted ratio for a client who smokes is 13.18 percentage points lower than for another client who is the same age but does not smoke.

The regression constant and coefficients are calculated by the method of least-squares, as in simple linear regression. Their magnitudes depend upon the units of measurement for the predicted and predictor variables and do not reflect the relative importance of each predictor. *Standardized regression coefficients* enable a researcher to determine this relative importance. In our example, the standardized coefficients are

−0.132 and −0.844 for 'age' and 'smoke', respectively.

Multiple regression is a very powerful technique. However, there are many pitfalls and a researcher needs to be aware of these and to understand the method thoroughly before he or she attempts to use it. Aspects to consider include: choice of predictor variables; interrelationships among the predictor variables and associated potential problems; choice of a subset of predictor variables to produce an adequate model and the procedure employed; checking the assumptions underlying a model; relationships between different models; and uses and misuses of a regression equation. Details on multiple linear regression may be found in Hays (1988), Krebs (1993), Howell (1997), and Katz (1999). Allison (1999) provides a clear and comprehensive discussion of this technique.

Use of regression analysis to analyse data from a completely randomized design or a clinical trial
Completely randomized designs (Section 18.1) may be represented by a regression model and the data may be analysed through regression analyses. The outcome variable is equivalent to the predicted variable, Y, and the factors are represented by predictor variables, X_i. Two common situations exist for a completely randomized one-factor design:

1. The treatments may be represented by values of a variable measured on a nominal scale (for example, type of therapy, type of equipment) and are represented by dummy variables that have values 0 or 1 (Nick and Hardin, 1999). As an example, three treatments would be represented by two dummy variables, X_1 and X_2, with values as follows:

Treatment	X_1	X_2
1	0	0
2	1	0
3	0	1

The data are analysed through a multiple linear regression of Y on X_1 and X_2.

2a. The treatments may be represented by values of a variable (X) measured on at least an interval scale (for example, dose of some drug, duration of an exercise session) and there is reason to believe that Y is linearly related to X. In this situation, a simple linear regression analysis of Y on X may be performed. Multiple linear regression might be applied when there is more than one factor.

2b. The treatments may be represented by values of a variable (X) measured on at least an interval scale, but the nature of the relationship between the outcome variable and the variable(s) reflecting treatment(s) is unknown; and then dummy variables are used as described in situation 1 above.

These analyses cope with unequal numbers of observations against each treatment or condition.

18.4.5 Use of statistical computing packages to perform regression analyses

The calculations required for regression analyses are very laborious and, therefore, are usually performed using one of the many available statistical computing packages. Most have a comprehensive choice for performing regression analyses, including the simple methods described in this section. Scatter diagrams, regression equations, confidence intervals (for the constant, slope and mean values of Y at specified values of X), prediction intervals for Y at given values of X, goodness-of-fit statistics, and analyses of residuals are some of the options provided.

The old adage 'garbage in, garbage out' is very pertinent in the context of regression methods. If a proposed regression model does not provide an adequate fit to the data, it might be tempting (because it is very easy to get the computer to do so) to fit a series of models that incorporate all possible combinations of the variables in the dataset, or to fit a curve that contains high powers of X. One of these models is likely to provide a good fit to the data. It might not, however, have any theoretical or experiential underpinning and, therefore, its contribution to knowledge or prediction of outcomes or behaviours would be very dubious.

It is advisable to check model assumptions through an analysis of standardized residuals. Such an analysis might identify problems (such as gross outliers or an inappropriate model) that are not discernible through the regression equation and associated statistics. Further, care should be taken not to request a predicted value for predictors with values outside the range of the available data. Most statistical computing packages will perform such predictions and very few print a warning that the fitted model is being extrapolated. A scatter diagram is always a good starting point for any regression analysis.

18.5 STATISTICAL CONTROL FOR EXTRANEOUS VARIABLES

Differences between characteristics of the participants is often a major source of variation in clinical trials. In completely randomized designs, this variation is one component of unassignable variation or experimental error (Section 18.1.1) and influences the power of hypothesis tests on differences between the effects of treatments or conditions. Repeated measures designs were introduced in Section 18.1.6 as one method for controlling the variability between people to reduce experimental error and, hence, to increase the power of hypothesis tests. Randomized block designs and matched-subject designs were described in Section 18.1.7 as alternatives to repeated measures when it is impractical to measure outcomes on one person under several treatments or conditions. However, these designs require larger numbers of potential participants to achieve a match on pertinent characteristics. Variation due to different participants may also be controlled through a statistical procedure called *analysis of covariance*.

Analysis of covariance (ANCOVA) is a combination of ANOVA and linear regression. It requires a researcher to collect information on at least one additional variable that is known, from prior research or experience, to be related to the outcome variable in a study. This variable is called a *covariate* because its values vary with values of the outcome variable. A large variation in participant characteristics is usually reflected in a large variation in values of a covariate. Age and length of time since diagnosis of a disease are frequently used as covariates in community-based randomized controlled trials.

Information on a covariate is collected before the start of a clinical trial, or during the trial if it is known that its values are not affected by the treatments being assessed. The relationship between this covariate and an outcome variable is represented by an additional term in the statistical model for the study design (Section 18.1). The relationship is used for two purposes. First, the covariate is identified as a source of variation in the outcome values and its contribution is removed from the variation due to experimental error. Second, it is used to adjust mean outcome values on each treatment for chance differences in mean values on the covariate due to the random assignment of participants to treatments.

ANCOVA is based on the usual assumptions associated with a study design (Section 18.1), plus two additional assumptions: (1) the covariate is linearly related to the outcome variable, and (2) the slope of the linear relationship is the same for every treatment or condition in a study. A linear model is usually a simplification of the real situation (Section 18.4.2), but it often provides an adequate representation to be useful in reducing the variation due to experimental error. The second assumption may be tested as part of the analysis.

Space precludes a detailed discussion of ANCOVA. It is a powerful technique and is available in most statistical computing packages. When baseline scores on an outcome variable are used as a covariate in a randomized controlled trial, the statistical power of the study may be enhanced (Everitt, 1996). However, there are potential problems with its use. A situation may arise in which the covariate is associated not only with the outcome variable but also with an intervention variable (i.e. the covariate and that intervention variable are confounded). Here, the effect of the intervention is indistinguishable from the association between the covariate and the outcome variable; consequently, it is inadvisable to draw any conclusions as to the effect of the intervention. ANCOVA can also lead to difficulties if used in quasi-experimental designs that lack randomization to intervention groups. Here, ANCOVA can serve to decrease, rather than enhance, statistical power (Owen and Froman, 1998). The researcher is strongly recommended to read a more detailed account of the technique before using it; for example, Myers and Well (1995) or Howell (1997).

18.6 DETERMINING SAMPLE SIZE

Determining the required sample size is an important consideration in studies that involve inferential statistics. Many such studies produce inconclusive findings by virtue of having too few participants to reject the null hypothesis (Ottenbacher and Maas, 1999). Calculating the required sample size is an early task in the planning of descriptive and explanatory studies. It requires the researcher to provide some fundamental information about the study design and the primary variables of interest. This section discusses some of the procedures that are routinely used for calculating sample size. Several texts contain tables, nomograms or power curves for this purpose (Friedman et al., 1982; Kraemer and Thiemann, 1987; Hulley and Cummings, 1988; Altman, 1991a; Cohen, 1992; Machin et al., 1997) and some computing packages now provide this facility. Most procedures assume that the data are obtained by drawing a simple random sample from the population(s) of interest (Section 8.3.1). They provide a guideline to required sample sizes for other random sampling methods. Sample size calculations in two group studies for binary, ordered categorical, and continuous outcomes are discussed by Campbell et al. (1995). The special case of sample size in cluster randomization is dealt with by Hsieh (1988), Donner (1992) and Kerry and Bland (1998).

In general, larger sample sizes lead to more precise estimates of population parameters and their differences (Armitage and Berry, 1994), and more powerful statistical tests (Section 13.4.8); however, they do not in themselves guarantee absence of bias (Section 8.5.1). It is theoretically possible, therefore, to achieve any specified degree of precision or power. In practice, however, a study is subject to resource constraints (for example, with regard to money, time, personnel, equipment and facilities) which may limit the study to a smaller sample size than that indicated by statistical considerations. The procedures discussed in this section can be reversed to provide estimates of the achievable precision or power for random samples of different sizes (Armitage and Berry, 1994). A researcher intending to use a smaller sample size can explore whether or not precision might be improved through a careful choice of design (Lipsey, 1998). If this is not feasible, one should consider whether or not the study will make an important contribution to practice or knowledge, notwithstanding the small sample size (Friedman et al., 1982). Studies with low statistical power may not detect beneficial interventions or important relationships between variables.

Non-response, incomplete information and attrition over time are features of most research studies. The *intended* sample size can be increased to allow for these potential losses, so that the actual achieved sample size might provide the desired precision or power. This adjustment does not guarantee that an adequate sample size will be *achieved*, and does not remove the possibility of bias relating to characteristics of the lost cases. Neither does it allow for overoptimistic estimates of effects.

We have assumed that the reader is familiar with the normal distribution and its properties, and with basic inferential statistics (Chapter 13).

18.6.1 Determining sample size for estimating parameters

Descriptive studies are performed to collect information on conditions, attitudes, opinions, beliefs or other characteristics in a population.

An objective might be to determine the mean value of some characteristic, or the proportion of a population that possesses some specific characteristic. Under certain assumptions, a population parameter may be estimated using a confidence interval, which is a range of values that contains the parameter with a stated degree of confidence (Sections 13.3 and 13.5). The interval is calculated from the data in a random sample drawn from the population of interest, and its width reflects the precision with which a parameter is estimated. Hence, confidence intervals provide a simple mechanism for determining an adequate sample size for many descriptive studies.

The most frequently used methods are based on a normal distribution and a confidence level of 90%, 95% or 99%.

Estimating a mean

Based on a random sample from the population and an assumption that individual values follow a normal distribution, a confidence interval for the population mean value is given by:

$$\bar{x} - z\left(\frac{\sigma}{\sqrt{n}}\right) \text{ to } \bar{x} + z\left(\frac{\sigma}{\sqrt{n}}\right)$$

which leads to:

$$n \geqslant \left(\frac{z\sigma}{w}\right)^2$$

where:

n is an adequate size for a random sample from the population;

σ is the standard deviation for individual values in the population;

w is the half width of the confidence interval and reflects the required precision for the estimate of the population mean; i.e. the confidence interval is $\bar{x} - w$ to $\bar{x} + w$

z is a standardized score and is related to the level of confidence associated with the interval:

level of confidence	z
90%	1.645
95%	1.960
99%	2.576

The sample size is affected by:

- the required precision (w), with higher precision equating to smaller w
- the specified level of confidence
- the population standard deviation σ.

In practice, σ is unknown but might be estimated from a pilot study, previous studies involving similar variables, or from an assumption that values of the variable of interest follow a normal distribution (when the expected difference between the maximum and minimum values of that variable is equated to 6σ). Table 18.24 presents some examples of sample sizes for varying values of w, confidence level and standard deviation.

When n is greater than 30, the formula is applicable for values from non-normal distributions (see Section 13.2.2). When n represents a high proportion of the population (5% or more) an adjustment is often made to the sample size; see Section 8.5.1 (Moser and Kalton, 1971; Daniel, 1991).

Estimating the difference between two means

Based on independent, random samples from two populations with equal standard deviations (or on two independent subgroups of a random sample from one population) and an assumption that the difference in sample mean values follows a normal distribution, an adequate number of cases (n) per sample may be calculated from:

Table 18.24 *Adequate sample sizes for estimating a population mean; varying values of precision, confidence level and standard deviation*

Precision (w)	Confidence level 95% (z = 1.960) Standard deviation (σ)		Confidence level 99% (z = 2.576) Standard deviation (σ)	
	1	2	1	2
0.2	96	385	166	664
0.4	24	96	42	166
0.6	11	43	19	74
0.8	6	24	11	42

$$n \geqslant 2\left(\frac{z\sigma}{w}\right)^2$$

where:

n is an adequate size for a random sample from *each* population (or from *each* subgroup of a random sample from one population);

σ is the standard deviation for individual values in the two populations;

w reflects the required precision for the estimate of the difference in population means and is the half width of the confidence interval:

$(\bar{x}_1 - \bar{x}_2) - w$ to $(\bar{x}_1 - \bar{x}_2) + w$
$\bar{x}_1, \bar{x}_2$ are sample mean values

z is a standardized score and is related to the level of confidence associated with the interval (see the subsection above on 'Estimating a mean').

It can be seen that the required precision (*w*), the specified level of confidence and the common population standard deviation (σ) affect the sample size. An estimate for σ might be obtained from a pilot study or from previous research. Alternatively, precision might be defined in terms of an *effect size statistic* (*d*), which is a standardized difference based on a number of standard deviations (i.e. $w = d\sigma$) (see Section 17.3.1). Using this option, the formula for calculating sample size from each population (or each subgroup) simplifies to:

$$n \geqslant 2\left(\frac{z}{d}\right)^2$$

Values of *d* may be interpreted as small (0.2), moderate (0.5) and large (0.8), following guidelines in Cohen (1992). Table 18.25 presents some examples of sample size for varying values of *d* and confidence levels of 95% and 99%.

The formula is applicable for values from non-normal distributions (see Section 13.2.2) when *n* is greater than 30. When *n* represents a high proportion of each population (5% or more) an adjustment is made to the sample size; see Section 8.5.1 (Moser and Kalton, 1971; Daniel, 1991).

Table 18.25 Adequate sample size (from each of two populations or from each subgroup of one population) for estimating the difference between two mean values; varying standardized differences and confidence levels of 95% and 99%

Standardized difference ($d = w/\sigma$)	Confidence level 95% ($z = 1.960$)	Confidence level 99% ($z = 2.576$)
0.8	13	21
0.7	16	28
0.6	22	37
0.5	31	54
0.4	48	83
0.3	86	148
0.2	193	332

Estimating a proportion

Based on a random sample from a population and an assumption that the sample proportion of cases with a particular attribute follows a normal distribution (Section 13.2.2), a confidence interval for the population proportion is given by:

$$p - z\sqrt{\frac{\pi(1-\pi)}{n}} \text{ to } p + z\sqrt{\frac{\pi(1-\pi)}{n}}$$

which leads to:

$$n \geqslant \frac{z^2\pi(1-\pi)}{w^2}$$

where:

n is an adequate size for a random sample from the population;

π is the proportion of cases with a particular attribute in the population;

p is the proportion of cases with a particular attribute in the sample;

w is the half width of the confidence interval and reflects the required precision for the estimate of the population proportion, i.e. confidence interval for π is $p - w$ to $p + w$;

z is a standardized score and is related to the level of confidence associated with the interval (see the subsection on 'Estimating a mean').

Table 18.26 *Adequate sample sizes for estimating a population proportion with 95% confidence; varying precision*

The unknown population proportion (π)	Precision (w)			
	.01	.05	.1	.2
.5	9604	385	97	25
.4	9220	369	93	24
.3	8068	323	81	21
.2	6147	246	62	16
.1	3458	139	35	9
.05	1825	73	19	5

The sample size depends upon the required precision (w), the specified confidence level and the value of the population parameter being estimated (π). Choice of the required precision (w) might be based on the purpose for making the estimate, or on past research. However, what value do we substitute in the formula for π, the unknown population proportion? The calculated sample size is relatively stable for proportions in the range .1 to .9 (Moser and Kalton, 1971) and, therefore, a 'reasonable guess' will suffice. If this strategy is thought to be impractical, using a value of .5 will produce a larger sample size than is necessary for other values of π (de Vaus, 1991). Table 18.26 presents some examples of sample sizes for varying values of w and a 95% confidence level.

Estimating the difference between two proportions

The formula for determining an adequate sample size to estimate the difference between two population proportions is based on the following assumptions:

- Random samples of the same size are drawn from the two populations of interest (or two independent subgroups in a random sample from one population).
- The difference in sample proportions of cases with a particular attribute follows a normal distribution (or the sample size is large enough for this approximation to hold; Section 13.2.2).

Under these assumptions, an adequate sample size from each population may be calculated from:

$$n \geqslant \frac{z^2(\pi_1(1-\pi_1)+\pi_2(1-\pi_2))}{w^2}$$

where:

n is an adequate size for random samples from each of the two populations;

π_1 is the proportion of cases with a particular attribute in the first population;

π_2 is the proportion of cases with a particular attribute in the second population;

w reflects the required precision for the estimate of the difference in population proportions and is the half width of the associated confidence interval:

$(p_1 - p_2) - w$ to $(p_1 - p_2) + w$

p_1, p_2 are proportions of cases with a particular attribute in the two random samples;

z is a standardized score and is related to the level of confidence associated with the interval (see the subsection on 'Estimating a mean').

It can be seen that a potential problem with this calculation is that it incorporates values for the two population proportions. If the researcher does not have 'reasonable estimates', then a strategy is to substitute a value of .5 for both π_1 and π_2. This produces a maximum sample size for a given confidence level and precision (see comments under 'Estimating a proportion'). Some illustrative sample sizes are shown in Table 18.27.

18.6.2 Determining sample size for hypothesis testing

Most explanatory studies and many descriptive studies involve hypothesis tests on a difference in mean values of some variable across two (or more) groups or points in time, or on the difference in proportions of cases with some particular

Table 18.27 *Adequate sample sizes for estimating the difference between two population proportions with 95% confidence (a random sample of the given size is drawn from each of the two populations)*

Population proportions		Precision (w)	
π_1	π_1	0.1	0.2
.9	.8	97	25
.9	.7	116	29
.9	.6	127	32
.7	.6	173	44
.7	.5	177	45
.5	.5	193	49
.5	.4	189	48
.5	.3	177	45
.3	.2	143	36
.3	.1	116	29

Table 18.28 *Values frequently used for determining sample sizes. The quantities z_a and z_b are standardized scores associated with the given significance level and power, respectively. It has been assumed that the null hypothesis is tested against a non-directional alternative hypothesis (Section 13.4.4)*

Significance level	z_a	Power	z_b	$z_a + z_b$	$(z_a + z_b)^2$
.05	1.960	.8	0.842	2.802	7.851
.05	1.960	.9	1.282	3.242	10.511
.01	2.576	.8	0.842	3.418	11.683
.01	2.576	.9	1.282	3.858	14.884

$$n \geqslant \frac{2(z_a + z_b)^2 \sigma^2}{\delta^2}$$

where:

- n is an adequate size for a random sample from each population;
- σ is the standard deviation for individual values in the populations;
- δ reflects the difference in population means deemed important to detect;
- z_a, z_b are standardized scores associated with the required significance level and power, respectively.

characteristic in two (or more) subgroups. The aim is to determine a sample size such that an observed difference in the sample data – which is equal in magnitude to a practically or clinically important difference in the population – is discerned as statistically significant, at stated levels of significance and power (Section 13.4.8). The chosen level of significance for a hypothesis test is the probability of rejecting a true null hypothesis and the power is the probability of rejecting a false null hypothesis. The most frequently used levels of significance are .05 and .01, and of power .8 and .9.

In the following subsections, we consider sample size for simple hypothesis tests that are based on a normal distribution. Table 18.28 shows some values that are useful for the calculation of sample size.

Comparison of population means (independent cases)

Based on independent, random samples from two populations with equal standard deviations (or on two independent subgroups of a random sample from one population), and an assumption that the difference in sample means follows a normal distribution, an adequate number of cases per sample may be calculated from:

Use of equal sample sizes provides maximum power for a given total sample size (Armitage and Berry, 1994; Campbell *et al.*, 1995). The significance level, power, common population standard deviation (σ) and the minimum difference to be detected (δ) affect the sample size. Usually, σ is unknown and is estimated from a pilot study or obtained from previous research on the same variable. As long as the resultant n is greater than about 30, the effect of using an estimate for σ will be small (Armitage and Berry, 1994). The difference δ might be a published minimum clinical important difference or a difference that is judged by the researcher to be important in practice.

The standardized difference or effect size statistic (d) provides an alternate method for determining n, whereby δ is stated in terms of

$\sigma(\delta = d\sigma)$. The formula for calculating sample size for each population simplifies to:

$$n \geqslant \frac{2(z_a + z_b)^2}{d^2}$$

Table 18.29 presents sample sizes for frequently used values of d, power and significance level. It can be seen that the magnitude of difference between two means that is considered important to detect has most effect on the sample size. If the sample size is small ($n < 30$), a correction factor is often applied to the formula (Campbell et al., 1995).

Lehr (1992) proposes the following as a simple formula that gives an approximate sample size, which is an overestimate for small values of d:

$$n \geqslant \frac{16}{d^2}$$

Comparison of population means (repeated measures or paired cases)

When the researcher is interested in change over time, the data usually comprise paired measurements, or measurements repeated at different time points on the same cases. In this situation, an adequate sample size is given by:

$$n \geqslant \frac{(z_a + z_b)^2 \sigma^2}{\delta^2}$$

or

$$n \geqslant \frac{(z_a + z_b)^2}{d^2}$$

where the notation and assumptions are the same as for determining sample size for comparisons of independent means. Sample sizes for typical values of d, significance level, and power are given in Table 18.30. The sample sizes indicated are for paired measurements. Therefore, if the required sample size is 32, this is the minimum number of cases that would be needed for a study in which two repeated measurements were taken on each case (as each case provides two measurements). However, for a study in which measurements are to be taken from matched cases, a minimum of 64 would be needed (since each case only provides one measurement).

As with independent samples, the magnitude of difference that is considered important to detect has most effect on the sample size.

Unequal group sizes

In a randomized controlled trial, patient allocation may be unrestricted (i.e. it may produce unequal numbers of patients in each group; Section 7.2.2). Such a situation may sometimes be helpful to the researcher. For example, it may be desirable to gain a more precise estimate of treatment response for the new therapy than for the standard therapy, since such information may already exist for the standard therapy. Randomizing more patients to the experimental

Table 18.29 Adequate sample size (from each population) for estimating the difference between two independent mean values; varying standardized differences, significance levels and power. It has been assumed that the null hypothesis is tested against a non-directional alternative hypothesis (Section 13.4.4)

Significance level	Power	Standardized difference ($d = \delta/\sigma$)		
		0.8	0.5	0.2
.05	.8	25	63	393
.05	.9	33	85	526
.01	.8	37	94	585
.01	.9	47	120	745

Table 18.30 Adequate sample size for estimating the difference between paired mean values; varying standardized differences, significance levels and power (with a non-directional alternative hypothesis)

Significance level	Power	Standardized difference ($d = \delta/\sigma$)		
		0.8	0.5	0.2
.05	.8	13	32	197
.05	.9	17	43	263
.01	.8	19	47	293
.01	.9	24	60	373

Table 18.31 *The approximate effect on power of unequal randomization to two treatment groups, for a fixed sample size, and assuming that the level of significance is set at .05 and that power is set at .95 for 1:1 allocation*

Allocation ratio	Power
1:1	.95
3:2	.94
2:1	.93
3:1	.88
4:1	.82
9:1	.58

Table 18.32 *Adequate sample size per group for comparisons of two population proportions (π_2 and π_2; $\pi_1 > \pi_2$), at a .05 level of significance*

π_1	Power .8 π_2				Power .9 π_2			
	.7	.5	.3	.1	.7	.5	.3	.1
.9	62	20	10	5	82	26	12	6
.7		94	24	10		125	31	12
.5			94	20			125	26
.3				62				82

arm of the study will have this effect. It is important, however, to consider the consequences of unequal randomization for the power of the study. It can be seen from Table 18.31 that there is little loss of power until an allocation ratio of 3:1, at which point power falls off quite rapidly (Pocock, 1979).

Comparisons of population proportions (independent cases)

A comparison of population proportions might be performed through a Pearson's chi-square test of independence (Section 14.1.1). Armitage and Berry (1994) give an exact formula for calculating sample size for each group to detect a difference between two population proportions (π_1 and π_2) at stated levels of significance and power. This is a rather complicated formula. A simpler formula, for an approximate sample size for each group, may bc found in Campbell and Machin (1993). Table 18.32 gives adequate sample sizes per group for varying values of π_1, π_2 and power, at a .05 level of significance, using the exact formula.

18.6.3 Determining sample size for nonparametric methods

Whereas sample size determination is relatively easy for parametric methods, it is much harder for nonparametric techniques that require far less restrictive assumptions (Sprent, 1993). Using computer simulation techniques, various studies have demonstrated:

- a slight power advantage for the parametric *t* test compared with the Wilcoxon rank sum test, when values in the populations follow normal distributions
- moderate to very large power advantages for the Wilcoxon rank sum test compared with the *t* test, when values in the populations follow non-normal distributions (with increasing advantage for larger sample sizes)
- greater effects of outliers or extreme values on Type I error rates for parametric tests compared with nonparametric tests (MacDonald, 1999)
- fewer rejections of the null hypothesis for differences in the wrong direction, e.g. positive when the population difference was negative (this is sometimes referred to as a Type III error)
- more pronounced benefits of non parametric tests for unequal sample sizes.

One strategy, then, for determining sample size for a nonparametric test such as the Wilcoxon rank sum (Section 14.2.6) is to use the formula for the equivalent parametric *t* test (Section 14.2.5) and apply a multiplicative factor of 1/0.95 (since the relative efficiency of the Wilcoxon rank sum test is about 95% when all assumptions for the *t* test are met). This strategy is likely to overestimate the required sample size. It is a suitable approach when there is reason to believe that individual values of the variable of interest might follow a highly skewed distribution, or when there is doubt that the level of measurement exceeds ordinal.

A second strategy is to use the approximation proposed by Campbell *et al.* (1995) for ordered categorical data. The corresponding formula for determining sample size for a Wilcoxon rank sum test (a comparison of median values across two groups, A and B) is based on the following assumptions:

1. The data represent values on a *k*-point ordinal scale. For example, a frequently used five-point Likert scale is denoted by 1 through 5, representing 'strongly disagree', 'disagree', 'neither', 'agree' and 'strongly agree', respectively.
2. Approximately equal numbers of all data values are anticipated at each scale point, across both groups (adjacent scale points might be combined to satisfy this requirement, although this effectively reduces the number of scale points on which the data have been measured).
3. The odds ratio (OR) is the odds of an individual value in one group being at a given point, or lower, on the measurement scale compared with the other group (see Section 17.3.2 for a discussion of odds ratios).
4. The odds ratio is constant for each pair of adjacent scale points (excluding the highest scale point).

An adequate sample size per group, for a Wilcoxon rank sum test, at a .05 level of significance, with power .8, is given by:

$$n \geqslant \frac{C}{(\log_e(OR))^2}$$

where:
- *n* is an adequate size for a sample of independent cases from each population;
- *C* is a constant that depends on the number of points in the measurement scale (see Table 18.33);
- $\log_e$ is the natural logarithm;
- *OR* is the anticipated odds ratio at each scale point (except the highest).

Table 18.33 *Adequate sample sizes and values for C associated with a Wilcoxon rank sum test, with a non-directional alternative hypothesis, significance level .05 and power .80; data values measured according to different numbers of scale points*

Number of scale points	C	Odds ratio (OR)					
		0.2	0.5	0.8	1.2	1.6	2.0
2	62.7	25	131	1260	1887	284	131
3	52.9	21	111	1063	1592	240	111
4	50.2	20	105	1009	1511	228	105
5	49.0	19	102	985	1475	222	102
>5	47.0	19	98	944	1414	213	98

The odds associated with a particular scale point is given by:

$$\frac{\text{probability that a value is at the stated point or a lower scale point}}{\text{probability that a value is at a higher scale point}}$$

The odds ratio at a particular scale point is given by:

$$\frac{\text{odds associated with that scale point for values in group A}}{\text{odds associated with that scale point for values in group B}}$$

An odds ratio of 1 denotes no difference between the two groups. The odds ratio might be estimated from a table of the response frequencies at each scale point in a pilot study, from previous research, or by considering the difference between response frequencies across the two groups. Table 18.33 gives approximate sample sizes for various values of OR and numbers of scale points.

A larger sample size is needed for a reduced number of scale points, since there is less information to discriminate between scores in the two groups.

18.6.4 Determining sample size for reliability coefficients

There are two issues to consider when determining sample size for a reliability study: the total sample size, and its apportioning to (1) subjects and (2) either raters (for inter-rater reliability) or time points (for intra-rater reliability). In many studies, practical constraints might limit the number of raters and subject tolerance might limit the number of occasions on which repeat measurements are feasible. These considerations led Walter *et al.* (1998) to develop a formula for the required number of subjects, given a stated number of raters or time points. Although this work assumes that components of reliability are given by between-subject and within-subject variation only (i.e. uses a model based on a one-way ANOVA) and is concerned with hypothesis testing rather than estimation, the resultant sample sizes provide guidelines for ICC(2,1) and ICC(3,1) models (Section 18.3.2). This work provides a guide as to the number of subjects required to estimate the 'true' reliability coefficient of an instrument of either .7 or .6, using different numbers of raters or time points (Table 18.34).

18.6.5 Adjusting the sample size to allow for non-responders and attrition

The formulae given in the preceding sections for the calculation of adequate sample sizes do not include allowances for non-response or attrition over time. For example, a random sample of 93 cases was recommended to estimate a population proportion (of about .4 in value) to within .1 units, with 95% confidence (Table 18.26). In the context of a particular study, a response rate of 60% from a questionnaire might be deemed good and 50% adequate (Section 15.5.1). To achieve 93 returns, we might be advised to administer 93/.60 = 155 questionnaires if we anticipate a good response rate, or 93/.50 = 186 questionnaires if we anticipate an adequate response rate.

Many clinical trials are set up to investigate change over time and to compare change across study groups (as in the Low Back Pain Study). An attrition rate around 10% is not uncommon at each occasion on which measurements are made after the initial baseline measurement. Two independent, random samples of size 63 (making a total of 126) would be needed to detect a standardized difference of 0.5 between the means of two sampled populations, at a significance level of .05 and with power .80 (Table 18.29). This sample size would also enable a standardized difference of 0.35 to be detected across time for paired means *within* each of the two groups at the same significance and power levels. Comparisons within subjects are more precise than comparisons between subjects (Sections 18.1.6 and 18.1.7). It is advisable to consider adequate sample sizes for important differences both between and within groups.

If we wish to detect a standardized mean difference of 0.5 across two groups at the second occasion on which measurements are taken (e.g. 4 weeks after baseline), we might be advised to use 63/.90 = 70 participants in each group at baseline (assuming 10% attrition, significance level .05, power .80).

To detect this difference between group means at a third occasion (e.g. 12 weeks after baseline), we might use $63/(.90)^2 = 78$ participants in each group at baseline (assuming 10% attrition at each time point after baseline, significance level .05, power .80).

18.6.6 Deciding what variables to use to determine sample size

Many studies involve the measurement of several variables on each participant (e.g. pain affect,

Table 18.34 *Adequate number of subjects, in most studies, to determine the reliability of an instrument with 'true' reliability exceeding either .7 or .6, and with either two, three or four raters*

'True' reliability exceeding	Number of raters or time points	Adequate number of subjects
.7	2	19
.7	3	13
.7	4	12
.6	2	40
.6	3	27
.6	4	22

pain intensity, self-rated change, and Aberdeen Back Pain Scale scores for participants in the Low Back Pain Study). It may be possible to calculate the required sample size for each variable and to select the largest. This strategy might produce higher power than necessary for some variables and entails a fair amount of work at the design stage. However, it should be remembered that '[i]f it is too much work to calculate sample size for 20 outcome measures, it will also be too much work to analyse the data' (Tate *et al.*, 1999, p. 491). Ultimately, the comparative importance of the variables and resource limitations may affect the decision to use this maximum sample size.

Another frequently used strategy is to determine sample size for the most important variable only. Here, the variable chosen as 'most important' should be the one that is of greatest relevance to the study and its context, not the one that is most parsimonious in terms of sample size.

It is also necessary to consider what proposed analyses are to be performed on the data – in particular, whether analyses of subgroups are planned (e.g. comparisons across male and female, or across participants with rheumatoid arthritis and osteoarthritis). If such analyses are inherent in a study's main objectives, sample size calculations are performed for these subgroup comparisons. A similar argument may be made for interaction effects in clinical trials (Section 18.1.9).

18.7 CONCLUSION

This chapter constitutes a brief encounter with a few of the more advanced techniques used to analyse data from clinical trials, surveys and reliability studies. An aim has been to introduce basic concepts and principles underlying these techniques, and to give examples of their use. Further details of these techniques may be found in more specialized texts.

REFERENCES

Aaronson, L S and Burman, M E (1994) Use of health records in research: reliability and validity issues. *Research in Nursing and Health*, **17**, 67–73.

Aaronson, N K, Muller, M, Cohen, P D, Essink-Bot, M L, Fekkes, M, Sanderman, R, Sprangers, M A, te Velde, A and Verrips, E (1998) Translation, validation, and norming of the Dutch language version of the SF-36 Health Survey in community and chronic disease populations. *Journal of Clinical Epidemiology*, **51**, 1055–1068.

Abrams, K R and Scragg, A M (1996) Quantitative methods in nursing research. *Journal of Advanced Nursing*, **23**, 1008–1015.

Abramson, J H (1990) *Survey Methods in Community Medicine: Epidemiological Studies, Programme Evaluation, Clinical Trials*, 4th edn. Churchill Livingstone, Edinburgh.

Abreu, B C, Peloquin, S M and Ottenbacher, K (1998) Competence in scientific inquiry and research. *American Journal of Occupational Therapy* **52**, 751–759.

Ackroyd, S and Hughes, J A (1992) *Data Collection in Context*, 2nd edn. Longman, London.

Admi, H (1995) The life history: a viable approach to nursing research. *Nursing Research*, **44**, 186–188.

Ahern, K J (1999) Ten tips for reflexive bracketing. *Qualitative Health Research*, **9**, 407–411.

Allison, P D (1999) *Multiple Regression: A Primer*. Pine Forge Press, Thousand Oaks.

Altman, D G (1991a) *Practical Statistics for Medical Research*. Chapman & Hall, London.

Altman, D G (1991b) Randomisation. *British Medical Journal*, **302**, 1481–1482.

Altman, D G (1998) Confidence intervals for the number needed to treat. *British Medical Journal*, **317**, 1309–1312.

Altman, D G and Bland, J M (1994) Quartiles, quintiles, centiles, and other quantiles. *British Medical Journal*, **309**, 996.

Altman, D G and Bland, J M (1995) Absence of evidence is not evidence of absence. *British Medical Journal*, **311**, 485.

Altman, D G and Bland, J M (1997) Units of analysis. *British Medical Journal*, **314**, 1874.

Altman, D G and Bland, J M (1998) Generalisation and extrapolation. *British Medical Journal*, **317**, 409–410.

Altman, D G and Bland, J M (1999a) Treatment allocation in controlled trials: why randomise? *British Medical Journal*, **318**, 1209.

Altman, D G and Bland, J M (1999b) How to randomise. *British Medical Journal*, **319**, 703–704.

Altman, D G and Bland, J M (1983) Measurement in medicine: the analysis of method comparison studies. *Statistician*, **32**, 307–317.

Altman, D G, Gore, S M, Gardner, M J and Pocock, S J (1989) Statistical guidelines for contributors to medical journals. In: *Statistics with Confidence: Confidence Intervals and Statistical Guidelines* (ed. Gardner, M J and Altman, D G). British Medical Journal, London, pp. 88–100.

Anderson, J M (1991) The phenomenological perspective. In: *Qualitative Nursing Research: A Contemporary Dialogue* (ed. Morse J M). Sage Publications, Newbury Park, pp. 25–38.

Andrews, K (1991) The limitations of randomized controlled trials in rehabilitation research. *Clinical Rehabilitation*, **5**, 5–8.

Antman, E M, Lau, J, Kupelnick, B, Mosteller, F and Chalmers, T C (1992) A comparison of the results of meta-analyses of randomized control trials and recommendations of clinical experts: treatments for myocardial infarction. *Journal of the American Medical Association*, **268**, 240–248.

APA (1994) *Publication Manual of the American Psychological Association*, 4th edn. American Psychological Association, Washington.

Appelbaum, P S, Roth, L H, Lidz, C W, Benson, P and Winslade, W (1987) False hopes and best data: consent to research and the therapeutic misconception. *Hastings Center Report*, **17**(2), 20–24.

Arber, S (1993) Designing samples. In: *Researching Social Life* (ed. Gilbert, N). Sage Publications, London, pp. 68–92.

Archbold, P (1986) Ethical issues in qualitative research. In: *From Practice to Grounded Theory: Qualitative Research in Nursing* (ed. Chenitz, W C and Swanson, J M). Addison-Wesley, Menlo Park, pp. 155–163.

Arksey, H and Knight, P (1999) *Interviewing for Social Scientists*. Sage Publications, London.

Armitage, P and Berry, G (1994) *Statistical Methods in Medical Research*, 3rd edn. Blackwell Scientific Publications, Oxford.

Avis, M (1995) Valid arguments? A consideration of the concept of validity in establishing the credibility of research findings. *Journal of Advanced Nursing*, **22**, 1203–1209.

Avis, M (1998) Objectivity in nursing research: observations and objections. *International Journal of Nursing Studies*, 35, 141–145.

Babbie, E (1989) *The Practice of Social Research*, 5th edn. Wadsworth Publishing, Belmont.

Babbie, E (1990) *Survey Research Methods*, 2nd edn. Wadsworth Publishing, Belmont.

Backman, C L and Harris, S R (1999) Case studies, single-subject research, and N of 1 randomized trials: comparisons and contrasts. *American Journal of Physical Medicine and Rehabilitation*, 78, 170–176.

Backman, C L, Harris, S R, Chisholm, J M and Monette, A D (1997) Single-subject research in rehabilitation: a review of studies using AB, withdrawal, multiple baseline, and alternating treatments designs. *Archives of Physical Medicine and Rehabilitation*, **78**, 1145–1153.

Baer, D M (1977) Perhaps it would be better not to know everything. *Journal of Applied Behavior Analysis*, **10**, 167–172.

Bailey, C A (1996) *A Guide to Field Research*. Pine Forge Press, Thousand Oaks.

Bailey, D M (1997) *Research for the Health Professional: A Practical Guide*, 2nd edn. F A Davis, Philadelphia.

Baillie, L (1995) Ethnography and nursing research: a critical appraisal. *Nurse Researcher*, 3(2), 5–21.

Barlow, D H and Hersen, M (1984) *Single Case Experimental Designs: Strategies for Studying Behavior Change*, 2nd edn. Pergamon Press, New York.

Barnard, S and Hartigan, G (1998) *Clinical Audit in Physiotherapy: From Theory into Practice*. Butterworth-Heinemann, Oxford.

Barnett, V (1991) *Sample Survey Principles and Methods*. Edward Arnold, London.

Barriball, K L and While, A E (1999) Non-response in survey research: a methodological discussion and development of an explanatory model. *Journal of Advanced Nursing*, 30, 677–686.

Bartko, J J (1976) On various intraclass correlation reliability coefficients. *Psychological Bulletin*, **83**, 762–765.

Bartko, J J and Carpenter, W T (1976) On the methods and theory of reliability. *Journal of Nervous and Mental Disease*, **163**, 307–317.

Beauchamp, T L and Childress, J F (1994) *Principles of Biomedical Ethics*, 4th edn. Oxford University Press, New York.

Bechtel, W (1988) *Philosophy of Science: An Overview for Cognitive Science*. Lawrence Erlbaum, Hillsdale.

Beck, A T, Ward, C H, Mendelson, M, Mock, J and Erbaugh, J (1961) An inventory for measuring depression. *Archives of General Psychiatry*, **4**, 561–571.

Beck, C T (1999) Facilitating the work of a meta-analyst. *Research in Nursing and Health*, **22**, 523–530.

Beech, I (1999) Bracketing in phenomenological research. *Nurse Researcher*, 6(3), 35–51.

Beery, K (1989) *Development Test of Visual Motor Integration*, rev. edn. Follett Publishing, Chicago.

Behi, R and Nolan, M (1996a) Causality and control: threats to internal validity. *British Journal of Nursing*, **5**, 374–377.

Behi, R and Nolan, M (1996b) Quasi-experimental research designs. *British Journal of Nursing*, 5, 1079–1081.

Behi, R and Nolan, M (1996c) Single-case experimental designs 1: using idiographic research. *British Journal of Nursing*, 5, 1334–1337.

Behi, R and Nolan, M (1997) Single-case experimental designs 2: common examples. *British Journal of Nursing*, 6, 116–119.

Belson, W A and Duncan, J A (1962) A comparison of the check-list and the open response questioning systems. *Applied Statistics*, **11**, 120–132.

Bengali, M K and Ottenbacher, K J (1998) The effect of autocorrelation on the results of visually analyzing data from single-subject designs. *American Journal of Occupational Therapy*, **52**, 650–655.

Benner, P (1994) The tradition and skill of interpretive phenomenology in studying health, illness and caring practices. In: *Interpretive Phenomenology: Embodiment, Caring and Ethics in Health and Illness* (ed. Benner, P). Sage Publications, Thousand Oaks, pp. 99–127.

Benoliel, J Q (1996) Grounded theory and nursing knowledge. *Qualitative Health Research*, 6, 406–428.

Benson, D and Hughes, J A (1983) *The Perspective of Ethnomethodology*. Longman, London.

Bird, S, Nicholls, G and White, E (1995) An overview of the research methodologies available to the occupational therapist and an outline of the research process. *British Journal of Occupational Therapy*, 58, 510–516.

Bithell, C (1994) Single subject experimental design: a case for concern? *Physiotherapy*, **80**, 85–67.

Bjordal, J M and Greve, G (1998) What may alter the conclusions of reviews? *Physical Therapy Reviews*, **3**, 121–132.

Blackwood, B and Lavery, G (1998) The crossover study design and its clinical application. *Nurse Researcher*, **5**(4), 5–14.

Blaikie, N (1991) A critique of the use of triangulation in social research. *Quality and Quantity*, **25**, 115–136.

Blaikie, N (1993) *Approaches to Social Enquiry*. Polity Press, Cambridge.

Blair, R C and Higgins, J J (1985) Comparison of the power of the paired samples *t* test to that of Wilcoxon's signed-ranks test under various populations. *Psychological Bulletin*, **97**, 119–128.

Blalock, H M (1972) *Social Statistics*, 2nd edn. McGraw-Hill Kogakusha, Tokyo.

Bland, C J, Meurer, L N and Maldonado, G (1995) A systematic approach to conducting a non-statistical meta-analysis of research literature. *Academic Medicine*, **70**, 642–653.

Bland, J M and Altman, D G (1986) Statistical methods for assessing agreement between two methods of clinical measurement. *Lancet*, **1**, 307–310.

Bland, J M and Altman, D G (1990) A note on the use of the intraclass correlation coefficient in the evaluation of agreement between two methods of measurement. *Computers in Biology and Medicine*, **20**, 337–340.

Bland, J M and Altman, D G (1994a) One and two sided tests of significance. *British Medical Journal*, **309**, 248.

Bland, J M and Altman, D G (1994b) Some examples of regression towards the mean. *British Medical Journal*, **309**, 780.

Bland, J M and Altman, D G (1994c) Matching. *British Medical Journal*, **309**, 1128.

Bland, J M and Altman, D G (1995) Multiple significance tests: the Bonferroni method. *British Medical Journal*, **310**, 170.

Bland, J M and Altman, D G (1997) Cronbach's alpha. *British Medical Journal*, **314**, 572.

Bland, J M and Altman, D G (1998) Bayesians and frequentists. *British Medical Journal*, **317**, 1151.

Bland, J M and Kerry, S M (1997) Trials randomised in clusters. *British Medical Journal*, **315**, 600.

Bland, M (1995) *An Introduction to Medical Statistics*, 2nd edn. Oxford University Press, Oxford.

Blettner, M, Sauerbrei, W, Schlehofer, B, Scheuchenpflug, T and Friedenreich, C (1999) Traditional reviews, meta-analyses and pooled analyses in epidemiology. *International Journal of Epidemiology*, **28**, 1–9.

Bloom, M and Fischer, J (1982) *Evaluating Practice: Guidelines for the Accountable Professional*. Prentice-Hall, Englewood Cliffs.

Bobrovitz, C D and Ottenbacher, K J (1998) Comparison of visual inspection and statistical analysis of single-subject data in rehabilitation research. *American Journal of Physical Medicine and Rehabilitation*, **77**, 94–102.

Bogdewic, S P (1992) Participant observation. In: *Doing Qualitative Research* (ed. Crabtree, B F and Miller, W L). Sage Publications, Newbury Park, pp. 45–69.

Bond, S and Bond, J (1982) A Delphi survey of clinical nursing research priorities. *Journal of Advanced Nursing*, **7**, 565–575.

Boniface, D R (1995) *Experiment Design and Statistical Methods for Behavioural and Social Research*. Chapman & Hall, London.

Bork, C (1993) Populations, samples, and statistical significance. In: *Research in Physical Therapy* (ed. Bork, C E). J B Lippincott, Philadelphia, pp. 207–222.

Bottorff, J L (1994) Using videotaped recordings in qualitative research. In: *Critical Issues in Qualitative Research Methods* (ed. Morse J M). Sage Publications, Thousand Oaks, pp. 244–261.

Bourque, L B and Fielder, E P (1995) *How to Conduct Self-Administered and Mail Surveys*. Sage Publications, Thousand Oaks.

Bowers, D (1996) *Statistics from Scratch: An Introduction for Health Care Professionals*. John Wiley, Chichester.

Bowling, A (1997) *Research Methods in Health: Investigating Health and Health Services*. Open University Press, Buckingham.

Boyle, J S (1994) Styles of ethnography. In: *Critical Issues in Qualitative Research Methods* (ed. Morse, J M). Sage Publications, Thousand Oaks, pp. 159–185.

Bradburn, N M and Sudman, S (1980) *Improving Interview Method and Questionnaire Design*. Jossey-Bass, San Francisco.

Bradford Hill, A and Hill, I D (1991) *Bradford Hill's Principles of Medical Statistics*, 12th edn. Edward Arnold, London.

Bradley, S (1995) Methodological triangulation in

healthcare research. *Nurse Researcher*, 3(2), 81–89.

Breakwell, G M and Wood, P (1995) Diary techniques. In: *Research Methods in Psychology* (ed. Breakwell, G M, Hammond, S and Fife-Schaw, C). Sage Publications, London, pp. 293–301.

Brennan, P and Croft, P (1994) Interpreting the results of observational research: chance is not such a fine thing. *British Medical Journal*, 309, 727–730.

Brennan, P and Silman, A (1992) Statistical methods for assessing observer variability in clinical measures. *British Medical Journal*, 304, 1491–1494.

Brewer, J and Hunter, A (1989) *Multimethod Research: A Synthesis of Styles*. Sage Publications, Newbury Park.

Britten, N (2000) Qualitative interviews in health care research. In: *Qualitative Research in Health Care*, 2nd edn (ed. Pope, C and Mays, N). British Medical Journal, London, pp. 11–19.

Britten, N and Fisher, B (1993) Qualitative research and general practice. *British Journal of General Practice*, 43, 270–271.

Bryant, T N and Machin, D (1997) Statistical methods. In: *Rehabilitation Studies Handbook* (ed. Wilson, B A and McLellan, D L). Cambridge University Press, Cambridge, pp. 189–204.

Bryman, A (1988) *Quantity and Quality in Social Research*. Unwin Hyman, London.

Bryman, A and Burgess, R G (1994) Reflections on qualitative data analysis. In: *Analyzing Qualitative Data* (ed. Bryman, A and Burgess, R G). Routledge, London, pp. 216–226.

Bullinger, M (1995) German translation and psychometric testing of the SF-36 Health Survey: preliminary results from the IQOLA Project – International Quality of Life Assessment. *Social Science and Medicine*, 41, 1359–1366.

Bulmer, M (1979) Concepts in the analysis of qualitative data. *Sociological Review*, 27, 651–677.

Burgess, R G (1984) *In the Field: An Introduction to Field Research*. Unwin Hyman, London.

Burman, E (1994a) Interviewing. In: *Qualitative Methods in Psychology: a Research Guide* (ed. Banister, P, Burman, E, Parker, I, Taylor, M and Tindall, C). Open University Press, Buckingham, pp. 49–71.

Burman, E (1994b) Feminist research. In: *Qualitative Methods in Psychology: a Research Guide* (ed.

Banister, P, Burman, E, Parker, I, Taylor, M and Tindall C). Open University Press, Buckingham, pp. 121–141.

Burnand, B, Paccaud, F and Santos-Eggimann, B (1991) What are the minimal methodological requirements for a good trial? II. The statistician's view. In: *Physiotherapy: Controlled Trials and Facts* (ed. Schlapbach, P and Gerber, N J). Karger, Basel, pp. 9–17.

Burns, N and Grove, S K (1997) *The Practice of Nursing Research: Conduct, Critique and Utilization*, 3rd edn. W B Saunders, Philadelphia.

Bury, T and Mead, J (1998) *Evidence-Based Healthcare: A Practical Guide for Therapists*. Butterworth-Heinemann, Oxford.

Busk, P L and Marascuilo, L A (1992) Statistical analysis in single-case research: issues, procedures, and recommendations, with applications to multiple behaviors. In: *Single-Case Research Design and Analysis: New Directions for Psychology and Education* (ed. Kratochwill, T R and Levin, J R). Lawrence Erlbaum, Hillsdale, pp. 159–185.

Busk, P L and Serlin, R C (1992) Meta-analysis for single-case research. In: *Single-Case Research Design and Analysis: New Directions for Psychology and Education* (ed. Kratochwill, T R and Levin, J R). Lawrence Erlbaum, Hillsdale, pp. 187–212.

Calder, J (1996) Statistical techniques. In: *Data Collection and Analysis* (ed. Sapsford, R and Jupp, V). Sage Publications, London, pp. 225–261.

Campbell, D T and Fiske, D W (1959) Convergent and discriminant validation by the Multitrait-Multimethod Matrix. *Psychological Bulletin*, 56, 81–105.

Campbell, D T and Stanley, J C (1963) *Experimental and Quasi-Experimental Designs for Research*. Rand McNally College Publishing, Chicago.

Campbell, M J, Julious, S A and Altman, D G (1995) Estimating sample sizes for binary, ordered categorical, and continuous outcomes in two group comparisons. *British Medical Journal*, 311, 1145–1148.

Campbell, M J and Machin, D (1993) *Medical Statistics: A Commonsense Approach*, 2nd edn. John Wiley, Chichester.

Campbell, M K and Grimshaw, J M (1998) Cluster randomised trials: time for improvement. *British Medical Journal*, 317, 1171–1172.

Canelón, M F (1995) Job site analysis facilitates work

reintegration. *American Journal of Occupational Therapy*, **49**, 461–467.

Cannon, S (1989) Social research in stressful settings: difficulties for the sociologist studying the treatment of breast cancer. *Sociology of Health and Illness*, **11**, 62–77.

Carey, M A (1994) The group effect in focus groups: planning, implementing, and interpreting focus group research. In: *Critical Issues in Qualitative Research Methods* (ed. Morse, J M). Sage Publications, Thousand Oaks, pp. 225–241.

Carey, M A and Smith, M W (1994) Capturing the group effect in focus groups: a special concern in analysis. *Qualitative Health Research*, **4**, 123–127.

Carmines, E G and Zeller, R A (1994) Reliability and validity assessment. In: *Basic Measurement* (ed. Lewis-Beck, M J). Sage Publications, Thousand Oaks, pp. 1–58.

Carpenter, C (1997) Conducting qualitative research in physiotherapy: a methodological example. *Physiotherapy*, **83**, 547–552.

Carr, E K (1991) Observational methods in rehabilitation research. *Clinical Rehabilitation*, **5**, 89–94.

Carr, L T (1994) The strengths and weaknesses of quantitative and qualitative research: what method for nursing? *Journal of Advanced Nursing*, **20**, 716–721.

Carter, D (1996) Barriers to the implementation of research findings in practice. *Nurse Researcher*, **4**(2), 30–40.

Chalmers, A F (1982) *What Is This Thing Called Science? An Assessment of the Nature and Status of Science and Its Methods*, 2nd edn. Open University Press, Milton Keynes.

Chalmers, I and Altman, D G (1995) *Systematic Reviews*. British Medical Journal, London.

Chalmers, T C, Levin, H, Sacks, H S, Reitman, D, Berrier, J and Nagalingam, R (1987) Meta-analysis of clinical trials as a scientific discipline. 1: Control of bias and comparison with large co-operative trials. *Statistics in Medicine*, **6**, 315–325.

Chapman, M and Mahon, B (1986) *Plain Figures*. HMSO, London.

Charlton, B G (1995) Mega-trials: methodological issues and clinical implications. *Journal of the Royal College of Physicians of London*, **29**, 96–100.

Charlton, B G and Walston, F (1998) Individual case studies in clinical research. *Journal of Evaluation in Clinical Practice*, **4**, 147–155.

Charmaz, K (1995) Grounded theory. In: *Rethinking Methods in Psychology* (ed. Smith, J A, Harré, R, Van Langenhove, L). Sage Publications, London, pp. 27–49.

Cherulnik, P D (1983) *Behavioral Research: Assessing the Validity of Research Findings in Psychology*. Harper & Row, New York.

Chesson, R (1993) How to design a questionnaire – a ten-stage strategy. *Physiotherapy*, **79**, 711–713.

Child, D (1990) *The Essentials of Factor Analysis*, 2nd edn. Cassell, London.

Chinn, S (1991a) Ranges, confidence intervals, and related quantities: what they are and when to use them. *Thorax*, **46**, 391–393.

Chinn, S (1991b) Repeatability and method comparison. *Thorax*, **46**, 454–456.

Chow, S L (1996) *Statistical Significance: Rationale, Validity and Utility*. Sage Publications, London.

Clarke, M J and Stewart, L A (1995) Obtaining data from randomised controlled trials: how much do we need for reliable and informative meta-analyses? In: *Systematic Reviews* (ed. Chalmers, I and Altman, D G). British Medical Journal, London, pp. 37–47.

Clarke, M J and Stewart, L A (1997) Meta-analyses using individual patient data. *Journal of Evaluation in Clinical Practice*, **3**, 207–212.

Clarke, R and Croft, P (1998) *Critical Reading for the Reflective Practitioner: A Guide for Primary Care*. Butterworth-Heinemann, Oxford.

Cleveland, W S and McGill, R (1984) Graphical perception: theory, experimentation, and application to the development of graphical methods. *Journal of the American Statistical Association*, **79**, 531–554.

Cliff, N (1996) *Ordinal Methods for Behavioral Data Analysis*. Lawrence Erlbaum, Mahwah.

Clifford, C (1997) *Nursing and Health Care Research*, 2nd edn. Prentice Hall, London.

Cobb, A K and Hamera, E (1986) Illness experience in a chronic disease – ALS. *Social Science and Medicine*, **23**, 641–650.

Cochran, W G (1952) The chi-square test of goodness-of-fit. *Annals of Mathematical Statistics*, **23**, 345–345.

Coggon, D (1995) *Statistics in Clinical Practice*. British Medical Journal, London.

Cohen, J (1960) A coefficient of agreement for nominal scales. *Educational and Psychological Measurement*, **20**, 37–46.

Cohen, J (1968) Weighted kappa: nominal scale agreement with provision for scaled disagreement or partial credit. *Psychological Bulletin*, **70**, 213–220.

Cohen, J (1992) A power primer. *Psychological Bulletin*, **112**, 155–159.

Cohen, L and Manion, L (1994) *Research Methods in Education*, 4th edn. Routledge, London.

Cole, B, Finch, E, Gowland, C and Mayo, N (1994) *Physical Rehabilitation Outcome Measures*. Canadian Physiotherapy Association, Toronto.

Collins, R, Gray, R, Godwin, J and Peto, R (1987) Avoidance of large biases and large random errors in the assessment of moderate treatment effects: the need for systematic overviews. *Statistics in Medicine*, **6**, 245–250.

Collins, R, Peto, R, Gray, R and Parish, S (1996) Large-scale randomized evidence: trials and overviews. In: *Oxford Textbook of Medicine, Vol 1* (ed. Weatherall, D J, Ledingham, J G G and Warrell, D A). Oxford University Press, Oxford, pp. 21–32.

Colquhoun, D and Kellehear, A (1993) *Health Research in Practice*. Chapman & Hall, London.

Conger, A J (1980) Integration and generalization of kappas for multiple raters. *Psychological Bulletin*, **88**, 322–328.

Conover, W J (1999) *Practical Nonparametric Statistics*, 3rd edn. John Wiley, New York.

Converse, J M and Presser, S (1994) Survey questions: handcrafting the standardized questionnaire. In: *Research Practice* (ed. Lewis-Beck, M S). Sage Publications, Thousand Oaks, pp. 89–161.

Cook, D J, Mulrow, C D and Haynes, R B (1997) Systematic reviews: synthesis of best evidence for clinical decisions. *Annals of Internal Medicine*, **126**, 376–380.

Cook, R J and Sackett, D L (1995) The number needed to treat: a clinically useful measure of treatment effect. *British Medical Journal*, **310**, 452–454.

Cook, T D and Campbell, D T (1979) *Quasi-Experimentation: Design and Analysis Issues for Field Settings*. Houghton Mifflin, Boston.

Coolican, H (1990) *Research Methods and Statistics in Psychology*. Hodder & Stoughton, London.

Cooper, H (1998) *Synthesizing Research: A Guide for Literature Reviews*, 3rd edn. Sage Publications, Thousand Oaks.

Cooper, H M and Lindsay, J J (1998) Research synthesis and meta-analysis. In: *Handbook of Applied Social Research Methods* (ed. Bickman, L

and Rog, D J). Sage Publications, Thousand Oaks, pp. 315–337.

Corbin, J (1986) Coding, writing memos, and diagramming. In: *From Practice to Grounded Theory: Qualitative Research in Nursing* (ed. Chenitz, W C and Swanson, J M). Addison-Wesley, Menlo Park, pp. 102–120.

Cormack, D F S and Benton, D C (1996) Asking the research question. In: *The Research Process in Nursing*, 3rd edn (ed. Cormack, D F S). Blackwell Science, Oxford, pp. 53–63.

Corner, J (1991) In search of more complete answers to research questions. Quantitative versus qualitative research methods: is there a way forward? *Journal of Advanced Nursing*, **16**, 718–727.

Cornwell, J (1984) *Hard-Earned Lives: Accounts of Health and Illness from East London*. Tavistock Publications, London.

Cowman, S (1993) Triangulation: a means of reconciliation in nursing research. *Journal of Advanced Nursing*, **18**, 788–792.

Coyne, I T (1997) Sampling in qualitative research. Purposeful and theoretical sampling; merging or clear boundaries? *Journal of Advanced Nursing*, **26**, 623–630.

Cresswell, J W (1994) *Research Design: Qualitative and Quantitative Approaches*. Sage Publications, Thousand Oaks.

Crisp, J, Pelletier, D, Duffield, C, Adams, A and Nagy, S (1997) The Delphi method? *Nursing Research*, **46**, 116–118.

Crombie, I K and Davies, H T O (1996) *Research in Health Care: Design, Conduct and Interpretation of Health Services Research*. John Wiley, Chichester.

Crombie, I K and McQuay, H J (1998) The systematic review: a good guide rather than a guarantee. *Pain*, **76**, 1–2.

Cronbach, L J (1951) Coefficient alpha and the internal structure of tests. *Psychometrika*, **16**, 297–334.

Crowley, P (1996) Using an overview. *Baillière's Clinical Obstetrics and Gynaecology*, **10**, 585–597.

Cuff, E C and Payne, G C E (1984) *Perspectives in Sociology*, 2nd edn. Allen & Unwin, London.

Cummings, S R, Ernster, V and Hulley, S B (1988) Designing a new study: I. Cohort studies. In: *Designing Clinical Research: An Epidemiologic Approach* (ed. Hulley, S B and Cummings, S R). Williams & Wilkins, Baltimore, pp. 63–74.

Czaja, R and Blair, J (1996) *Designing Surveys: A Guide to Decisions and Procedures*. Pine Forge Press, Thousand Oaks.

Daly, F, Hand, D J, Jones, M C, Lunn, A D and McConway, K J (1995) *Elements of Statistics*. Addison-Wesley, Wokingham.

Daly, J, McDonald, I and Willis, E (1992) *Researching Health Care: Designs, Dilemmas, Disciplines*. Routledge, London.

Dancy, J (1985) *An Introduction to Contemporary Epistemology*. Basil Blackwell, Oxford.

Daniel, W W (1990) *Applied Nonparametric Statistics*, 2nd edn. PWS-Kent, Boston.

Daniel, W W (1991) *Biostatistics: A Foundation for Analysis in the Health Sciences*, 5th edn. John Wiley, New York.

Davey Smith, G and Egger, M (1998) Meta-analysis: unresolved issues and future developments. *British Medical Journal*, 316, 221–225.

Davies, P L and Gavin, W J (1999) Measurement issues in treatment effectiveness studies. *American Journal of Occupational Therapy*, 53, 363–372.

Davis, A (1995) The experimental method in psychology. In: *Research Methods in Psychology* (ed. Breakwell, G M, Hammond, S and Fife-Schaw, C). Sage Publications, London, pp. 50–68.

Day, R A (1998) *How to Write and Publish a Scientific Paper*, 5th edn. Cambridge University Press, Cambridge.

Delucchi, K L (1993) On the use and misuse of chi-square. In: *A Handbook for Data Analysis in the Behavioral Sciences: Statistical Issues* (ed. Keren, G and Lewis, C). Lawrence Erlbaum, Hillsdale, pp. 295–320.

Denzin, N K (1971) Symbolic interactionism and ethnomethodology. In: *Understanding Everyday Life* (ed. Douglas, J D). Routledge & Kegan Paul, London, pp. 259–284.

Denzin, N K (1989a) *Interpretive Interactionism*. Sage Publications, Newbury Park.

Denzin, N K (1989b) *The Research Act: A Theoretical Introduction to Sociological Methods*, 3rd edn. Prentice Hall, Englewood Cliffs.

DePoy, E and Gitlin, L N (1998) *Introduction to Research: Understanding and Applying Multiple Strategies*, 2nd edn. Mosby, St Louis.

DeProspero, A and Cohen, S (1979) Inconsistent visual analysis of intrasubject data. *Journal of Applied Behavior Analysis*, 12, 573–579.

DeSantis, L and Ugarizza, D N (2000) The concept of theme as used in qualitative nursing research. *Western Journal of Nursing Research*, 22, 351–372.

DerSimonian, R and Laird, N (1986) Meta-analysis in clinical trials. *Controlled Clinical Trials*, 7, 177–188.

De Souza, L H (1997) One case at a time. *Physiotherapy*, 83, 107–108.

De Souza, L H (1999) The development of a scale of the Guttman type for the assessment of mobility disability in multiple sclerosis. *Clinical Rehabilitation*, 13, 476–481.

de Vaus, D A (1991) *Surveys in Social Research*, 3rd edn. UCL Press, London.

DeVellis, R F (1991) *Scale Development: Theory and Applications*. Sage Publications, Thousand Oaks.

de Vet, H C W, de Bie, R A, van der Heijden, G J M G, Verhagen, A P, Sijpkes, P and Knipschild, P G (1997) Systematic reviews on the basis of methodological criteria. *Physiotherapy*, 83, 284–289.

Dey, I (1993) *Qualitative Data Analysis: A User-Friendly Guide for Social Scientists*. Routledge, London.

Di Fabio, R P (1999) Significance of relationships. *Journal of Orthopaedic and Sports Physical Therapy*, 29, 572–573.

DiCenso, A, Cullum, N (1998) Implementing evidence-based nursing: some misconceptions. *Evidence-Based Nursing*, 1, 38–40.

Dickersin, K, Scherer, R and Lefebvre, C (1994) Identifying relevant studies for systematic reviews. *British Medical Journal*, 309, 1286–1291.

Diers, D (1979) *Research in Nursing Practice*. J B Lippincott, Philadelphia.

Dijkers, M P J M and Creighton, C L (1994) Data cleaning in occupational therapy research. *Occupational Therapy Journal of Research*, 14, 144–156.

Dillman, D A (1978) *Mail and Telephone Surveys: The Total Design Method*. John Wiley, New York.

Dingwall, R (1980) Ethics and ethnography. *Sociological Review*, 28, 871–891.

Dingwall, R (1997) Accounts, interviews and observations. In: *Context and Method in Qualitative Research* (ed. Miller, G and Dingwall R). Sage Publications, London, pp. 51–65.

Dixon, R A, Munro, J F and Silcocks, P B (1997) *The Evidence-Based Medicine Workbook. Critical Appraisal for Clinical Problem Solving*. Butterworth-Heinemann, Oxford.

Dohan, D and Sánchez-Jankowski, M (1998) Using

computers to analyze ethnographic field data: theoretical and practical considerations. *Annual Review of Sociology*, **24**, 477–498.

Dolan, P, Cookson, R and Ferguson, B (1999) Effect of discussion and deliberation on the public's views of priority setting in health care: focus group study. *British Medical Journal*, **318**, 916–919.

Domholdt, E (1993) *Physical Therapy Research: Principles and Applications*. W B Saunders, Philadelphia.

Donner, A (1992) Sample size requirements for stratified cluster randomization designs. *Statistics in Medicine*, **11**, 743–750.

Doyal, L (1993) On discovering the nature of knowledge in a world of relationships. In: *Nursing: Art and Science* (ed. Kitson, A). Chapman & Hall, London, pp. 1–10.

Droogan, J and Cullum, N (1998) Systematic reviews in nursing. *International Journal of Nursing Studies*, **35**, 13–22.

Droogan, J and Song, F (1996) The process and importance of systematic reviews. *Nurse Researcher*, **4**(1), 15–26.

Drummond, A (1996) *Research Methods for Therapists*. Chapman & Hall, London.

Duff, R S and Hollingshead, A B (1968) *Sickness and Society*. Harper & Row, New York.

Duffy, M E (1987) Methodological triangulation: a vehicle for merging quantitative and qualitative methods. *Image: Journal of Nursing Scholarship*, **19**, 130–133.

Dukes, W F (1965) N=1. *Psychological Bulletin*, **64**, 74–79.

Dunn, G (1989) *Design and Analysis of Reliability Studies: The Statistical Evaluation of Measurement Errors*. Edward Arnold, London.

Dworkin, S F and Whitney, C W (1992) Relying on objective and subjective measures of chronic pain: guidelines for use and interpretation. In: *Handbook of Pain Assessment* (ed. Turk, D C and Melzack, R). Guilford Press, New York, pp. 429–446.

Easterbrook, P J, Berlin, J A, Gopalan, R and Matthews, D R (1991) Publication bias in published research. *Lancet*, **337**, 867–872.

Egger, M and Davey Smith, G (1995) Misleading meta-analysis. *British Medical Journal*, **310**, 752–754.

Egger, M and Davey Smith, G (1997) Meta-analysis: potentials and promise. *British Medical Journal*. **315**, 1371–1374.

Egger, M and Davey Smith, G (1998) Meta-analysis bias in location and selection of studies. *British Medical Journal*, **316**, 61–66.

Egger, M, Davey Smith, G and Phillips, A N (1997a) Meta-analysis: principles and procedures. *British Medical Journal*, **315**, 1533–1537.

Egger, M, Davey Smith, G, Schneider, M and Minder, M (1997b) Bias in meta-analysis detected by a simple, graphical test. *British Medical Journal*, **315**, 629–634.

Elwood, J M (1998) *Critical Appraisal of Epidemiological Studies and Clinical Trials*, 2nd edn. Oxford University Press, Oxford.

Endacott, R, Clifford, C M and Tripp, J H (1999) Can the needs of the critically ill child be identified using scenarios? Experiences of a modified Delphi study. *Journal of Advanced Nursing*, **30**, 665–676.

Engebretson, J C and Wardell, D W (1997) Development of a pacifier for low-birth-weight infants' nonnutritive sucking. *Journal of Obstetric, Gynecologic and Neonatal Nursing*, **26**, 660–664.

Erlandson, D A, Harris, E L, Skipper, B L and Allen, S D (1993) *Doing Naturalistic Research: A Guide to Methods*. Sage Publications, Newbury Park.

Evans, D and Evans, M (1996) *A Decent Proposal: Ethical Review of Clinical Research*. John Wiley, Chichester.

Evans, J (1994) Physiotherapy as a clinical science: the role of single case research designs. *Physiotherapy Theory and Practice*, **10**, 65–68.

Everitt, B S (1996) *Making Sense of Statistics in Psychology: A Second-Level Course*. Oxford University Press, Oxford.

Everitt, B S (1998) *The Cambridge Dictionary of Statistics*. Cambridge University Press, Cambridge.

Eysenck, H J (1995) Problems with meta-analysis. In: *Systematic Reviews* (ed. Chalmers, I and Altman, D G). British Medical Journal, London, pp. 64–74.

Eysenck, H J and Eysenck, S G B (1975) *The Eysenck Personality Questionnaire*. Hodder & Stoughton, Sevenoaks.

Faith, M S, Allison, D B and Gorman, B S (1996) Meta-analysis of single-case research. In: *Design and Analysis of Single-Case Research* (ed. Franklin, R D, Allison, D B and Gorman, B S). Lawrence Erlbaum, Mahwah, pp. 245–277.

Farmer, R and Miller, D (1991) *Lecture Notes on Epidemiology and Public Health Medicine*, 3rd edn. Blackwell Scientific Publications, Oxford.

Farsides, C C S (1989) It's a hard life bein' a guinea

pig – the problem of human experimentation. In: *By What Right? Studies in Medicine, Ethics and the Law* (ed. de Cruz, P and McNaughton, D). Penrhos Publications, Newcastle under Lyme, pp. 35–52.

Fawcett, J and Downs, F S (1992) *The Relationship of Theory and Research*, 2nd edn. F A Davis, Philadelphia.

Feldman, A B, Haley, S M and Coryell, J (1990) Concurrent and construct validity of the Pediatric Evaluation of Disability Inventory. *Physical Therapy*, **70**, 602–610.

Ferketich, S and Verran, J (1994) An overview of data transformation. *Research in Nursing and Health*, **17**, 393–396.

Ferrans, C E (1990) Development of a quality of life index for patients with cancer. *Oncology Nursing Forum*, **17**, 15–21.

Festinger, L (1957) *A Theory of Cognitive Dissonance*. Stanford University Press, Stanford.

Fetterman, D M (1998) *Ethnography: Step by Step*, 2nd edn. Sage Publications, Thousand Oaks.

Field, P A and Morse, J M (1996) *Nursing Research: The Application of Qualitative Approaches*, 2nd edn. Chapman & Hall, London.

Fielding, N (1993) Qualitative interviewing. In: *Researching Social Life* (ed. Gilbert, N). Sage Publications, London, pp. 135–153.

Fielding, N G and Fielding, J L (1986) *Linking Data*. Sage Publications, Newbury Park.

Fielding, N G and Lee, R M (1991) *Using Computers in Qualitative Research*. Sage Publications, London.

Fielding, N G and Lee, R M (1998) *Computer Analysis and Qualitative Research*. Sage Publications, London.

Fife-Schaw, C (1995a) Surveys and sampling issues. In: *Research Methods in Psychology* (ed. Breakwell, G M, Hammond, S and Fife-Schaw, C). Sage Publications, London, pp. 99–115.

Fife-Schaw, C (1995b) Questionnaire design. In: *Research Methods in Psychology* (ed. Breakwell, G M, Hammond, S and Fife-Schaw, C). Sage Publications, London, pp. 174–193.

Finch, J (1984) 'It's great to have someone to talk to': the ethics and politics of interviewing women. In: *Social Researching: Politics, Problems, Practice* (ed. Bell, C and Roberts, C). Routledge & Kegan Paul, London, pp. 70–87.

Finch, J (1987) The vignette technique in survey research. *Sociology*, **21**, 105–114.

Fink, A (1995a) *The Survey Handbook*. Sage Publications, Thousand Oaks.

Fink, A (1995b) *How to Ask Survey Questions*. Sage Publications, Thousand Oaks.

Fink, A and Kosecoff, J (1998) *How to Conduct Surveys: A Step-by-Step Guide*, 2nd edn. Sage Publications, Thousand Oaks.

Finlay, L (1998) Reflexivity: an essential component for all research? *British Journal of Occupational Therapy*, **61**, 453–456.

Finn, R H (1972) Effects of some variations in rating scale characteristics on the means and reliabilities of ratings. *Educational and Psychological Measurement*, **32**, 255–265.

Fleiss, J L (1971) Measuring nominal scale agreement among many raters. *Psychological Bulletin*, **76**, 378–382.

Foddy, W (1993) *Constructing Questions for Interviews and Questionnaires: Theory and Practice in Social Research*. Cambridge University Press, Cambridge.

Foddy, W (1996) The in-depth testing of survey questions: a critical appraisal of methods. *Quality and Quantity*, **30**, 361–370.

Ford, J S and Reutter, L I (1990) Ethical dilemmas associated with small samples. *Journal of Advanced Nursing*, **15**, 187–191.

Foster, P (1996) Observational research. In: *Data Collection and Analysis* (ed. Sapsford, R and Jupp, V). Sage Publications, London, pp. 57–93.

Fowler, F J (1993) *Survey Research Methods*, 2nd edn. Sage Publications, Newbury Park.

Fowler, F J (1995) *Improving Survey Questions: Design and Evaluation*. Sage Publications, Thousand Oaks.

Fowler, F J and Mangione, T W (1990) *Standardized Survey Interviewing: Minimizing Interviewer-Related Error*. Sage Publications, Newbury Park.

Francis, G (1997) The use of a patient diary in health-care research. *British Journal of Therapy and Rehabilitation*, **5**, 362–364.

Franklin, R D, Gorman, B S, Beasley, T M and Allison, D B (1996) Graphical display and visual analysis. In: *Design and Analysis of Single-Case Research* (ed. Franklin, R D, Allison, D B and Gorman, B S). Lawrence Erlbaum, Mahwah, pp. 119–158.

Freedman, B (1987) Equipoise and the ethics of clinical research. *New England Journal of Medicine*, **317**, 141–145.

Freemantle, N and Geddes, J (1998) Understanding and interpreting systematic reviews and meta-analyses. Part 2: meta-analyses. *Evidence-Based Mental Health*, **1**, 102–104.

Freiman, J A, Chalmers, T C, Smith, H and Kuebler, R R (1978) The importance of beta, the type II error and sample size in the design and interpretation of the randomized controlled trial: survey of 71 'negative' trials. *New England Journal of Medicine*, **299**, 690–694.

French, S (1993) *Practical Research: A Guide for Therapists*. Butterworth-Heinemann, Oxford.

French, S, Sim, J (1993) *Writing: A Guide for Therapists*. Butterworth-Heinemann, Oxford.

French, S and Swain, J (1997) Changing disability research: participating and emancipatory research with disabled people. *Physiotherapy*, **83**, 26–32.

Frey, J H and Oishi, S B (1995) *How to Conduct Interviews by Telephone and in Person*. Sage Publications, Thousand Oaks.

Friedman, L M, Furberg, C D and DeMets, D L (1982) *Fundamentals of Clinical Trials*. John Wright, Boston.

Fulton, T R (1996) Nurses' adoption of a patient-controlled analgesia approach. *Western Journal of Nursing Research*, **18**, 383–396.

Gahan, C and Hannibal, M (1998) *Doing Qualitative Analysis Using QSR NUD.IST*. Sage Publications, London.

Gardner, M J and Altman, D G (1989a) *Statistics with Confidence: Confidence Intervals and Statistical Guidelines*. British Medical Journal, London.

Gardner, M J and Altman D G (1989b) Calculating confidence intervals for proportions and their differences. In: *Statistics with Confidence: Confidence Intervals and Statistical Guidelines* (ed. Gardner, M J and Altman, D G). British Medical Journal, London, pp. 28–33.

Garfinkel, H (1967) *Studies in Ethnomethodology*. Prentice-Hall, New York.

Geddes, J, Freemantle, N, Streiner, D and Reynolds, S (1998) Understanding and interpreting systematic reviews and meta-analyses. Part 1: rationale, search strategy, and describing results. *Evidence-Based Mental Health*, **1**, 68–69.

Geertz, C (1973) Thick description: toward an interpretive theory of culture. In: *The Interpretation of Cultures: Selected Essays* (ed. Geertz, C). Basic Books, New York, pp. 3–30.

Gibbon, B (1995) Validity and reliability of assessment tools. *Nurse Researcher*, **2**(4), 48–55.

Gibbons, J D (1985) *Nonparametric Statistical Inference*, 2nd edn. Marcel Dekker, New York.

Gibson, V (1995) An analysis of the use of diaries as a data collection method. *Nurse Researcher*, **3**(1), 66–73.

Gigerenzer, G (1993) The superego, the ego, and the id in statistical reasoning. In: *A Handbook for Data Analysis in the Behavioral Sciences: Methodological Issues* (ed. Keren, G and Lewis, C). Lawrence Erlbaum, Hillsdale, pp. 311–339.

Gilchrist, V J (1992) Key informant interviews. In: *Doing Qualitative Research* (ed. Crabtree, B F and Miller, W L). Sage Publications, Newbury Park, pp. 70–89.

Gill, N E, Behnke, M, Conlon, M, McNeely, J B and Anderson, G C (1988) Effect of nonnutritive sucking on behavioral state in preterm infants before feeding. *Nursing Research*, **37**, 347–350.

Gilliss, C L (1994) Randomized clinical trials. In: *Exploring Collaborative Research in Primary Care* (ed. Crabtree, B F, Miller, W L, Addison, R B, Gilchrist, V J and Kuzel, A). Sage Publications, Thousand Oaks, pp. 37–44.

Gillon, R (1986) *Philosophical Medical Ethics*. John Wiley, Chichester.

Gissane, C (1998) Understanding and using descriptive statistics. *British Journal of Occupational Therapy*, **61**, 267–272.

Glaser, B G (1978) *Theoretical Sensitivity*. Sociology Press, Mill Valley.

Glaser, B G (1992) *Emergence versus Forcing: Basics of Grounded Theory Analysis*. Sociology Press, Mill Valley.

Glaser, B and Strauss, A (1967) *The Discovery of Grounded Theory: Strategies for Qualitative Research*. Aldine, Chicago.

Glass, G V (1976) Primary, secondary, and meta-analysis of research. *Educational Researcher*, **5**, 3–8.

Gold, R (1958) Roles in sociological field observation. *Social Forces*, **36**, 217–223.

Golden, C J, Sawicki, R F and Franzen, M D (1990) Test construction. In: *Handbook of Psychological Assessment*, 2nd edn (ed. Goldstein, G and Hersen, M). Pergamon Press, New York, pp. 21–40.

Gonnella, C (1989) Single-subject experimental paradigm as a clinical decision tool. *Physical Therapy*, **69**, 601–609.

Goodman, C M (1987) The Delphi technique: a critique. *Journal of Advanced Nursing*, **12**, 729–734.

Gorman, B S and Allison, D B (1996) Statistical alternatives for single-case designs. In: *Design and Analysis of Single-Case Research* (ed. Franklin, R D, Allison, D B and Gorman, B S). Lawrence Erlbaum, Mahwah, pp. 159–214.

Gould, D (1996) Using vignettes to collect data for nursing research studies: how valid are the findings? *Journal of Clinical Nursing*, 5, 207–212.

Grady, K E and Wallston, B S (1988) *Research in Health Care Settings*. Sage Publications, Newbury Park.

Graham, H (1983) Do her answers fit his questions? Women and the survey method. In: *The Public and the Private* (ed. Gamarnikow, E, Morgan, D, Purvis, J and Taylorson, D). Heinemann, London, pp. 132–146.

Grant, J S and David, L L (1997) Selection and use of content experts for instrument development. *Research in Nursing and Health*, 20, 269–274.

Gravetter, F J and Wallnau, L B (1988) *Statistics for the Behavioral Sciences*, 2nd edn. West Publishing, St Paul.

Gray, B H (1975) *Human Subjects in Medical Experimentation: A Sociological Study of the Conduct and Regulation of Clinical Research*. John Wiley, New York.

Gray, J A M (1997) *Evidence-Based Healthcare: How to Make Health Policy and Management Decisions*. Churchill Livingstone, Edinburgh.

Graziano, A M and Raulin, M L (1993) *Research Methods: A Process of Inquiry*, 2nd edn. HarperCollins, New York.

Grbich, C (1999) *Qualitative Research in Health: An Introduction*. Sage Publications, London.

Green, B, Jones, M, Hughes, D and Williams, A (1999) Applying the Delphi technique in a study of GPs' information requirements. *Health and Social Care in the Community*, 7, 198–205.

Green, H and Britten, N (1998) Qualitative research and evidence based medicine. *British Medical Journal*, 316, 1230–1232.

Green, J M (1996) Warning that reminders will be sent increased response rate. *Quality and Quantity*, 30, 449–450.

Greene, J and D'Oliveira, M (1982) *Learning to Use Statistical Tests in Psychology: A Student's Guide*. Open University Press, Milton Keynes.

Greener, J and Grimshaw, J (1996) Using meta-analysis to summarise evidence within systematic reviews. *Nurse Researcher*, 4(1), 27–38.

Greenhalgh, T (1997) *How to Read a Paper: The Basics of Evidence Based Medicine*. British Medical Journal, London.

Guba, E G and Lincoln, Y S (1981) *Effective Evaluation: Improving the Usefulness of Evaluation Reports through Responsive and Naturalist Approaches*. Jossey-Bass, San Francisco.

Guttman, L (1944) A basis for scaling quantitative data. *American Sociological Review*, 9, 139–150.

Haas, M (1991a) Statistical methodology for reliability studies. *Journal of Manipulative and Physiological Therapeutics*, 14, 119–132.

Haas, M (1991b) The reliability of reliability. *Journal of Manipulative and Physiological Therapeutics*, 14, 199–208.

Haas, M (1995) How to evaluate intraexaminer reliability using an interexaminer reliability study design. *Journal of Manipulative and Physiological Therapeutics*, 18, 10–15.

Haber, A and Runyon, R P (1977) *General Statistics*, 3rd edn. Addison-Wesley, London.

Haber, J (1994) Sampling. In: *Nursing Research: Methods, Critical Appraisal, and Utilization*, 3rd edn (ed. LoBiondo-Wood, G and Haber, J). Mosby, St Louis, pp. 286–312.

Hagemaster, J N (1992) Life history: a qualitative method of research. *Journal of Advanced Nursing*, 17, 1122–1128.

Hakim, C (1987) *Research Design: Strategies and Choices in the Design of Social Research*. Allen & Unwin, London.

Haley, S M and Osberg, J S (1989) Kappa coefficient calculation using multiple ratings per subject: a special communication. *Physical Therapy*, 69, 970–974.

Hall, E J (1963) A system for the notation of proxemic behavior. *American Anthropologist*, 65, 1003–1026.

Hammersley, M (1990) *Reading Ethnographic Research: A Critical Guide*. Longman, London.

Hammersley, M and Atkinson, P (1995) *Ethnography: Principles in Practice*, 2nd edn. Routledge, London.

Hammond, S (1995) Using psychometric tests. In: *Research Methods in Psychology* (ed. Breakwell, G M, Hammond, S and Fife-Schaw, C). Sage Publications, London, pp. 194–212.

Hansson, M O (1998) Balancing the quality of consent. *Journal of Medical Ethics*, 24, 182–187.

Harding, S (1986) *The Science Question in Feminism*. Open University Press, Milton Keynes.

Hart, E and Bond, M (1995) *Action Research for*

Health and Social Care. Open University Press, Buckingham.

Harth, S C and Thong, Y H (1995) Parental perceptions and attitudes about informed consent in clinical research involving children. *Social Science and Medicine*, **40**, 1573–1577.

Hartmann, D P (1977) Considerations in the choice of interobserver reliability estimates. *Journal of Applied Behavior Analysis*, **10**, 103–116.

Hays, W L (1988) *Statistics*, 4th edn. Holt, Rinehart & Winston, New York.

Heacock, P, Souder, E and Chastain, J (1996) Subjects, data and videotapes. *Nursing Research*, **45**, 336–338.

Headland, T N, Pike, K L and Harris, M (1990) *Emics and Etics: The Insider/Outside Debate*. Sage Publications, Newbury Park.

Hedges, L V and Vevea, J L (1998) Fixed- and random-effects models in meta-analysis. *Psychological Methods*, **3**, 486–504.

Hedrick, T E, Bickman, L and Rog, D J (1993) *Applied Research Design: A Practical Guide*. Sage Publications, Newbury Park.

Heise, D R (1970) The semantic differential and attitude research. In: *Attitude Measurement* (ed. Summers, G F). Rand McNally, Chicago, pp. 235–253.

Held, D (1980) *Introduction to Critical Theory: Horkheimer to Habermas*. Hutchinson, London.

Henerson, M E, Morris, L L and Fitz-Gibbon, C T (1987) *How to Measure Attitudes*. Sage Publications, Newbury Park.

Henry, G T (1990) *Practical Sampling*. Sage Publications, Newbury Park.

Henry, G T (1995) *Graphing Data: Techniques for Displaying and Analysis*. Sage Publications, Thousand Oaks.

Herman, J (1998) Shortcomings of the randomized controlled trial: a view from the boondocks. *Journal of Evaluation in Clinical Practice*, **4**, 283–286.

Hevey, D and McGee, H M (1998) The effect size statistic. *Journal of Health Psychology*, **3**, 163–170

Hewison, A (1995) Nurses' power in interaction with patients. *Journal of Advanced Nursing*, **21**, 75–82.

Hewlett, S (1996) Consent to clinical research – adequately voluntary or substantially influenced? *Journal of Medical Ethics*, **22**, 232–237.

Hicks, C M (1998) The randomised controlled trial: a critique. *Nurse Researcher*, **6**(1), 19–32.

Hicks, C M (1999) *Research Methods for Clinical Therapists: Applied Project Design and Analysis*, 3rd edn. Churchill Livingstone, Edinburgh.

Hillier, V and Gibbs, A (1996) Calculations to determine sample size. *Nurse Researcher*, **3**(4), 27–34.

Hinds, P S and Young, K J (1987) A triangulation of methods and paradigms to study nurse-given wellness care. *Nursing Research*, **36**, 195–198.

Hinds, P S, Scandrett-Hibden, S and McAuley, L S (1990) Further assessment of a method to estimate reliability and validity of qualitative research findings. *Journal of Advanced Nursing*, **15**, 430–435.

Hodges, J L and Lehmann, E L (1964) *Basic Concepts of Probability and Statistics*. Holden-Day, San Francisco.

Hoel, P (1962) *Introduction to Mathematical Statistics*, 3rd edn. Wiley, New York.

Hoinville, G, Jowell, R, Airey, C, Brook, L, Courtenay, G, Hedges, B, Kalton, G, Morton-Williams, J, Walker, D and Wood, D (1978) *Survey Research Practice*. Heinemann Educational Books, London.

Hojem, M A and Ottenbacher, K J (1988) Empirical investigation of visual-inspection versus trend-line analysis of single-subject data. *Physical Therapy*, **68**, 983–988.

Hollis, S and Campbell, F (1999) What is meant by intention to treat analysis? Survey of published randomised controlled trials. *British Medical Journal*, **319**, 670–674.

Holloway, I (1997) *Basic Concepts for Qualitative Research*. Blackwell Science, Oxford.

Holloway, I and Wheeler, S (1996) *Qualitative Research for Nurses*. Blackwell Science, Oxford.

Holstein, J A and Gubrium, J F (1994) Phenomenology, ethnomethodology, and interpretive practice. In: *Handbook of Qualitative Research* (ed. Denzin, N K and Lincoln, Y S). Sage Publications, Thousand Oaks, pp. 262–272.

Holstein, J A and Gubrium, J F (1997) Active interviewing. In: *Qualitative Research: Theory, Method and Practice* (ed. Silverman, D). Sage Publications, London, pp. 113–129.

Holsti, O (1969) *Content Analysis for the Social Sciences and Humanities*. Addison-Wesley, Reading.

Holter, I M and Schwartz-Barcott, D (1993) Action research: what is it? How has it been used and how can it be used in nursing? *Journal of Advanced Nursing*, **18**, 298–304.

Homan, R (1991) *The Ethics of Social Research*. Longman, London.

Hornsby-Smith, M (1993) Gaining access. In: *Researching Social Life* (ed. Gilbert, N). Sage Publications, London, pp. 52–67.

Howell, D C (1997) *Statistical Methods for Psychology*, 4th edn. Duxbury Press, Belmont.

Howson, C and Urbach, P (1989) *Scientific Reasoning: The Bayesian Approach*. Open Court, La Salle.

Hsieh, F Y (1988) Sample size formulae for intervention studies with the cluster as unit of randomization. *Statistics in Medicine*, 8, 1195–1201.

Huck, S W and Cormier, W H (1996) *Reading Statistics and Research*. HarperCollins, New York.

Hughes, C C (1992) 'Ethnography': what's in a word – process? product? promise? *Qualitative Health Research*, 2, 439–450.

Hughes, J A (1990) *The Philosophy of Social Research*, 2nd edn. Longman, London.

Hugman, R (1991) *Power in Caring Professions*. Macmillan, London.

Hulley, S B and Cummings, S R (1988) *Designing Clinical Research*. Williams & Wilkins, Baltimore.

Hulley, S B, Feigal, D, Martin, M and Cummings, S R (1988a) Designing a new study: IV. Experiments. In: *Designing Clinical Research: An Epidemiologic Approach* (ed. Hulley, S B and Cummings, S R). Williams & Wilkins, Baltimore, pp. 110–127.

Hulley, S B, Newman, T B and Cummings, S R (1988b) Getting started: the anatomy and physiology of research. In: *Designing Clinical Research: An Epidemiologic Approach* (ed. Hulley, S B and Cummings, S R). Williams & Wilkins, Baltimore, pp. 1–11.

Humphreys, L (1970) *Tearoom Trade: A Study of Homosexual Encounters in Public Places*. Duckworth, London.

Hunter, M A and May, R B (1993) Some myths concerning parametric and nonparametric tests. *Canadian Psychology*, 34, 384–389.

Hurlburt, R T (1994) *Comprehending Behavioral Statistics*. Brooks/Cole Publishing, Pacific Grove.

Hyland, M E, Bott, J, Singh, S and Kenyon, C A P (1994) Domains, constructs and the development of the breathing problems questionnaire. *Quality of Life Research*, 3, 245–256.

Jadad, A (1998) *Randomised Controlled Trials: A User's Guide*. British Medical Journal, London.

Jadad, A R, Moher, M, Browman, G P, Booker, L, Sigouin, C, Fuentes, M and Stevens, R (2000) Systematic reviews and meta-analyses on treatment of asthma: critical evaluation. *British Medical Journal*, 320, 537–540.

Jadad, A R, Moore, R A, Carroll, D, Jenkinson, C, Reynolds, D J, Gavaghan, D J and McQuay, H J (1996) Assessing the quality of reports of randomized clinical trials: is blinding necessary? *Controlled Clinical Trials*, 17, 1–12.

Jelinek, M (1992) The clinician and the randomised controlled trial. In: *Researching Health Care: Designs, Dilemmas, Disciplines* (ed. Daly, J, McDonald, I and Willis, E). Routledge, London, pp. 76–89.

Jenkins, S, Price, C J and Straker, L (1998) *The Researching Therapist: A Practical Guide to Planning, Performing and Communicating Research*. Churchill Livingstone, New York.

Jette, A M (1987) The Functional Status Index: reliability and validity of a self-report functional disability measure. *Journal of Rheumatology*, 14(suppl), 15–19.

Johannessen, T (1991) Controlled trials in single subjects: 1. Value in clinical medicine. *British Medical Journal*, 303, 173–174.

Johnston, J M and Pennypacker, H S (1993) *Strategies and Tactics of Behavioral Research*, 2nd edn. Lawrence Erlbaum, Hillsdale.

Johnstone, M-J (1994) *Bioethics: A Nursing Perspective*, 2nd edn. W B Saunders / Baillière Tindall, Sydney.

Jones, B, Jarvis, P, Lewis, J A and Ebbutt, A F (1996) Trials to assess equivalence: the importance of rigorous methods. *British Medical Journal*, 313, 36–39.

Jones, J and Hunter, D (2000) Using the Delphi and nominal group technique in health services research. In: *Qualitative Research in Health Care*, 2nd edn (ed. Pope, C and Mays, N). British Medical Journal, London, pp. 40–49.

Jones, S (1985a) Depth interviewing. In: *Applied Qualitative Research* (ed. Walker, R). Gower, Aldershot, pp. 45–55.

Jones, S (1985b) The analysis of depth interviews. In: *Applied Qualitative Research* (ed. Walker, R). Gower, Aldershot, pp. 56–70.

Jordan, K, Ong, B N and Croft, P (1998) *Mastering Statistics: A Guide for Health Service Professionals and Researchers*. Stanley Thornes, Cheltenham.

Jorgensen, D L (1989) *Participant Observation: A*

Methodology for Human Studies. Sage Publications, Newbury Park.

Jüni, P, Witschi, A, Bloch, R and Egger, M (1999) The hazards of scoring the quality of clinical trials for meta-analysis. *Archives of Internal Medicine*, **282**, 1054–1060.

Katz, M H (1999) *Multivariable Analysis: A Practical Guide for Clinicians*. Cambridge University Press, Cambridge.

Kavanaugh, K and Ayres, L (1998) 'Not as bad as it could have been': assessing and mitigating harm during research interviews on sensitive topics. *Research in Nursing and Health*, **21**, 91–97.

Kazdin, A E (1982) *Single-Case Research Designs: Methods for Clinical and Applied Settings*. Oxford University Press, New York.

Kazdin, A E (1984) Statistical analyses for single-case experimental designs. In: *Single Case Experimental Designs: Strategies for Studying Behavior Change*, 2nd edn (ed. Barlow, D H and Hersen, M). Pergamon Press, New York, pp. 185–324.

Kazdin, A E (1992) *Research Design in Clinical Psychology*, 2nd edn. Allyn & Bacon, Boston.

Kazis, L E, Anderson, J J and Meenan, R F (1989) Effect sizes for interpreting changes in health status. *Medical Care*, **27**, S179–S189.

Keating, J and Matyas, T A (1998) Unreliable inferences from reliable measurements. *Australian Journal of Physiotherapy*, **44**, 5–10.

Kellehear, A (1996) Unobtrusive methods in delicate situations. In: *Ethical Intersections: Health Research, Methods and Researcher Responsibility* (ed. Daly, J). Allen & Unwin, St Leonards, pp. 97–105.

Kelly, A (1985) Action research: what is it and what can it do? In: *Issues in Educational Research: Qualitative Methods* (ed. Burgess, R G). Falmer Press, London, pp. 129–151.

Kelman, H C (1967) Human use of human subjects: the problem of deception in social psychological experiments. *Psychological Bulletin*, **67**, 1–11.

Keppel, G and Saufley, W H (1980) *Introduction to Design and Analysis*. W H Freeman, San Francisco.

Kerlinger, F N (1986) *Foundations of Behavioral Research*, 3rd edn. Harcourt Brace Jovanovich College Publishers, Fort Worth.

Kernan, W N, Viscoli, C M, Makuch, R W, Brass, L M and Horwitz, R I (1999) Stratified randomization for clinical trials. *Journal of Clinical Epidemiology*, **52**, 19–26.

Kerry, S M and Bland, J M (1998) Sample size in cluster randomisation. *British Medical Journal*, **316**, 549.

Kidder, L H and Judd, C M (1986) *Research Methods in Social Relations*, 5th edn. CBS Publishing, New York.

Kimmel, A J (1988) *Ethics and Values in Applied Social Research*. Sage Publications, Newbury Park.

Kimmel, A J (1996) *Ethical Issues in Behavioral Research: A Survey*. Blackwell Publishers, Oxford.

Kirk, J and Miller, M L (1986) *Reliability and Validity in Qualitative Research*. Sage Publications, Newbury Park.

Kitzinger, J (1994a) Focus groups: methods or madness? In: *Challenge and Innovation: Methodological Advances in Social Research on HIV/AIDS* (ed. Boulton, M). Taylor & Francis, London, pp. 159–175.

Kitzinger, J (1994b) The methodology of focus groups: the importance of interaction between research participants. *Sociology of Health and Illness*, **16**, 103–121.

Kitzinger, J (2000) Focus groups with users and providers of health care. In: *Qualitative Research in Health Care* (ed. Pope, C and Mays, N), 2nd edn. British Medical Journal, London, pp. 20–29.

Kitzinger, J and Barbour, R S (1999) Introduction: the challenge and promise of focus groups. In: *Developing Focus Group Research: Politics, Theory and Practice* (ed. Barbour, R S and Kitzinger, J. Sage Publications, London, pp. 1–20.

Kline, P (1993) *The Handbook of Psychological Testing*. Routledge, London.

Kline, P (1994) *An Easy Guide to Factor Analysis*. Routledge, London.

Knafl, K A and Breitmayer, B J (1991) Triangulation in qualitative research: issues of conceptual clarity and purpose. In: *Qualitative Nursing Research: A Contemporary Dialogue* (ed. Morse, J M). Sage Publications, Newbury Park, pp. 226–239.

Knapp, T R (1990) Treating ordinal scales as interval scales: an attempt to resolve the controversy. *Nursing Research*, **39**, 121–123.

Knapp, T R, Kimble, L P and Dunbar, S B (1998) Distinguishing between the stability of a construct and the stability of an instrument in trait/state measurement. *Nursing Research*, **47**, 60–62.

Koch, T (1994) Establishing rigour in qualitative research: the decision trail. *Journal of Advanced Nursing*, **19**, 976–986.

Koes, B W and Hoving, J L (1998) The value of the

randomized clinical trial in the field of physiotherapy. *Manual Therapy*, 3, 179–186.

Kosslyn, S M (1985) *Elements of Graphic Design*. W H Freeman, New York.

Kraemer, H C and Thiemann, S (1987) *How Many Subjects? Statistical Power Analysis in Research*. Sage Publications, Newbury Park.

Kratochwill, T R (1978) Foundations of time-series research. In: *Single Subject Research: Strategies for Evaluating Change* (ed. Kratochwill, T R). Academic Press, New York, pp. 1–100.

Kratochwill, T R and Levin, J R (1992) *Single-Case Research Design and Analysis: New Directions for Psychology and Education*. Lawrence Erlbaum, Hillsdale.

Krebs, D E (1984) Intraclass correlation coefficients: use and calculation. *Physical Therapy*, 64, 1581–1589.

Krebs, D E (1993) A general, multivariate approach to research design and inferential statistical analysis. In: *Research in Physical Therapy* (ed. Bork, C E). J B Lippincott, Philadelphia, pp. 277–316.

Krefting, L (1991) Rigor in qualitative research: the assessment of trustworthiness. *American Journal of Occupational Therapy*, 45, 214–222.

Kremer, B (1990) Learning to say no: keeping feminist research for ourselves. *Women's Studies International Forum*, 13, 463–467.

Krosnick, J A (1999) Survey research. *Annual Review of Psychology*, 50, 537–567.

Krueger, R A (1994) *Focus Groups: A Practical Guide for Applied Research*, 2nd edn. Sage Publications, Thousand Oaks.

Krueger, R A (1998) *Moderating Focus Groups*. Sage Publications, Thousand Oaks.

Kvale, S (1996) *InterViews: An Introduction to Qualitative Research Interviewing*. Sage Publications, Thousand Oaks.

Labovitz, S (1970) The assignment of numbers to rank order categories. *American Sociological Review*, 35, 515–524.

Lagakos, S W and Pocock, S J (1984) Randomization and stratification in cancer clinical trials: an international survey. In: *Cancer Clinical Trials: Methods and Practice* (ed. Buyse, M E, Staquet, M J and Sylvester, R J). Oxford University Press, Oxford, pp. 277–286.

Lancaster, T, Shepperd, S and Silagy, C (1997) Systematic reviews and meta-analysis. In: *Assessment and Evaluation of Health and Medical Care* (ed. Jenkinson, C). Open University Press, Buckingham, pp. 171–185.

Landis, J R and Koch, G G (1977) The measurement of observer agreement for categorical data. *Biometrics*, 33, 159–174.

Lassman, P (1974) Phenomenological perspectives in sociology. In: *Approaches to Sociology: An Introduction to Major Trends in British Sociology* (ed. Rex, J). Routledge & Kegan Paul, London, pp. 125–144.

Last, J M (1988) *A Dictionary of Epidemiology*, 2nd edn. Oxford University Press, New York.

Laupacis, A, Sackett, D L and Roberts, R S (1988) An assessment of clinically useful measures of the consequences of treatment. *New England Journal of Medicine*, 318, 1728–1733.

LaValley, M (1997) A clinician's guide to meta analysis. *Arthritis Care and Research*, 10, 208–213.

Lavrakas, P J (1993) *Telephone Survey Methods: Sampling, Selection and Supervision*, 2nd edn. Sage Publications, Newbury Park.

Layte, R and Jenkinson, C (1997) Social surveys. In: *Assessment and Evaluation of Health and Medical Care* (ed. Jenkinson, C). Open University Press, Buckingham, pp. 47–63.

LeComte, M D and Goetz, J P (1982) Problems of reliability and validity in ethnographic research. *Review of Educational Research*, 52, 31–60.

Lee, R M (1993) *Doing Research on Sensitive Topics*. Sage Publications, London.

Lehmann, E L and D'Abrera, H J M (1975) *Nonparametrics: Statistical Methods Based on Ranks*. McGraw-Hill, New York.

Lehr, R (1992) Sixteen s-squared over d-squared: a relation for crude sample size estimates. *Statistics in Medicine*, 11, 1099–1102.

Leininger, M M (1985a) Nature, rationale and importance of qualitative research methods in nursing. In: *Qualitative Research Methods in Nursing* (ed. Leininger, M M). Grune & Stratton, Orlando, pp. 1–25.

Leininger, M M (1985b) Ethnoscience method and componential analysis. In: *Qualitative Research Methods in Nursing* (ed. Leininger, M M). Grune & Stratton, Orlando, pp. 237–249.

Levine, G and Parkinson, S (1994) *Experimental Methods in Psychology*. Lawrence Erlbaum, Hillsdale.

Levine, R J (1988) *Ethics and Regulation of Clinical Research*, 2nd edn. Yale University Press, New Haven.

Lewis, J A (1991) Controlled trials in single subjects: 2. Limitations of use. *British Medical Journal*, **303**, 175–176.

Lewis, J A and Machin, D (1993) Intention to treat – who should use ITT? *British Journal of Cancer*, **68**, 647–650.

Li Wan Po, A (1998) *Dictionary of Evidence-Based Medicine*. Radcliffe Medical Press, Oxford.

Liehr, P R and Marcus, M T (1994) Qualitative approaches to research. In: *Nursing Research: Methods, Critical Appraisal, and Utilization*, 3rd edn (ed. LoBiondo-Wood, G and Haber, J). Mosby, St Louis, pp. 253–285.

Light, R J (1987) Accumulating evidence from independent studies: what we can win and what we can lose. *Statistics in Medicine*, 6, 221–228.

Likert, R (1932) *A Technique for the Measurement of Attitudes (Archives of Psychology No 140)*. Columbia University Press, New York.

Lilford, R J and Jackson, J (1995) Equipoise and the ethics of randomization. *Journal of the Royal Society of Medicine*, **88**, 552–559.

Lilford, R J, Thornton, J G and Braunholtz, D (1995) Clinical trials and rare diseases: a way out of a conundrum. *British Medical Journal*, **311**, 1621–1625.

Lincoln, Y S and Guba, E G (1985) *Naturalistic Inquiry*. Sage Publications, Newbury Park.

Lindeman, C A (1975) Delphi survey of priorities in clinical nursing research. *Nursing Research*, **24**, 434–441.

Lipsey, M W (1998) Design sensitivity: statistical power for applied experimental research. In: *Handbook of Applied Social Research Methods* (ed. Bickman, L and Rog, D J). Sage Publications, Thousand Oaks, pp. 39–68.

Lipson, J G (1994) Ethical issues in ethnography. In: *Critical Issues in Qualitative Research Methods* (ed. Morse J M). Sage Publications, Thousand Oaks, pp. 333–355.

Litwin, M S (1995) *How to Analyze Survey Reliability and Validity*. Sage Publications, Thousand Oaks.

Lloyd, J (1998) Rheumatoid arthritis. In: *Rheumatological Physiotherapy* (ed. David, C and Lloyd, J). Mosby, London, pp. 65–81.

LoBiondo-Wood, G and Haber, J (1994) Reliability and validity. In: *Nursing Research: Methods, Critical Appraisal, and Utilization*, 3rd edn (ed LoBiondo-Wood, G and Haber, J). Mosby, St Louis, pp. 365–384.

Locke, S (1998) Qualitative research and data analysis. *British Journal of Therapy and Rehabilitation*, 5, 357–361.

Loewenthal, K M (1996) *An Introduction to Psychological Tests and Scales*. UCL Press, London.

Lofland, J (1976) *Doing Social Life: The Qualitative Study of Human Action in Natural Settings*. John Wiley, New York.

Lund, E and Gram, I T (1998) Response rate according to title and length of questionnaire. *Scandinavian Journal of Social Medicine*, 26, 154–160.

McCain, L J and McCleary, R (1979) The statistical analysis of the simple interrupted time-series quasi-experiment. In: *Quasi-Experimentation: Design and Analysis Issues for Field Settings* (ed. Cook, T D and Campbell, D T). Houghton Mifflin, Boston, pp. 233–293.

McCall, J (1996) *Statistics: A Guide for Therapists*. Butterworth-Heinemann, Oxford.

McCarthy, M (1998) Interviewing people with learning disabilities about sensitive topics: a discussion of ethical issues. *British Journal of Learning Disabilities*, **26**, 140–145.

MacDonald, P (1999) Power, Type I, and Type III error rates of parametric and nonparametric statistical tests. *Journal of Experimental Education*, **67**, 367–379.

McDowell, I and Newell, C (1996) *Measuring Health: A Guide to Rating Scales and Questionnaires*, 2nd edn. Oxford University Press, New York.

McGuire, D B (1984) The measurement of clinical pain. *Nursing Research*, 33, 152–156.

McKenna, H P (1994) The Delphi technique: a worthwhile research approach for nursing? *Journal of Advanced Nursing*, 19, 1221–1225.

McQuay, H J (1991) N of 1 trials. In: *Advances in Pain Research and Therapy, Vol 18* (ed. Portenoy, M and Laska, E). Raven Press, New York, pp. 179–192.

McQuay, H J and Moore, R A (1999) Methods of therapeutic trials. In: *Textbook of Pain*, 4th edn (ed. Wall, P D and Melzack, R). Churchill Livingstone, Edinburgh, pp. 1125–1138.

Machin, D, Campbell, M J, Fayers, P M and Pinol, A P Y (1997) *Sample Size Tables for Clinical Studies*, 2nd edn. Blackwell Science, Oxford.

Maclaren, W M (1998) Statistical inference: some basic concepts. *British Journal of Therapy and Rehabilitation*, 5, 424–430.

Madonald, K and Tipton, C (1993) Using documents.

In: *Researching Social Life* (ed. Gilbert, N). Sage Publications, London, pp. 187–200.

Madsen, P and Conte, J R (1980) Single subject research in occupational therapy: a case illustration. *American Journal of Occupational Therapy*, 34, 263–267.

Maher, C (1993) Pitfalls in reliability studies: some suggestions for change. *Australian Journal of Physiotherapy*, 39, 5–7.

Maisel, R and Persell, C H (1996) *How Sampling Works*. Pine Forge Press, Thousand Oaks.

Mangione, T W (1998) Mail surveys. In: *Handbook of Applied Social Research Methods* (ed. Bickman, L and Rog, D J). Sage Publications, Thousand Oaks, pp. 399–427.

Mant, J and Jenkinson, C (1997) Case control and cohort studies. In: *Assessment and Evaluation of Health and Medical Care* (ed. Jenkinson, C). Open University Press, Buckingham, pp. 31–46.

Mantel, N (1963) Chi-square tests with one degree of freedom: extensions of the Mantel-Haenszel procedure. *American Statistical Association Journal*, 58, 690–700.

Marshall, C and Rossman, G B (1999) *Designing Qualitative Research*, 3rd edn. Sage Publications, Thousand Oaks.

Mason, J (1996) *Qualitative Researching*. Sage Publications, London.

Mason, R L, Gunst, R F and Hess, J L (1989) *Statistical Design and Analysis of Experiments: With Applications to Engineering and Science*. John Wiley, New York.

Massarik, F (1981) The interviewing process re-examined. In: *Human Inquiry: A Sourcebook of New Paradigm Research* (ed. Reason, P and Rowan, J). John Wiley, Chichester, pp. 201–206.

Matyas, T A and Greenwood, K M (1996) Serial dependency in single-case time series. In: *Design and Analysis of Single-Case Research* (ed. Franklin, R D, Allison, D B and Gorman, B S). Lawrence Erlbaum, Mahwah, pp. 215–243.

Maxwell, J A (1996) *Qualitative Research Design: An Interactive Approach*. Sage Publications, Thousand Oaks.

May, B (1991) Pain. In: *The Psychology of Health* (ed. Pitts, M and Phillips, K). Routledge, London, pp. 91–105.

May, K A (1991) Interview techniques in qualitative research: concerns and challenges. In: *Qualitative Nursing Research: A Contemporary Dialogue*, rev.

edn (ed. Morse, J M). Sage Publications, Newbury Park, pp. 188–201.

May, R B, Masson, M E J and Hunter, M A (1990) *Application of Statistics in Behavioral Research*. Harper & Row, New York.

Maykut, P and Morehouse, R (1994) *Beginning Qualitative Research: A Philosophic and Practical Guide*. Falmer Press, London.

Mays, N and Pope, C (1995) Rigour and qualitative research. *British Medical Journal*, 311, 109–112.

Mead, R (1988) *The Design of Experiments: Statistical Principles for Practical Applications*. Cambridge University Press, Cambridge.

Melia, K M (1987) *Learning and Working: The Occupational Socialization of Nurses*. Tavistock Publications, London.

Melia, K M (1996) Rediscovering Glaser. *Qualitative Health Research*, 6, 368–378.

Merton, R K, Fiske, M and Kendall, P L (1956) *The Focused Interview: A Manual of Problems and Procedures*. Free Press, Glencoe.

Meyer, J (2000) Using qualitative methods in health related action research. *British Medical Journal*, 320, 178–181.

Meyer, J E (1993) New paradigm research in practice: the trials and tribulations of action research. *Journal of Advanced Nursing*, 18, 1066–1072.

Mies, M (1993) Towards a methodology for feminist research. In: *Social Research: Philosophy, Politics and Practice* (ed. Hammersley, M). Sage Publications, London, pp. 64–82.

Miles, M B and Huberman, A M (1994) *Qualitative Data Analysis: An Expanded Sourcebook*, 2nd edn. Sage Publications, Thousand Oaks.

Miles-Tapping, C, Dyck, A, Brunham, S, Simpson, E and Barber, L (1990) Canadian therapists' priorities for clinical research: a Delphi study. *Physical Therapy*, 70, 448–454.

Millman, M and Moss Kanter, R (1975) *Another Voice: Feminist Perspectives on Social Life and Social Science*. Anchor Books, New York.

Minichiello, V, Aroni, R, Timewell, E and Alexander, L (1990) *In-Depth Interviewing: Researching People*. Longman Cheshire, Melbourne.

Mitchell, G D (1979) *A New Dictionary of Sociology*. Routledge & Kegan Paul, London.

Mitchell, J C (1983) Case and situational analysis. *Sociological Review*, 31, 187–211.

Mitchell, S K (1979) Interobserver agreement, reliability, and generalizability of data collected in observational studies. *Psychological Bulletin*, **86**, 376–390.

Moher, D and Olkin, I (1995) Meta-analysis of randomized controlled trials: a concern for standards. *Journal of the American Medical Association*, **274**, 1962–1964.

Moher, D, Jadad, A R, Nichol, G, Penman, M, Tugwell, P and Walsh, S (1995) Assessing the quality of randomized controlled trials: an annotated bibliography of scales and checklists. *Controlled Clinical Trials*, **16**, 62–73.

Montgomery, D C (1991) *Design and Analysis of Experiments*, 3rd edn. John Wiley, New York.

Morgan, D L (1988) *Focus Groups as Qualitative Research*. Sage Publications, Newbury Park.

Morgan, D L (1996) Focus groups. *Annual Review of Sociology*, **22**, 129–152.

Morgan, D L and Spanish, M T (1985) Social interaction and the cognitive organisation of health-relevant knowledge. *Sociology of Health and Illness*, **7**, 401–422.

Morley, S (1996) Single case research. In: *Behavioural and Mental Health Research: A Handbook of Skills and Methods*, 2nd edn (ed. Parry, G and Watts, F N). Psychology Press, Hove, pp. 277–314.

Morris, J A and Gardner, M J (1989) Calculating confidence intervals for relative risks, odds ratios, and standardised ratios and rates. In: *Statistics with Confidence: Confidence Intervals and Statistical Guidelines* (ed. Gardner, M J and Altman, D G). British Medical Journal, London, pp. 50–63.

Morse, J M (1995) The significance of saturation. *Qualitative Health Research*, **5**, 147–149.

Morse, J M (1998a) Validity by committee. *Qualitative Health Research*, **8**, 443–445.

Morse, J M (1998b) What's wrong with random selection? *Qualitative Health Research*, **8**, 733–734.

Moser, C A and Kalton, G (1971) *Survey Methods in Social Investigation*, 2nd edn. Heinemann Educational Books, London.

Mosteller, F and Colditz, G A (1996) Understanding research synthesis (meta-analysis). *Annual Review of Public Health*, **17**, 1–23.

Müller, R and Büttner, P (1994) A critical discussion of intraclass correlation coefficients. *Statistics in Medicine*, **13**, 2465–2476.

Mulrow, C D (1987) The medical review article: state of the science. *Annals of Internal Medicine*, **106**, 485–488.

Mulrow, C D (1994) Rationale for systematic reviews. *British Medical Journal*, **309**, 597–599.

Munhall, P L (1988) Ethical considerations in qualitative research. *Western Journal of Nursing Research*, **10**, 150–162.

Munro, B H (1997) *Statistical Methods for Health Care Research*, 3rd edn. Lippincott, Philadelphia.

Murdoch, J and Barnes, J A (1974) *Statistical Tables*, 2nd edn. Macmillan. London.

Murrell, W (1889) *Massotherapeutics or Massage as a Mode of Treatment*. H K Lewis, London.

Myers, J L and Well, A D (1995) *Research Design and Statistical Analysis*. Lawrence Erlbaum, Hillsdale.

Naglieri, J A (1988) *Draw a Person: A Quantitative Scoring System*. Psychological Corporation / Harcourt Brace Jovanovich, San Antonio.

Naylor, C D (1997) Meta-analysis and the meta-epidemiology of clinical research. *British Medical Journal*, **315**, 617–619.

Neave, H R and Worthington, P L (1988) *Distribution-Free Tests*. Routledge, London.

Nevill, A M and Atkinson, G (1997) Assessing agreement between measurements recorded on a ratio scale in sports medicine and sports science. *British Journal of Sports Medicine*, **31**, 314–318.

Newell, D J (1992a) Intention-to-treat analysis: implications for quantitative and qualitative research. *International Journal of Epidemiology*, **21**, 837–841.

Newell, D J (1992b) Randomised controlled trials in health care research. In: *Researching Health Care: Designs, Dilemmas, Disciplines* (ed. Daly, J, McDonald, I and Willis, E). Routledge, London, pp. 47–61.

Newell, R (1993) Questionnaires. In: *Researching Social Life* (ed. Gilbert, N). Sage Publications, London, pp. 94–115.

Newell, R (1996) The reliability and validity of samples. *Nurse Researcher*, **3**(4), 16–26.

Newell, R (1998) Single case experimental design: controlling the study. *Nurse Researcher*, **5**(4), 25–39.

Newman, T B, Browner, W S, Cummings, S R and Hulley, S B (1988a) Designing a new study: II. Cross-sectional and case-control studies. In: *Designing Clinical Research: An Epidemiologic Approach* (ed. Hulley, S B and Cummings, S R). Williams & Wilkins, Baltimore, pp. 75–86.

Newman, T B, Browner, W S and Hulley, S B (1988b) Enhancing causal inference in observational studies. In: *Designing Clinical Research: An*

Epidemiologic Approach (ed. Hulley, S B and Cummings, S R). Williams & Wilkins, Baltimore, pp. 98–109.

NHSCRD (1996) *Undertaking Systematic Reviews of Research on Effectiveness: CRD Guidelines for those Carrying out or Commissioning Reviews.* National Health Service Centre for Reviews and Dissemination. University of York, York.

Nick, T G and Hardin, J M (1999) Regression modeling strategies: an illustrative case study from medical rehabilitation outcomes research. *American Journal of Occupational Therapy*, 53, 459–470.

Nolan, B (1994) *Data Analysis: An Introduction.* Polity Press, Cambridge.

Norman, G R and Streiner, D L (1994) *Biostatistics: The Bare Essentials.* Mosby, St Louis.

Norušis, M J (1997) *SPSS 7.5 Guide to Data Analysis.* Prentice-Hall, Upper Saddle River.

Noseworthy, J H, Ebers, G C, Vandervoort, M K, Farquhar, R E, Yetisir, E and Roberts, R (1994) The impact of blinding on the results of a randomized, placebo-controlled multiple sclerosis clinical trial. *Neurology*, 44, 16–20.

Nourbakhsh, M R and Ottenbacher, K J (1994) The statistical analysis of single-subject data: a comparative evaluation. *Physical Therapy*, 74, 768–776.

Nunnally, J C (1967) *Psychometric Theory.* McGraw-Hill, New York.

Nunnally, J C and Bernstein, I H (1994) *Psychometric Theory*, 3rd edn. McGraw-Hill, New York.

Nyamathi, A and Shuler, P (1990) Focus group interview: a research technique for informed nursing practice. *Journal of Advanced Nursing*, 15, 1281–1288.

O'Connell, D C and Kowal, S (1995) Basic principles of transcription. In: *Rethinking Methods in Psychology* (ed. Smith, J A, Harré, R and Van Langenhove, L). Sage Publications, London, pp. 93–105.

O'Hear, A (1989) *An Introduction to the Philosophy of Science.* Clarendon Press, Oxford.

O'Neill, S A (1999) Living with obsessive-compulsive disorder: a case study of a woman's construction of self. *Counselling Psychology Quarterly*, 12, 73–86.

Oakes, M (1986) *Statistical Inference: A Commentary for the Social and Behavioural Sciences.* John Wiley, Chichester.

Oakley, A (1981) Interviewing women: a contradiction in terms. In: *Doing Feminist Research* (ed. Roberts, H). Routledge & Kegan Paul, London, pp. 30–61.

Oakley, A (1989) Who's afraid of the randomized controlled trial? Some dilemmas of the scientific method and 'good' research practice. *Women and Health*, 15(4), 25–59.

Olkin, I (1995) Statistical and theoretical considerations in meta-analysis. *Journal of Clinical Epidemiology*, 48, 133–146.

Ong, B N (1993) *The Practice of Health Services Research.* Chapman & Hall, London.

Oppenheim, A N (1992) *Questionnaire Design, Interviewing and Attitude Measurement*, rev. edn. Pinter Publishers, London.

Orne, M T (1962) On the social psychology of the psychological experiment, with particular reference to demand characteristics and their implications *American Psychologist*, 17, 776–783.

Orona, C J (1997) Temporality and identity loss due to Alzheimer's disease. In: *Grounded Theory in Practice* (ed. Strauss, A and Corbin, J). Sage Publications, Thousand Oaks, pp. 171–196.

Osgood, C E, Suci, G J and Tannenbaum, P H (1957) *The Measurement of Meaning.* University of Illinois Press, Urbana.

Ottenbacher, K J (1986a) *Evaluating Clinical Change: Strategies for Occupational and Physical Therapists.* Williams & Wilkins, Baltimore.

Ottenbacher, K J (1986b) Reliability of accuracy of visually analyzing graphed data from single-subject designs. *American Journal of Occupational Therapy*, 40, 464–469.

Ottenbacher, K J (1995) The chi-square test: its use in rehabilitation research. *Archives of Physical Medicine and Rehabilitation*, 76, 678–681.

Ottenbacher, K J and Barrett, K A (1989) Measures of effect size in the reporting of rehabilitation research. *American Journal of Physical Medicine and Rehabilitation*, 68, 52–58.

Ottenbacher, K J and Maas, F (1999) How to detect effects: statistical power and evidence-based practice in occupational therapy research. *American Journal of Occupational Therapy*, 53, 181–188.

Ottenbacher, K J and York, J (1984) Strategies for evaluating clinical change: implications for practice and research. *American Journal of Occupational Therapy*, 38, 647–659.

Øvretveit, J (1998) *Evaluating Health Interventions: An Introduction to Evaluation of Health*

Treatments, Services, Policies and Organizational Interventions. Open University Press, Buckingham.

Owen, S V and Froman, R D (1998) Uses and abuses of the analysis of covariance. *Research in Nursing and Health*, 21, 557–562.

Pallikkathayil, L, Crighton, F and Aaronson, L S (1998a) Balancing ethical quandaries with scientific rigor: part 1. *Western Journal of Nursing Research*, 20, 388–393.

Pallikkathayil, L, Crighton, F and Aaronson, L S (1998b) Balancing ethical quandaries with scientific rigor: part 2. *Western Journal of Nursing Research*, 20, 501–507.

Pappworth, M H (1967) *Human Guinea Pigs: Experimentation on Man.* Routledge & Kegan Paul, London.

Parker, I (1994) Qualitative research. In: *Qualitative Methods in Psychology: A Research Guide* (ed. Banister, P, Burman, E, Parker, I, Taylor, M and Tindall, C). Open University Press, Buckingham, pp. 1–16.

Parry, A (1991) Physiotherapy and methods of inquiry: conflict and resolution. *Physiotherapy*, 77, 435–438.

Parry, A W (1995) Single-subject research in clinical practice. *British Journal of Therapy and Rehabilitation*, 2, 40–43

Parsonson, B S and Baer, D M (1978) The analysis and presentation of graphic data. In: *Single Subject Research: Strategies for Evaluating Change* (ed. Kratochwill, T R). Academic Press, New York, pp. 101–165.

Payton, O D (1993) Single-subject, behavioral, and sequential medical trials research. In: *Research in Physical Therapy* (ed. Bork, C E). J B Lippincott, Philadelphia, pp. 125–142.

Payton, O D (1994) *Research: The Validation of Clinical Practice*, 3rd edn. F A Davis, Philadelphia.

Pellegrino, E D (1995) The limitation of empirical research in ethics. *Journal of Clinical Ethics*, 6, 161–162.

Penslar, R L (1995) *Research Ethics: Cases and Materials.* Indiana University Press, Bloomington.

Perneger, T V (1998) What's wrong with Bonferroni adjustments. *British Medical Journal*, 316, 1236–1238.

Perrin, T (1998) Single-system methodology: a way forward in dementia care? *British Journal of Occupational Therapy*, 61, 448–452.

Peters, D J (1996) Qualitative inquiry. Expanding rehabilitation medicine's research repertoire: a commentary. *American Journal of Physical Medicine and Rehabilitation*, 75, 144–148.

Pett, M A (1997) *Nonparametric Statistics in Health Care Research.* Sage Publications, Thousand Oaks.

Plager, K A (1994) Hermeneutic phenomenology: a methodology for family health and health promotion study in nursing. In: *Interpretive Phenomenology: Embodiment, Caring and Ethics in Health and Illness* (ed. Benner, P). Sage Publications, Thousand Oaks, pp. 65–83.

Platt, J (1981a) Evidence and proof in documentary research: 1. Some specific problems of documentary research. *Sociological Review*, 29, 31–52.

Platt, J (1981b) Evidence and proof in documentary research: 2. Some shared problems of documentary research. *Sociological Review*, 29, 53–66.

Plummer, K (1983) *Documents of Life: An Introduction to the Problems and Literature of a Humanistic Method.* Allen & Unwin, London.

Plummer, K (1995) Life story research. In: *Rethinking Methods in Psychology* (ed. Smith, J A, Harré, R and Van Langenhove, L). Sage Publications, London, pp. 50–63.

Plutchik, R (1974) *Foundations of Experimental Research*, 2nd edn. Harper & Row, New York.

Pocock, S J (1979) Allocation of patients to treatment in clinical trials. *Biometrics*, 35, 183–197.

Pocock, S J (1983) *Clinical Trials: A Practical Approach.* John Wiley, Chichester.

Pocock, S J and Simon, R (1975) Sequential treatment assignment with balancing for prognostic factors in the controlled clinical trial. *Biometrics*, 31, 103–115.

Polgar, S and Thomas, S A (1995) *Introduction to Research in the Health Sciences*, 3rd edn. Churchill Livingstone, Melbourne.

Polit, D F and Hungler, B P (1995) *Nursing Research: Principles and Methods*, 5th edn. J B Lippincott, Philadelphia.

Polit, D F and Hungler, B P (1997) *Essentials of Nursing Research: Methods, Appraisal, and Utilization*, 4th edn. J B Lippincott, Philadelphia.

Pope, C and Mays, N (2000) Observational methods in health care settings. In: *Qualitative Research in Health Care*, 2nd edn (ed. Pope, C and Mays, N). British Medical Journal, London, pp. 30–39.

Pope, C, Ziebland, S and Mays, N (2000) Analysing qualitative data. In: *Qualitative Research in Health*

Care, 2nd edn (ed. Pope, C and Mays, N). British Medical Journal, London, pp. 75–88.

Pope, D and Croft, P (1996) Surveys using general practice registers: who are the non-responders? *Journal of Public Health Medicine*, 18, 6–12.

Popper, K R (1972) *Conjectures and Refutations: The Growth of Scientific Knowledge*, 4th edn. Routledge & Kegan Paul, London.

Popper, K R (1979) *Objective Knowledge: An Evolutionary Approach*, rev. edn. Clarendon Press, Oxford.

Portney, L G and Watkins, M P (1993) *Foundations of Clinical Research: Applications to Practice*. Appleton & Lange, Norwalk.

Price, B (1996) Illness careers: the chronic illness experience. *Journal of Advanced Nursing*, 24, 275–279.

Price, C (1996a) How to produce clear tables and figures. Part 1. *Australian Journal of Physiotherapy*, 42, 67–70.

Price, C (1996b) How to produce clear tables and figures. Part 2. *Australian Journal of Physiotherapy*, 42, 163–167.

Price, D D and Harkins, S W (1992) Psychophysical approaches to pain measurement and assessment. In: *Handbook of Pain Assessment* (ed. Turk, D C and Melzack, R). Guilford Press, New York, pp. 111–134.

Price, D D, McGrath, P A, Rafii, A and Buckingham, B (1983) The validation of visual analogue scales as ratio scale measures for chronic and experimental pain. *Pain*, 17, 45–56.

Procter, M (1993a) Measuring attitudes. In: *Researching Social Life* (ed. Gilbert, N). Sage Publications, London, pp. 116–134.

Procter, M (1993b) Analysing other researchers' data. In: *Researching Social Life* (ed. Gilbert, N). Sage Publications, London, pp. 255–269.

Quine, W V (1964) *Word and Object*. MIT Press, Cambridge.

Ramos, M C (1989) Some ethical implications of qualitative research. *Research in Nursing and Health*, 12, 57–63.

Rankin, G and Stokes, M (1998) Reliability of assessment tools in rehabilitation: an illustration of appropriate statistical analyses. *Clinical Rehabilitation*, 12, 187–199.

Reason, P (1988) Introduction. In: *Human Inquiry in Action: Developments in New Paradigm Research* (ed. Reason, P). Sage Publications, London, pp. 1–17.

Reason, P and Heron, J (1995) Co-operative inquiry. In: *Rethinking Methods in Psychology* (ed. Smith, J A, Harré, R and Van Langenhove, L). Sage Publications, London, pp. 122–142.

Reason, P and Rowan, J (1981a) *Human Inquiry: A Sourcebook of New Paradigm Research*. John Wiley, Chichester.

Reason, P and Rowan, J (1981b) Issues of validity in new paradigm research. In: *Human Inquiry. A Sourcebook of New Paradigm Research* (ed. Reason, P and Rowan, J). John Wiley, Chichester, pp. 239–250.

Reboussin, D M and Morgan, T M (1996) Statistical considerations in the use and analysis of single-subject designs. *Medicine and Science in Sports and Exercise*, 28, 639–644.

Reckase, M D (1990) Scaling techniques. In: *Handbook of Psychological Assessment*, 2nd edn (ed. Goldstein, G and Hersen, M). Pergamon Press, New York, pp. 41–56.

Redfern, S J and Norman, I J (1994) Validity through triangulation. *Nurse Researcher*, 2, 41–56.

Reed, A (1990) An investigation into the problems involved in teaching electrotherapy and their possible solutions using the Delphi technique. *Physiotherapy Theory and Practice*, 6, 9–16.

Reed, J (1992) Secondary data in nursing research. *Journal of Advanced Nursing*, 17, 877–883.

Reed, J and Payton, V R (1997) Focus groups: issues of analysis and interpretation. *Journal of Advanced Nursing*, 26, 765–771.

Reichardt, C S and Mark, M M (1998) Quasi-experimentation. In: *Handbook of Applied Social Research Methods* (ed. Bickman, L and Rog, D J). Sage Publications, Thousand Oaks, pp. 193–228.

Reid, A O (1992) Computer management strategies for text data. In: *Doing Qualitative Research* (ed. Crabtree, B F and Miller, W L). Sage Publications, Newbury Park, pp. 125–145.

Reid, N (1988) The Delphi technique: its contribution to the evaluation of professional practice. In: *Professional Competence and Quality Assurance in the Caring Professions* (ed. Ellis, R). Croom Helm, London, pp. 230–254.

Reid, N (1993) *Health Care Research by Degrees*. Blackwell Scientific Publications, Oxford.

Rembold, C M (1998) Number needed to screen: development of a statistic for disease screening. *British Medical Journal*, 317, 307–312.

Rice, N and Leyland, A (1996) Multilevel models:

applications to health data. *Journal of Health Services Research and Policy*, **1**, 154–164.

Richards, L (1998) Closeness to data: the changing goals of qualitative data handling. *Qualitative Health Research*, 8, 319–328.

Richards, T J and Richards, L (1994) Using computers in qualitative research. In: *Handbook of Qualitative Research* (ed. Denzin, N K and Lincoln, Y S). Sage Publications, Thousand Oaks, 445–462.

Riddoch, J and Lennon, S (1991) Evaluation of practice: the single case study approach. *Physiotherapy Theory and Practice*, 7, 3–11.

Riddoch, J and Lennon, S (1994) Single subject experimental design: one way forward? *Physiotherapy*, 80, 215–218.

Rigge, M (1995) Users' involvement in clinical audit. A speech to the Partners in Care Conference, Wednesday 1 March 1995; a conference of the Royal Medical Colleges and the Patients Forum at the Royal College of Physicians, London. *Journal of Evaluation in Clinical Practice*, 1, 67–70.

Rimm, E B, Stampfer, M J, Colditz, G A, Giovannucci, E and Willett, W C (1990) Effectiveness of various mailing strategies among nonrespondents in a prospective cohort study. *American Journal of Epidemiology*, **131**, 1068–1071.

Riolo-Quinn, L (1990) Across the great divide. *Clinical Management*, 10, 30–35.

Roberts, C and Sibbald, B (1998) Randomising groups of patients. *British Medical Journal*, 316, 1898–1900.

Roberts, H, Pearson, J C and Dengler, R (1993) Impact of a postcard versus a questionnaire as a first reminder in a postal lifestyle survey. *Journal of Epidemiology and Community Health*, 47, 334–335.

Roberts, I and Schierhout, G (1997) The private life of systematic reviews. *British Medical Journal*, 315, 686–687.

Robertson, V J and Lee, V L (1994) Some misconceptions about single subject designs in physiotherapy. *Physiotherapy*, 80, 762–766.

Robson, C (1993) *Real World Research: A Resource for Social Scientists and Practitioner-Researchers*. Blackwell Publishers, Oxford.

Roethlisberger, F J and Dickson, W J (1939) *Management and the Worker*. Harvard University Press, Cambridge.

Roland, M and Morris, R (1983) A study of the natural history of back pain. Part 1: Development

of a reliable and sensitive measure of disability in low back pain. *Spine*, 8, 141–144.

Roland, M and Torgerson, D (1998a) What are pragmatic trials? *British Medical Journal*, **316**, 285.

Roland, M and Torgerson, D (1998b) What outcomes should be measured? *British Medical Journal*, 317, 1075.

Roper, J M and Shapira, J (2000) *Ethnography in Nursing Research*. Sage Publications, Thousand Oaks.

Rose, K (1994) Unstructured and semi-structured interviewing. *Nurse Researcher*, 1(3), 23–32.

Rose, M J (1991) The statistical analysis of the intra-observer repeatability of four clinical measurement techniques. *Physiotherapy*, 77, 89–91.

Rose, M J, Reilly, J P, Pennie, B, Bowen-Jones, K, Stanley, I M and Slade, P D (1997) Chronic low back pain rehabilitation programs: a study of the optimum duration of treatment and a comparison of group and individual therapy. *Spine*, 22, 2246–2253.

Rosenberg, W and Donald, A (1995) Evidence based medicine: an approach to clinical problem-solving. *British Medical Journal*, 310, 1122–1126.

Rosenthal, R (1966) *Experimenter Effects in Behavioral Research*. Appleton-Century-Crofts, New York.

Rosenthal, R (1991) *Meta-Analytic Procedures for Social Research*. Sage Publications, Newbury Park.

Ross, L M, Hall, B A and Heater, S L (1998) Why are occupational therapists not doing more replication research? *American Journal of Occupational Therapy*, 52, 234–235.

Ross, M M, Rideout, E M and Carson, M M (1994) The use of the diary as a data collection technique. *Western Journal of Nursing Research*, **16**, 414–425.

Roth, J A (1963) *Timetables: Structuring the Passage of Time in Hospital Treatment and Other Careers*. Bobbs-Merrill, Indianapolis.

Roth, L M and Esdaile, S A (1999) Action research: a dynamic discipline for advancing professional goals. *British Journal of Occupational Therapy*, **62**, 498–506.

Rothstein, J M (1985) Measurement and clinical practice: theory and application. In: *Measurement in Physical Therapy* (ed. Rothstein, J M). Churchill Livingstone, New York, pp. 1–46.

Rothstein, J M (1993a) Reliability and validity: implications for research. In: *Research in Physical Therapy* (ed. Bork, C E). J B Lippincott, Philadelphia, pp. 18–36.

Rothstein, J M (1993b) The case for case reports. *Physical Therapy*, 73, 492–493.

Rothstein, J M (1995) Statistical words. *Physical Therapy*, 75, 82–83.

Rubin, H J and Rubin, I S (1995) *Qualitative Interviewing: The Art of Hearing Data*. Sage Publications, Thousand Oaks.

Rugg, D (1941) Experiments in question wording: II. *Public Opinion Quarterly*, 5, 91–92.

Ruse, M (1988) At what level of statistical uncertainty ought a random clinical trial to be interrupted? In: *The Use of Human Beings in Research* (ed. Spicker, S F, Alon, I, de Vries, A and Engelhardt, H T). Kluwer Academic Publishers, Dordrecht, pp. 189–222.

Rust, J and Golombok, S (1999) *Modern Psychometrics: The Science of Psychological Assessment*, 2nd edn. Routledge, London.

Ruta, D A, Garratt, A M, Wardlaw, D and Russell, I T (1994) Developing a valid and reliable measure of health outcome for patients with low back pain. *Spine*, 19, 1887–1896.

Ryle, G (1947) *The Concept of Mind*. Hutchinson, London.

Sackett, D L (1983) On some prerequisites for a successful clinical trial. In: *Clinical Trials: Issues and Approaches* (ed. Shapiro, S H and Louis, T A). Marcel Dekker, New York, pp. 65–79.

Sackett, D L and Haynes, R B (1997) Summarising the effects of therapy: a new table and some more terms. *Evidence-Based Medicine*, 2, 103–104.

Sackett, D L and Wennberg, J E (1997) Choosing the best design for each question. *British Medical Journal*, 315, 1636.

Sackett, D L, Gray, J A M, Haynes, R B and Richardson, W S (1996) Evidence based medicine: what it is and what it isn't. *British Medical Journal*, 312, 71–72.

Sackett, D L, Straus, S E, Richardson, W S, Rosenberg, W and Haynes, R B (2000) *Evidence-Based Medicine: How to Practice and Teach EBM*, 2nd edn. Churchill Livingstone, Edinburgh.

Sacks, H S, Berrier, J, Reitman, D, Ancona-Berk, V A and Chalmers, T C (1987) Meta-analysis of randomized controlled trials. *New England Journal of Medicine*, 316, 450–455.

Sánchez-Meca, J and Marín-Martínez, F (1997) Homogeneity tests in meta-analysis: a Monte Carlo comparison of statistical power and Type I error. *Quality and Quantity*, 31, 385–399.

Sandelowski, M (1986) The problem of rigor in qualitative research. *Advances in Nursing Science*, 8(3), 27–37.

Sandelowski, M (1994) Notes on transcription. *Research in Nursing and Health*, 17, 311–314.

Sandelowski, M (1995) Sample size in qualitative research. *Research in Nursing and Health*, 18, 179–183.

Sandelowski, M (1996) One is the liveliest number: the case orientation of qualitative research. *Research in Nursing and Health*, 19, 525–529.

Sandelowski, M (1998) The call to experts in qualitative research. *Research in Nursing and Health*, 21, 467–471.

Sapsford, R and Abbott, P (1996) Ethics, politics and research. In: *Data Collection and Analysis* (ed. Sapsford, R and Jupp, V). Sage Publications, London, pp. 317–342.

Sato, T (1996) Type I and Type II error in multiple comparisons. *Journal of Psychology*, 130, 293–302.

Sawilowsky, S S and Blair, R C (1992) A more realistic look at the robustness and Type II error properties of the *t* test to departures from population normality. *Psychological Bulletin*, 111, 352–360.

Schlesselman, J J (1982) *Case-Control Studies: Design, Conduct, Analysis*. Oxford University Press, New York.

Schmidt, K, Montgomery, L A, Bruene, D and Kenney, M (1997) Determining research priorities in pediatric nursing: a Delphi study. *Journal of Pediatric Nursing*, 12, 201–207.

Schmoll, B J (1987) Ethnographic inquiry in clinical settings. *Physical Therapy*, 67, 1895–1897.

Schmoll, B J (1993) Qualitative research. In: *Research in Physical Therapy* (ed. Bork, C E). J B Lippincott, Philadelphia, pp. 83–124.

Schulz, K F, Chalmers, I, Hayes, R J and Altman, D G (1995) Empirical evidence of bias: dimensions of methodological quality associated with estimates of treatment effects in controlled trials. *Journal of the American Medical Association*, 273, 408–412.

Schumann, H and Presser, S (1981) *Questions and Answers in Attitude Surveys*. Academic Press, New York.

Schwandt, T A (1997) *Qualitative Inquiry: A Dictionary of Terms*. Sage Publications, Thousand Oaks.

Schwartz, D and Lellouch, J (1967) Explanatory and pragmatic attitudes in therapeutic trials. *Journal of Chronic Diseases*, 20, 637–648.

Schwarz, N, Knäuper, B, Hippler, H-J, Noelle-Neumann, E and Clark, L (1991) Rating scales: numerical values may change the meaning of scale labels. *Public Opinion Quarterly*, 55, 570–582.

Scott, J (1990) *A Matter of Record: Documentary Sources in Social Research*. Polity Press, Cambridge.

Scott, S (1985) Feminist methods and qualitative research: a discussion of some of the issues. In: *Issues in Educational Research: Qualitative Methods* (ed. Burgess, R G). Falmer Press, London, pp. 67–85.

Seale, C (1999) *The Quality of Qualitative Research*. Sage Publications, London.

Seale, J and Barnard, S (1998) *Therapy Research: Principles and Practicalities*. Butterworth-Heinemann, Oxford.

Seale, J K and Barnard, S (1999) Ethical considerations in therapy research. *British Journal of Occupational Therapy*, 62, 371–375.

Seaman, C H C (1987) *Research Methods: Principles, Practice and Theory for Nursing*, 3rd edn. Appleton & Lange, Norwalk.

Seiler, L H and Hough, R L (1970) Empirical comparisons of the Thurstone and Likert techniques. In: *Attitude Measurement* (ed. Summers, G F). Rand McNally, Chicago, pp. 159–173.

Senn, S (1993) *Cross-Over Trials in Clinical Research*. John Wiley, Chichester.

Shaffer, J P (1995) Multiple hypothesis testing. *Annual Review of Psychology*, 46, 561–584.

Sharp, K (1998) The case for case studies in nursing research: the problem of generalization. *Journal of Advanced Nursing*, 27, 785–789.

Sheikh, K and Mattingly, S (1981) Investigating non-response bias in mail surveys. *Journal of Epidemiology and Community Health*, 35, 293–296.

Sheldon, M R, Fillyaw, M J and Thompson, W D (1996) The use and interpretation of the Friedman test in the analysis of ordinal-scale data in repeated measures designs. *Physiotherapy Research International*, 1, 221–228.

Shepard, K F, Jensen, G M, Schmoll, B J, Hack, L M and Gwyer, J (1993) Alternative approaches to research in physical therapy: positivism and phenomenology. *Physical Therapy*, 73, 88–101.

Shrout, P E and Fleiss, J L (1979) Intraclass correlations: uses in assessing rater reliability. *Psychological Bulletin*, 86, 420–428.

Sibbald, B and Roberts, C (1998) Crossover trials. *British Medical Journal*, 316, 1719.

Sidani, S (1998) Measuring the intervention in effectiveness research. *Western Journal of Nursing Research*, 20, 621–635.

Sieber, J E (1992) *Planning Ethically Responsible Research: A Guide for Students and Internal Review Boards*. Sage Publications, Newbury Park.

Siegel, S and Castellan, N J (1988) *Nonparametric Statistics for the Behavioral Sciences*, 2nd edn. McGraw-Hill, New York.

Siemonsma, P C and Walker, M F (1997) Practical guidelines for independent assessment in randomized controlled trials (RCTs) of rehabilitation. *Clinical Rehabilitation*, 11, 273–279.

Silva, F (1993) *Psychometric Foundations and Behavioral Assessment*. Sage Publications, Newbury Park.

Silverman, D (1985) *Qualitative Methodology and Sociology: Describing the Social World*. Gower, Aldershot.

Silverman, D (1993) *Interpreting Qualitative Data: Methods for Analysing Talk, Text and Interaction*. Sage Publications, London.

Silverman, D (2000) *Doing Qualitative Research: A Practical Handbook*. Sage Publications, London.

Silverman, W A (1985) *Human Experimentation. A Guided Step into the Unknown*. Oxford University Press, Oxford.

Sim, J (1986) Informed consent: ethical implications for physiotherapy. *Physiotherapy*, 72, 584–587.

Sim, J (1989) Methodology and morality in physiotherapy research. *Physiotherapy*, 75, 237–243.

Sim, J (1994) The ethics of single system (n=1) research. *Physiotherapy Theory and Practice*, 10, 211–222.

Sim, J (1995a) Sources of knowledge in physical therapy. *Physiotherapy Theory and Practice*, 11, 193–194.

Sim, J (1995b) The external validity of group comparative and single system studies. *Physiotherapy*, 81, 263–270.

Sim, J (1996) Client confidentiality: ethical issues in occupational therapy. *British Journal of Occupational Therapy*, 59, 56–61.

Sim, J (1997) *Ethical Decision Making in Therapy Practice*. Butterworth-Heinemann, Oxford.

Sim, J (1998) Collecting and analysing qualitative data: issues raised by the focus group. *Journal of Advanced Nursing*, 28, 345–352.

Sim, J and Arnell, P (1993) Measurement validity in physical therapy research. *Physical Therapy*, **73**, 102–115.

Sim, J and Reid, N (1999) Statistical inference by confidence intervals: issues of interpretation and utilization. *Physical Therapy*, **79**, 186–195.

Sim, J and Sharp, K (1998) A critical appraisal of the role of triangulation in nursing research. *International Journal of Nursing Studies*, **35**, 23–31.

Sim, J and Snell, J (1996) Focus groups in physiotherapy evaluation and research. *Physiotherapy*, **82**, 189–198.

Sim, J and Waterfield, J (1997) Validity, reliability and responsiveness in the assessment of pain. *Physiotherapy Theory and Practice*, **13**, 23–37

Simmonds, M J and Claveau, Y (1997) Measures of pain and physical function in patients with low back pain. *Physiotherapy Theory and Practice*, **13**, 53–65.

Simmons, S (1995) From paradigm to method in interpretive action research. *Journal of Advanced Nursing*, **21**, 837–844.

Skelton, J (1997) Coding and analysing data. In: *Research Methods in Primary Care* (ed. Carter, Y and Thomas, C). Radcliffe Medical Press, Oxford, pp. 63–71.

Smith, B A (1999) Ethical and methodologic benefits of using a reflexive journal in hermeneutic-phenomenologic research. *Image: Journal of Nursing Scholarship*, **31**, 359–363.

Smith, H W (1975) *Strategies of Social Research: The Methodological Imagination*. Prentice-Hall, London.

Smith, J A (1996) Beyond the divide between cognition and discourse: using interpretative phenomenological analysis in health psychology. *Psychology and Health*, **11**, 261–271.

Smith, J A, Harré, R and Van Langenhove, L (1995) Idiography and the case study. In: *Rethinking Psychology* (ed. Smith, J A, Harré, R and Van Langenhove, L). Sage Publications, London, pp. 59–69.

Smith, S (1996a) Ethnographic inquiry in physiotherapy research. 1. Illuminating the working culture of the physiotherapy assistant. *Physiotherapy*, **82**, 342–349.

Smith, S (1996b) Ethnographic inquiry in physiotherapy research. 2. The role of self in qualitative research. *Physiotherapy*, **82**, 349–352.

Smith, T (1999) *Ethics in Medical Research: A Handbook of Good Practice*. Cambridge University Press, Cambridge.

Spector, P E (1981) *Research Designs*. Sage Publications, Beverly Hills.

Spector, P E (1992) *Summated Rating Scale Construction: An Introduction*. Sage Publications, Newbury Park.

Spiegelhalter, D J, Myles, J P, Jones, D R and Abrams, K R (1999) An introduction to Bayesian methods in health technology assessment. *British Medical Journal*, **319**, 508–512.

Sprent, P (1993) *Applied Nonparametric Statistical Methods*, 2nd edn. Chapman & Hall, London.

SPSS (1999) *SPSS Base 9.0 User's Guide*. SPSS, Illinois.

Stake, R E (1994) Case studies. In: *Handbook of Qualitative Research* (ed. Denzin, N K and Lincoln, Y S). Sage Publications, Thousand Oaks, pp. 236–247.

Stake, R E (1995) *The Art of Case Study Research*. Sage Publications, Thousand Oaks.

Stanfield, J H and Katerndahl, D A (1994) Using human documents. In: *Exploring Collaborative Research in Primary Care* (ed. Crabtree, B F, Miller, W L, Addison, R B, Gilchrist, V J and Kuzel, A). Sage Publications, Thousand Oaks, pp. 77–86.

Staples, D (1991) Questionnaires. *Clinical Rehabilitation*, **5**, 259–264.

Sterling, Y M and McNally, J A (1992) Single-subject research for nursing practice. *Clinical Nurse Specialist*, **6**, 21–26.

Stern, J M and Simes, R J (1997) Publication bias: evidence of delayed publication in a cohort study of clinical research projects. *British Medical Journal*, **315**, 640–645.

Stevens, S S (1946) On the theory of scales of measurement. *Science*, **103**, 677–680.

Stevens, S S (1951) Mathematics, measurement, and psychophysics. In: *Handbook of Experimental Psychology* (ed. Stevens, S S). John Wiley, New York, pp. 1–49.

Stewart, A L and Ware, J E (1992) *Measuring Function and Well-Being: The Medical Outcomes Study Approach*. Duke University Press, Durham.

Stewart, D W (1984) *Secondary Research: Information Sources and Methods*. Sage Publications, Beverly Hills.

Stewart, D W and Shamdasani, P N (1990) *Focus Groups: Theory and Practice*. Sage Publications, Newbury Park.

Stoecker, R (1991) Evaluating and rethinking the case study. *Sociological Review*, **38**, 88–112.

Stratford, P W, Binkley, J, Solomon, P, Finch, E, Gill, C and Moreland, J (1996) Defining the minimum level of detectable change for the Roland-Morris Questionnaire. *Physical Therapy*, 76, 359–365.

Strauss, A and Corbin, J (1990) *Basics of Qualitative Research: Grounded Theory Procedures and Techniques*. Sage Publications, Newbury Park.

Strauss, A and Corbin, J (1997) *Grounded Theory in Practice*. Sage Publications, Thousand Oaks.

Strauss, A and Corbin, J (1998) *Basics of Qualitative Research: Techniques and Procedures for Developing Grounded Theory*, 2nd edn. Sage Publications, Thousand Oaks.

Strauss, A L (1987) *Qualitative Analysis for Social Scientists*. Cambridge University Press, Cambridge.

Streiner, D and Geddes, J (1998) Some useful concepts and terms used in articles about diagnosis. *Evidence-Based Mental Health*, 1, 6–7.

Streiner, D L and Norman, G R (1995) *Health Measurement Scales: A Practical Guide to Their Development and Use*, 2nd edn. Oxford University Press, Oxford.

Strong, J, Ashton, R, Chant, D and Cramond, T (1994) An investigation of the dimensions of chronic low back pain: the patients' perspectives. *British Journal of Occupational Therapy*, 57, 204–208.

Strong, P and Robinson, J (1990) *The NHS Under New Management*. Open University Press, Milton Keynes.

Sudman, S (1966) Probability sampling with quotas. *Journal of the American Statistical Association*, 61, 749–771.

Sudman, S and Bradburn, N M (1982) *Asking Questions: A Practical Guide to Questionnaire Design*. Jossey-Bass Publishers, San Francisco.

Sullivan, M, Karlsson, J and Ware, J E (1995) The Swedish SF-36 Health Survey – 1. Evaluation of data quality, scaling assumptions, reliability and construct validity across general populations in Sweden. *Social Science and Medicine*, 41, 1349–1358.

Sulmasy, D P, Lehmann, L S, Levine, D M and Faden, R R (1994) Patients' perceptions of the quality of informed consent for common medical procedures. *Journal of Clinical Ethics*, 5, 189–194.

Sumsion, T (1998) The Delphi technique: an adaptive research tool. *British Journal of Occupational Therapy*, 61, 153–156.

Susman, G I and Evered, R D (1978) An assessment of the scientific merits of action research. *Administrative Science Quarterly*, 23, 582–603.

Swingewood, A (1984) *A Short History of Sociological Thought*. Macmillan, London.

Swinscow, T D V and Campbell, M J (1996) *Statistics at Square One*, 9th edn. British Medical Journal, London.

Sword, W (1999) Accounting for presence of self: reflections on doing qualitative research. *Qualitative Health Research*, 9, 270–278.

Szatmari, P (1998) Some useful concepts and terms used in articles about treatment. *Evidence-Based Mental Health*, 1, 39–40.

Tabachnick, B G and Fidell, L S (1996) *Using Multivariate Statistics*, 3rd edn. HarperCollins, New York.

Tagg, S K (1985) Life story interviews and their interpretation. In: *The Research Interview: Uses and Approaches* (ed. Brenner, M, Brown, J and Canter, D). Academic Press, London, pp. 163–199.

Tak, S H, Nield, M and Becker, H (1999) Use of a computer software program for qualitative analyses – Part 2: advantages and disadvantages. *Western Journal of Nursing Research*, 21, 436–439.

Tarnow-Mordi, W O and Healy, M J R (1999) Distinguishing between 'no evidence of effect' and 'evidence of no effect' in randomised controlled trials and other comparisons. *Archives of Disease in Childhood*, 80, 210–211.

Task Force on Standards for Measurement in Physical Therapy (1991) Standards for tests and measurements in physical therapy practice. *Physical Therapy*, 71, 589–622.

Tate, D G, Findley, T, Dijkers, M, Nobunaga, A I and Karunas, R B (1999) Randomized clinical trials in medical rehabilitation research. *American Journal of Physical Medicine and Rehabilitation*, 78, 486–499.

Tatsuoka, M (1993) Effect size. In: *A Handbook for Data Analysis in the Behavioral Sciences: Methodological Issues* (ed. Keren, G and Lewis, C). Lawrence Erlbaum, Hillsdale, pp. 461–479.

Taylor, M (1994) Action research. In: *Qualitative Methods in Psychology: A Research Guide* (ed. Banister, P, Burman, E, Parker, I, Taylor, M and Tindall, C). Open University Press, Buckingham, pp. 108–120.

Thomas, C, Greenfield, S and Carter, Y (1997) Questionnaire design. In: *Research Methods in*

Primary Care (ed. Carter, Y and Thomas, C). Radcliffe Medical Press, Oxford, pp. 49–61.

Thomas, R (1996) Statistical sources and databases. In: *Data Collection and Analysis* (ed. Sapsford, R and Jupp, V). Sage Publications, London, pp. 121–137.

Thompson, C (1999) If you could just provide me with a sample: examining sampling in qualitative and quantitative research papers. *Evidence-Based Nursing*, 2, 68–70.

Thompson, S G (1994) Why sources of heterogeneity in meta-analysis should be investigated. *British Medical Journal*, 309, 1351–1355.

Thompson, S G and Pocock, S J (1991) Can meta-analysis be trusted? *Lancet*, 338, 1127–1130.

Thurstone, L L and Chave, E J (1929) *The Measurement of Attitude: A Psychophysical Method and Some Experiments with a Scale for Measuring Attitude toward the Church*. University of Chicago Press, Chicago.

Tickle-Degnen, L (1998) Communicating with clients about treatment outcomes: the use of meta-analytic evidence in collaborative treatment planning. *American Journal of Occupational Therapy*, 52, 526–530.

Tindall, C (1994) Issues of evaluation. In: *Qualitative Methods in Psychology: A Research Guide* (ed. Banister, P, Burman, E, Parker, I, Taylor, M and Tindall, C). Open University Press, Buckingham, pp. 142–159.

Torgerson, D and Roberts, C (1999) Randomisation methods: concealment. *British Medical Journal*, 319, 375–376.

Tramèr, M R, Reynolds, D J M, Moore, R A and McQuay, H J (1997) Impact of covert duplicate publication on meta-analysis: a case study. *British Medical Journal*, 315, 635–640.

Treasure, T and MacRae, K D (1998) Minimisation: the platinum standard for trials? *British Medical Journal*, 317, 362–363.

Trinkoff, A M and Storr, C L (1997) Incorporating auxiliary variables into probability sampling designs. *Nursing Research*, 46, 182–185.

Trusted, J (1979) *The Logic of Scientific Inference: An Introduction*. Macmillan, London.

Tryon, W W (1982) A simplified time-series analysis for evaluating treatment interventions. *Journal of Applied Behavior Analysis*, 15, 423–429.

Tull, D S and Albaum, G S (1973) *Survey Research: A Decisional Approach*. Intertext Books, Aylesbury.

Turner, B A (1994) Patterns of crisis behaviour: a qualitative inquiry. In: *Analyzing Qualitative Data* (ed. Bryman, A and Burgess, R G). Routledge, London, pp. 195–215.

van der Linden, S, Bouter, L and Tugwell, P (1991) What are the minimal methodological requirements for a good trial? I. The clinician's view. In: *Physiotherapy: Controlled Trials and Facts* (ed. Schlapbach, P and Gerber, N J). Karger, Basel, pp. 1–8.

van der Ven, A H G S (1980) *Introduction to Scaling*. John Wiley, Chichester.

van der Zalm, J E and Bergum, V (2000) Hermeneutic-phenomenology: providing living knowledge for nursing practice. *Journal of Advanced Nursing*, 31, 211–218.

Van Sant, A F (1993) Nonparametric statistics. In: *Research in Physical Therapy* (ed. Bork, C E). J B Lippincott, Philadelphia, pp. 223–250.

van Tulder, M W, Assendelft, W J J, Koes, B W and Bouter, L M (1997) Method guidelines for systematic reviews in the Cochrane Collaboration Back Review Group for Spinal Disorders. *Spine*, 22, 2323–2330.

Vargas, S and Camilli, G (1999) A meta-analysis of research on sensory integration treatment. *American Journal of Occupational Therapy*, 53, 189–198.

Vaughn, S, Schumm, J S and Sinagub, J (1996) *Focus Group Interviews in Education and Psychology*. Sage Publications, Thousand Oaks.

Vogt, W P (1999) *Dictionary of Statistics and Methodology. A Nontechnical Guide for the Social Sciences*, 2nd edn. Sage Publications, Newbury Park.

Wade, D T (1992) *Measurement in Neurological Rehabilitation*. Oxford University Press, Oxford.

Wade, T C (1990) Patients may not recall disclosure of risk of death: implications for informed consent. *Medicine, Science and the Law*, 30, 259–262.

Wainwright, S P (1994) Analysing data using grounded theory. *Nurse Researcher*, 1(3), 43–49.

Walker, A M (1994) A Delphi study of research priorities in the clinical practice of physiotherapists. *Physiotherapy*, 80, 205–207.

Walter, S D, Eliasziw, M and Donner, A (1998) Sample size and optimal designs for reliability studies. *Statistics in Medicine*, 17, 101–110.

Wampold, B E and Furlong, M J (1981) The heuristics of visual inspection. *Behavioral Assessment*, 3, 79–92.

Ware, J E and Sherbourne, C D (1992) The SF-36 health status survey: 1, conceptual framework and item selection. *Medical Care*, 30, 473–483.

Waterfield, J and Sim, J (1996) Clinical assessment of pain by the visual analogue scale. *British Journal of Therapy and Rehabilitation*, 3, 94–97.

Webb, C (1984) Feminist methodology in nursing research. *Journal of Advanced Nursing*, 9, 249–256.

Webb, C (1989) Action research: philosophy, methods and personal experiences. *Journal of Advanced Nursing*, 14, 403–410.

Webb, C (1993) Feminist research: definitions, methodology, methods and evaluation. *Journal of Advanced Nursing*, 18, 416–423.

Webb, E J, Campbell, D T, Schwartz, R D and Sechrest, L (1966) *Unobtrusive Measures: Nonreactive Research in the Social Sciences*. Rand McNally, Chicago.

Weber, R P (1994) Basic content analysis. In: *Research Practice* (ed. Lewis-Beck, M S). Sage Publications, Thousand Oaks, pp. 251–338.

Wechsler, D (1974) *Wechsler Intelligence Scale for Children*, rev. edn. Psychological Corporation / Harcourt Brace Jovanovich, San Antonio.

Weitzman, E and Miles, M B (1995) *Computer Programs for Qualitative Data Analysis*. Sage Publications, Thousand Oaks.

West, P (1979) An investigation into the social construction and consequences of the label epilepsy. *Sociological Review*, 27, 719–741.

West, R R (1993) A look at the statistical overview (or meta-analysis). *Journal of the Royal College of Physicians of London*, 27, 111–115.

White, S J (1997) Evidence-based medicine and nursing: the new panacea? *British Journal of Nursing*, 6, 175–178.

Whitehead, A and Whitehead, J (1991) A general parametric approach to the meta-analysis of randomized clinical trials. *Statistics in Medicine*, 10, 1665–1677.

Whyte, W F (1982) Interviewing in field research. In: *Field Research: A Sourcebook and Field Manual* (ed. Burgess, R G). Allen & Unwin, London, pp. 111–122.

Wilde, V (1992) Controversial hypotheses on the relationship between researcher and informant in qualitative research. *Journal of Advanced Nursing*, 17, 234–242.

Wilkes, W C (1993) Comparison of means: one sample, two independent samples, paired observations. In: *Research in Physical Therapy* (ed.

Bork, C E). J B Lippincott, Philadelphia, pp. 251–276.

Williams, P L and Webb, C (1994) The Delphi technique: a methodological discussion. *Journal of Advanced Nursing*, 19, 180–186.

Williams, R D (1999) Use of focus groups with rural women of low socioeconomic status. *Applied Nursing Research*, 12, 45–50.

Wilson, A, Grimshaw, G, Baker, R and Thompson, J (1999) Differentiating between audit and research: postal survey of health authorities' views. *British Medical Journal*, 319, 1235.

Wilson, B A (1997) Research and evaluation in rehabilitation. In: *Rehabilitation Studies Handbook* (ed. Wilson, B A and McLellan, D L). Cambridge University Press, Cambridge, pp. 161–187.

Wilson, J and While, A E (1998) Methodological issues surrounding the use of vignettes in qualitative research. *Journal of Interprofessional Care*, 12, 79–87.

Wilson, K and Rose, K (1998) Patient recruitment and retention strategies in randomised controlled trials. *Nurse Researcher*, 6(1), 35–46.

Wilson, M (1996) Asking qquestions. In: *Data Collection and Analysis* (ed. Sapsford, R and Jupp, V). Sage Publications, London, pp. 94–120.

Wilson, S L (1995) Single case experimental designs. In: *Research Methods in Psychology* (ed. Breakwell, G M, Hammond, S and Fife-Schaw, C). Sage Publications, London, pp. 69–84.

Wilson-Barnett, J (1991) The experiment: is it worthwhile? *International Journal of Nursing Studies*, 28, 77–87.

Winer, B J, Brown, D R and Michels, K M (1991) *Statistical Principles in Experimental Design*, 3rd edn. McGraw-Hill, New York.

Winkler, R L (1993) Bayesian statistics: an overview. In: *A Handbook for Data Analysis in the Behavioral Sciences: Statistical Issues* (ed. Keren, G and Lewis, C). Lawrence Erlbaum, Hillsdale, pp. 201–232.

Wolcott, H F (1990) *Writing up Qualitative Research*. Sage Publications, Newbury Park.

Wolery, M and Harris, S R (1982) Interpreting results of single-subject research designs. *Physical Therapy*, 62, 445–452.

Wood, P (1995) Meta-analysis. In: *Research Methods in Psychology* (ed. Breakwell, G M, Hammond, S and Fife-Schaw, C). Sage Publications, London, pp. 386–399.

Wood-Dauphinee, S and Williams, J I (1989) Much

ado about reliability. *Physiotherapy Canada*, 41, 234–236.

Woodward, C A (1988) Questionnaire construction and question writing for research in medical education. *Medical Education*, 22, 347–363.

Worthington, A D (1995) Single case design experimentation. *British Journal of Therapy and Rehabilitation*, 2, 536–438, 555–557.

Wright, D B (1997) *Understanding Statistics: An Introduction for the Social Sciences*. Sage Publications, London.

Yin, R K (1984) *Case Study Research: Design and Methods*, rev. edn. Sage Publications, Newbury Park.

Zeller, R A and Carmines, E G (1980) *Measurement in the Social Sciences: The Link between Theory and Data*. Cambridge University Press, Cambridge.

Zimmerman, D H (1971) The practicalities of rule use. In: *Understanding Everyday Life* (ed. Douglas, J D). Routledge & Kegan Paul, London, pp. 221–238.

Zwick, R (1993) Pairwise comparison procedures for one-way analysis of variance designs. In: *A Handbook for Data Analysis in the Behavioral Sciences: Statistical Issues* (ed. Keren, G and Lewis, C). Lawrence Erlbaum, Hillsdale, pp. 43–71.

APPENDIX I: CASE STUDIES

CASE STUDY 1: THE STUDENT ATTITUDES STUDY

A brief outline is given for a small-scale hypothetical study based on the exploratory research question: what do health care students understand by 'self-inflicted' illness in terms of the notion of responsibility for health? A health psychologist, Teresa Ganz, is running the study.

Summary of background

Many illnesses are regarded as being in some sense 'self-inflicted', in so far as they may be caused or exacerbated by activities performed by the person affected by the condition, or by other individual lifestyle factors. The extent to which certain conditions are conceptualized in this way may have implications for the way in which health care is delivered to individual patients and, at a wider level, may play a part in moulding professional ideologies of care and aspects of health policy.

Research questions

1 What attitudes and beliefs do student health care professionals hold towards putatively 'self-inflicted' illness?
2 How are students' attitudes formulated, developed and expressed in the interaction that occurs in the teaching situation?
3 What professional orthodoxy, if any, exists on this topic in the health care professions?

Method

Participants

The sample was a convenience sample of approximately 15 nursing and occupational therapy students at a university. Two professions are represented in the sample because Dr Ganz anticipated that there might be points of comparison and contrast between these groups

of students, given their rather different patterns of professional education and socialization.

Design and data collection

This study uses a nonexperimental, naturalistic design, using three main sources of data:

1 One-to-one unstructured interviews with health care students, conducted according to a list of general topics in an interview guide. The interviews were audiotaped and subsequently transcribed.
2 Non-participant observation of small-group teaching sessions on areas of the curriculum likely to embrace or touch upon the notion of 'self-inflicted' illness.
3 A content analysis of core texts used by the students, so as to gather information on images of 'self-inflicted' illness as they are presented (in both manifest and latent form) within the academic and professional literature.

The design of this study is considered more fully in Chapter 5. Extracts from some of the unstructured interviews have been used to illustrate the recording and analysis of qualitative data (Chapters 10 and 11).

CASE STUDY 2: THE RHEUMATOID ARTHRITIS STUDY

A brief outline is given for a hypothetical study based on the descriptive research question: what therapeutic approaches do occupational therapists and physiotherapists use in the management of rheumatoid arthritis? The study is being coordinated by Angela Carella, a research assistant in a rehabilitation research unit.

Summary of background

Rheumatoid arthritis (RA) is a common inflammatory disease of the joints which affects around

1% of the population in the UK – about 1 in every 200 women compared with 1 in 600 men. Onset can be at any age, but with a peak onset in the fifth decade (Lloyd, 1998). Although many alternative treatments are available, there is no cure. This study aims to identify and describe current assessment and management of patients with RA by hospital-based occupational therapists (OTs) and physiotherapists (PTs).

Research questions

1 What are the characteristic patterns and modes of practice of occupational therapists and of physiotherapists for clients with rheumatoid arthritis?
2 What therapeutic strategies and approaches are adopted by occupational therapists and by physiotherapists with these clients?
3 What are the attitudes of occupational therapists and of physiotherapists to clients with rheumatoid arthritis and their care?

Method

Participants

Three convenience samples were used in the first phase of the study. These comprised eight OTs from local hospitals, eight PTs from local hospitals and 20 hospital-based therapists.

Phase 2 of the study employed a three-stage cluster sampling strategy. The regions of the UK were categorized as predominantly urban, predominantly rural or mixed urban and rural. Two regions were randomly chosen from each of these categories and five hospitals were randomly selected within each chosen region At each of these 30 hospitals, a random sample of eight therapists (occupational therapists or physiotherapists) working in musculoskeletal practice was selected, resulting in a total sample of 240 therapists. A total of 150 questionnaires were returned, and of these respondents 117 satisfied the condition of having seen patients with rheumatoid arthritis in the last 12 months.

Phase 3 of the study planned to use about five therapists, purposively chosen with regard to their responses on the study questionnaire.

Measures

A questionnaire was developed in Phase 1, which comprised both open-ended and closed-ended questions. The content was based on a review of previous studies, informal discussions with therapists who were experienced in the management of rheumatological conditions, and a scrutiny of key items of the professional literature to ascertain 'standard' practice.

Closed-ended questions were used to obtain information on the following key areas:

- area of practice
- typical caseload and referral sources
- means by which clients are assessed and their needs are identified
- particular aspects of treatment/management objectives
- specific assessment methods used in practice, such as standardized tools to measure pain intensity and psychological and physical functioning
- specific interventions used in practice, including different types of exercise, psychological techniques, electrotherapy, education, devices and appliances
- attitudes to certain statements about clients with RA
- biographical details.

Information sought by open-ended questions included:

- clinical features with which clients with RA usually present
- details of specific treatment/management programmes for clients with RA
- factors associated with *good* therapeutic outcome
- factors associated with *poor* therapeutic outcome
- any other issues associated with the treatment/management of clients with RA which were not covered by the questionnaire.

One final question asked the respondent whether he or she was willing to be contacted again; if so, the therapist's name and a contact telephone number or address were requested.

A filter question was used to exclude therapists who had not seen clients with a confirmed diagnosis of RA in the previous 12 months. This question was placed near the beginning of the questionnaire, following questions on biographical details and area and context of practice.

Design

There were three phases to the study. Phase 1 comprised development and piloting of a questionnaire. Two focus groups (one for OTs and the other PTs) were used to inform the response options on some of the closed-ended questions. The pilot was used to test the initial questionnaire for clarity and comprehensiveness. Appropriate changes were made to the questionnaire before Phase 2.

A cross-sectional, prospective survey was employed in Phase 2, with data collected via self-completed, postal questionnaires. In Phase 3 one-to-one unstructured interviews were used to explore any unexpected or unusual results from Phase 2.

The design of this study is considered more fully in Chapter 6. Items from the questionnaire have been used to illustrate issues in attitude measurement and questionnaire design in Chapter 15. Responses to some of the closed-ended questions have been used to demonstrate descriptive and inferential statistics (Chapters 12, 14 and 18). These analyses are illustrative only, and they will not in all cases necessarily represent the optimum way in which this study as a whole should be analysed.

CASE STUDY 3: THE LOW BACK PAIN STUDY

A brief outline is given for a hypothetical study based on the explanatory research question: is there a difference in effectiveness between an individual-based and a group-based cognitive-behavioural approach to the management of low back pain? The study is coordinated by a primary care physician, Joseph Buckley.

Summary of background

Low back pain (LBP) is one of the most common causes of morbidity in society. It is reported to afflict 14% of the UK population at any one point in time and between 58% and 80% of people at some point during their lifetime (Rose et al., 1997; Ruta et al., 1994). Its management and treatment impose high costs on health and medical services in all Western countries and it is a major cause of lost days at work. Physical therapy has long played a significant role in the management of patients with LBP (Simmonds and Claveau, 1997). More recently, cognitive-behavioural programmes have been developed based on a combination of psychosocial and behavioural models. These aim to reduce disability and facilitate improved psychological and physical functioning. They have been shown to be effective through meta-analysis (Rose et al., 1997). However, there is a need for the measurement of treatment efficacy to reflect the patient's functional ability on a day-to-day basis. This study aims to compare the effectiveness on functional ability of a cognitive-behavioural programme when delivered in two different contexts.

Definition of LBP

Pain, bilateral or unilateral, between the eleventh rib and the gluteal fold, with or without radiation to the lower limb, as far as the knee.

Research hypothesis

There is a difference in effectiveness between individual-based and group-based cognitive-behavioural approaches to the management of low back pain.

Method

Participants

A sample of 150 patients with chronic LBP was recruited through prospective accrual from the orthopaedic departments in three major hospitals and from primary care physicians, over a period of 12 months.

Referrals were accepted into the study if the following inclusion criteria were satisfied:

- aged between 18 and 65 years
- experienced constant benign LBP for a minimum period of 6 months
- received no treatment for LBP within the last 6 weeks
- condition stable over the previous 6 weeks
- could attend the clinic for a 3-hour session per week for 5 weeks.

Exclusion criteria were as follows:

- serious pathology or injury
- previous back surgery, or awaiting such injury
- physiotherapy or other treatment (other than medication or self-help measures) in the previous 6 weeks
- diagnosis of clinical depression or other specified psychiatric pathology.

Data were collected via self-completed, postal questionnaires, completed 1 week before attendance on a programme, and at 1 week and 12 weeks after completion of the programme. Self-addressed, stamped envelopes were included for return of the completed questionnaires. Postal and telephone reminders were used to increase the completion rate.

There were 130 completed questionnaires 1 week before beginning the programme, and 109 at 1 week and 98 at 12 weeks after completion of the programme.

Outcome measures

The following outcome variables were chosen to cover pain intensity, pain affect, dysfunction and self-rated change:

- A 10 cm visual analogue scale for pain intensity, anchored by 'no pain' and 'worst pain imaginable'. This scale has established reliability and validity for use with LBP patients (McDowell and Newell, 1996).
- A 10 cm visual analogue scale for pain affect (how much a person is affected by the pain). This scale is anchored by 'pain doesn't bother me' and 'pain couldn't

bother me more'. This scale has established reliability and validity for use with LBP patients (McDowell and Newell, 1996).
- Aberdeen Back Pain Scale, a condition specific measure of the effect of LBP on health status. It is a 19 question, multi-item scale that covers type, frequency, therapy and dysfunction. The responses are converted to produce a score between 0 and 100, with higher scores indicating higher effects of LBP on health. The scale has established reliability and validity in clinical settings and is sensitive to change over time (Ruta et al., 1994).
- A five-point, self-rating scale for symptomatic change at 12 weeks; with 1 through to 5 denoting 'symptoms considerably worse', 'symptoms slightly worse', 'symptoms unchanged', 'symptoms slightly better' and 'symptoms considerably better', respectively.

Other baseline measures:

- age, sex, marital status, employment status
- comorbidity
- duration of current episode of LBP
- duration of LBP
- previous treatment of LBP by health professionals (and perceived success)
- health locus of control.

Design

The therapeutic input was a cognitive-behavioural programme for the management of LBP, run at the clinic during one 3-hour session per week over a period of 5 weeks. A physiotherapist, an occupational therapist and a psychologist each delivered 1 hour per session.

A randomized controlled trial was performed, with willing and eligible participants being randomly assigned to one of two approaches for delivering the programme: group intervention (delivery of the programme to participants in groups of size 7 to 10) and individual intervention (delivery of the programme to individual participants). Patients were allotted randomly, and in equal numbers, to each approach.

Outcome measures were recorded at baseline (1 week before commencement on the programme), and at 1 week and 12 weeks after completion of the programme. Other variables were recorded at baseline only.

Following completion of the study, a subsample of participants from both arms of the study were interviewed to discover possible reasons why the treatment they received was or was not helpful, and to reveal any issues relating to adherence, treatment preference and treatment acceptability.

The design of this study is considered more fully in Chapter 5. Subsets of data from this case study have been used to demonstrate various statistical methods in Chapters 14 and 18. These analyses are illustrative only, and they will not in all cases necessarily represent the optimum way in which the study as a whole should be analysed.

APPENDIX II: ANALYSIS OF VARIANCE: MODELS

ONE-WAY ANALYSIS OF VARIANCE

In the home exercise example (Section 18.1.2), the study was designed to test the effects of three different approaches to goal setting upon adherence to home exercise sessions. The percentage adherence for a particular patient could be described explicitly in terms of symbols:

$$y_{ij} = \mu_i + \varepsilon_{ij}$$

$$\mu_i = \mu + \tau_i$$

where,

- y_{ij} is the percentage adherence for the jth patient following the ith goal-setting approach. $i = 1, 2, 3$, corresponding to none, therapist-set and collaboratively set goals, respectively;
- μ_i is a mean percentage adherence unique to the ith goal-setting approach;
- μ is a mean percentage adherence common to all approaches;
- τ_i is the unique effect of the ith approach to goal setting on percentage adherence;
- ε_{ij} is the contribution of error to the individual percentage adherence value for the jth patient following the ith approach to goal setting.

ONE-WAY REPEATED MEASURES ANOVA

For the rehabilitation example (Section 18.1.6), the model can be expressed in symbols as:

$$y_{ij} = \mu_j + \pi_i + (\pi\tau)_{ij} + \varepsilon_{ij}$$

$$\mu_j = \mu + \tau_j$$

where:

- y_{ij} is the Aberdeen Back Pain Scale (ABPS) score for the ith individual participant at the jth time period; $j = 1, 2, 3,$ corresponding to before, 1 week after and 12 weeks after the rehabilitation programme;
- μ_j is a mean ABPS score unique to the jth time period;
- μ is a mean ABPS score common to all time periods (and individuals);
- τ_j *is the effect of rehabilitation unique to the jth time period;*
- π_i is the effect of rehabilitation unique to the ith individual;
- $(\pi\tau)_{ij}$ is the effect of rehabilitation unique to the combination of the ith individual and the jth time period;
- ε_{ij} is the experimental error associated with the ith individual and the jth time period.

RANDOMIZED BLOCK DESIGN

The design and analysis for a randomized block design (Section 18.1.7) are expressed in the following model for outcome values:

$$y_{ij} = \mu_j + \beta_i + \varepsilon_{ij}$$

and

$$\mu_j = \mu + \tau_j$$

- y_{ij} is the outcome value for the jth treatment in the ith block;
- μ_j is a mean outcome value unique to the jth treatment (or condition);
- μ is a mean outcome value common to all treatments;
- τ_j is a unique effect of the jth treatment;
- β_i is a unique effect of the ith block;
- ε_{ij} is the experimental error associated with the ith block and the jth treatment.

COMPLETELY RANDOMIZED FACTORIAL DESIGNS

An example for a two-factor design (Section 18.1.9, subsection 'Model'): patients with low back pain were allotted randomly to one of six exercise programmes comprising all combinations of a group-based or an individual-based programme and durations of 1, 2 or 3 weeks. Health status was recorded by the Aberdeen Back Pain Scale (ABPS) after completion of a programme.

The ABPS score for a particular patient could be described as:

$$y_{ijk} = \mu + \tau_i + \beta_j + (\tau\beta)_{ij} + \varepsilon_{ijk}$$

where:

y_{ijk} is the ABPS score for the kth participant following the ith mode of delivery for the jth duration;

μ is a common mean ABPS score (irrespective of mode and duration);

τ_i is the unique effect that the ith mode of delivery has on ABPS scores; $i = 1$, 2, corresponding to group-based and individual-based, respectively;

β_j is the unique effect that the jth duration has on ABPS scores; $j = 1, 2, 3$, corresponding to durations of 1, 2 and 3 weeks, respectively;

$(\tau\beta)_{ij}$ is the unique effect of the particular combination of the ith mode of delivery for the jth duration on ABPS scores;

ε_{ijk} is the contribution of experimental error to the individual ABPS score for the kth participant following the ith mode of delivery over the jth duration.

When all effects are zero, this model reduces to:

$$y_{ijk} = \mu + \varepsilon_{ijk}.$$

INDEX